The cover image is of Dr. Desiree Persaud, our Residency Program Director of Anesthesiology at the University of Ottawa (2010 - Present). Dr. Persaud has received the

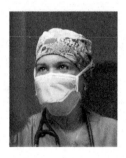

Canadian Anesthesiologists' Society Clinical Teacher Award (2007), the Dave Roberts Ottawa Memorial Award (2002, 2006, and 2008), and the Professional Association of Internes and Residents of Ontario (PAIRO) Teaching Travel Award (2000). She was also chosen as Teacher of the Year both at the University of Ottawa (2000) and at the University of Western Ontario (1998). Dr. Persaud has a keen interest in regional anesthesia and an infectious enthusiasm and commitment to patient care. She played a key role in engaging residents and staff in the production of our Anesthesia Primer.

| | |
|---:|:---|
| Editor: | Patrick Sullivan |
| Editorial Assistance: | Pamela Karzali |
| Graphic Illustrations: | Perry Ng |
| Simulation Centre Photography: | Mariane Tremblay |
| Photography: | Patrick Sullivan |
| Anestheisa Primer Videos: | Patrick Sullivan |
| University of Ottawa Videos: | Nikhil Rastogi |
| Simulation Centre Demonstrator: | DevinSydor |
| Print Layout: | Greg Kerr (www.eliquo.ca) |

www.anesthesiaprimer.com

Every effort has been made to ensure the accuracy of information describing generally accepted anesthetic practices and concerning drug indications, adverse reactions, and dosages. It is possible that this information may change or be erroneous. It is the reader's responsibility to review the manufacturer's package information data prior to administration. This is particularly important for new or infrequently used medications.

# Authors

**Takpal Birdi MD**
Resident Anesthesia,
University of Ottawa

**M. Dylan Bould MB ChB, MEd, FRCA**
Assistant Professor Anesthesia,
University of Ottawa

**Sandra Bromley MD**
Resident Anesthesia,
University of Ottawa

**Gregory Bryson MD, FRCPC**
Associate Professor Anesthesia,
University of Ottawa

**Alan Chaput PharmD, MSc, MD,FRCPC**
Assistant Professor Anesthesia,
University of Ottawa

**Ilia Charapov MD, FRCPC**
Assistant Professor Anesthesia,
University of Ottawa

**Natalie Clavel MD**
Resident Anesthesia,
University of Ottawa

**Michael Curran MD, FRCPC**
Assistant Professor Anesthesia,
University of Ottawa

**Janie Desrosier MD**
Resident Anesthesia,
University of Ottawa

**Marc Doré MD**
Resident Anesthesia,
University of Ottawa

**Daniel Dubois MD**
Resident Anesthesia,
University of Ottawa

**George Evans MD, FRCPC**
Assistant Professor Anesthesia,
University of Ottawa

**Holly Evans MD, FRCPC**
Assistant Professor Anesthesia,
University of Ottawa

**Ashleigh Farrell MD**
Resident Anesthesia,
University of Ottawa

**Amy Fraser MD, FRCPC**
Assistant Professor Anesthesia,
University of Ottawa

**Lillia Fung MD**
Resident Anesthesia,
University of Ottawa

**Teresa Furtak MD**
Resident Anesthesia,
University of Ottawa

**Catherine Gallant MD, FRCPC**
Assistant Professor Anesthesia,
University of Ottawa

**Christopher Hudson MD, FRCPC**
Assistant Professor Anesthesia,
University of Ottawa

**Jordan Hudson MD, FRCPC**
Assistant Professor Anesthesia,
University of Ottawa

**Jarmila Kim MD, FRCPC**
Assistant Professor Anesthesia,
University of Ottawa

**Leo M. Jeyaraj MD, FRCA**
Department of Anesthesiology,
University of Ottawa

**T. Doris Leung MD**
Resident Anesthesia,
University of Ottawa

**Anne Lui MD, FRCPC**
Assistant Professor Anesthesia,
University of Ottawa

**Jennifer Mihill MD**
Resident Anesthesia,
University of Ottawa

**Sarika Mann MD**
Resident Anesthesia,
University of Ottawa

**Sarah McIsaac MB ChB, Med**
Resident Anesthesia,
University of Ottawa

**Christopher Mercer MD**
Resident Anesthesia,
University of Ottawa

**Patti Murphy MD, FRCPC**
Assistant Professor Anesthesia,
University of Ottawa

**Viren N. Naik MD, MEd, FRCPC**
Associate Professor Anesthesia,
University of Ottawa

**Tim O'Connor MD**
Resident Anesthesia,
University of Ottawa

**Annie Pang MD**
Resident Anesthesia,
University of Ottawa

**John Penning MD, FRCPC**
Associate Professor Anesthesia,
University of Ottawa

**Desiree Persaud MD, FRCPC**
Associate Professor Anesthesia,
University of Ottawa

**Marie-Jo Plamondon MDCM**
Resident Anesthesia,
University of Ottawa

**Alim Punja MD**
Resident Anesthesia,
University of Ottawa

**Nikhil Rastogi MD, FRCPC**
Assistant Professor Anesthesia,
University of Ottawa

**Dennis Reid MD, FRCPC, FRCA**
Professor Anesthesia,
University of Ottawa

**Andrew Roberts MD**
Resident Anesthesia,
University of Ottawa

**Raylene Sauvé MD**
Resident Anesthesia,
University of Ottawa

**Ahmed Soliman MD**
Resident Anesthesia,
University of Ottawa

**Patrick Sullivan MD, FRCPC**
Associate Professor Anesthesia,
University of Ottawa

**Devin Sydor MD, FRCPC**
Simulation Fellow
University of Ottawa

**Melanie Toman MD**
Resident Anesthesia,
University of Ottawa

**Kimberly Walton MD, PhD**
Resident Anesthesia,
University of Ottawa

**Anna Wyand MD, FRCPC**
Assistant Professor Anesthesia,
University of Ottawa

**Janet Young MD**
Resident Anesthesia,
University of Ottawa

**Jordan Zacny MD**
Resident Anesthesia,
University of Ottawa

# Forward

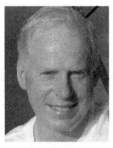

In the early 1990s, the University of Ottawa, Department of Anesthesiology published a textbook entitled *Anesthesia for Medical Students*. Its purpose was to provide a concise primary reference for students completing a two-week rotation in anesthesia. The nature of the specialty of anesthesiology makes it ideally suited as a means through which to impart the essential knowledge and skill set that all physicians should possess. In writing this text, the authors recognized that the majority of students would not be pursuing a career in anesthesiology. With this in mind, they identified learning objectives appropriate for students completing a rotation in anesthesia with a focus on the fundamental principles and skills, including preoperative assessment, securing intravenous access, airway management (mask ventilation and tracheal intubation), basic resuscitation skills, acute pain management, and safe use of local anesthetic agents.

*Anesthesia for Medical Students* was well received and soon became the primary anesthesia reference text for medical students across Canada. The concise straightforward approach to our specialty also made the text a popular choice for anesthesia, medical, and surgical residents, paramedics, respiratory therapists, nurses, and industry representatives.

In 2005, publication of the text ceased, as there was need for significant revisions and updates. Encouragingly, demand for the text continued, and in 2011, our department embarked on a revision of the original text. It is renamed the *Ottawa Anesthesia Primer*, recognizing that the content is suitable for medical care providers practicing in a wide variety of roles.

We are particularly excited to offer an accompanying electronic version of the Ottawa Anesthesia Primer. The ePrimer is available as an *iBook* that can be purchased for use on an iPad by downloading a free apple application called ibooks. It is also available as a digitally encrypted (DE) pdf for viewing on other electronic readers. The ePrimer offers URL links, video links, animated graphics and expanded case problem discussions. Selected URL addresses for additional resources are listed in the text.

I sincerely thank the anesthesia faculty and residents at the University of Ottawa who have volunteered their time to contribute to this project. Each chapter is the combined work of a resident in training under the guidance of one of our anesthesiologists. I am also grateful to Perry Ng and Mariane Tremblay at the University of Ottawa; Perry for his expertise in graphic illustration and Mariane for her photographic know-how. Finally, I would like to thank Pamela Kartzali for her excellent editorial insight and assistance.

We are eager to direct the proceeds of this project towards the Canadian Anesthesiologists' Society International Education Foundation (CAS IEF). The CAS has been a leader in supporting initiatives to improve anesthesia care in developing countries. Recent initiatives include supporting Dr. Enright's Lifebox campaign (www.lifebox.org), a global organization providing pulse oximeters to operating rooms in Third World countries. Dr. Angela Enright was President of the World Federation of Societies of Anaesthesiologists (WFSA) from 2008 to 2012, and a past President of the Canadian Anesthesiologists' Society (CAS). In 2010, she received the Order of Canada for her work with the Lifebox initiative. The CAS is currently leading an educational initiative called 'SAFE' to improve the delivery of obstetrical anesthesia care in Rwanda.

We hope you enjoy our Ottawa Anesthesia Primer and ePrimer.

Sincerely

Pat Sullivan MD

# Table of Contents

# Additional Resources for the Ottawa Anesthesia Primer

## Ottawa Anesthesia Primer Videos:

Technique of securing peripheral intravenous access:
http:/hml.med.uottawa.ca/Play/111

Examination of a patient's airway for ease of intubation and ventilation:
http:/hml.med.uottawa.ca/Play/104

Insertion technique using a classic laryngeal mask airway (LMA) device:
http:/hml.med.uottawa.ca/Play/106

Insertion technique using an AMBU laryngeal mask airway device (LMAD):
http:/hml.med.uottawa.ca/Play/100

Tracheal intubation technique using direct laryngoscopy:
http:/hml.med.uottawa.ca/Play/110

Gum elastic bougie assisted tracheal intubation with direct laryngoscopy:
http:/hml.med.uottawa.ca/Play/108

Tracheal intubation using Glidescope videolaryngoscopy:
http:/hml.med.uottawa.ca/Play/109

Tracheal intubation with a Storz C-Mac videolarygoscope:
http:/hml.med.uottawa.ca/Play/107

Tracheal intubation using a lighted stylet:
http:/hml.med.uottawa.ca/Play/113

Asleep tracheal intubation using a Storz Bonfils videoscope:
http:/hml.med.uottawa.ca/Play/105

Fiberoptic tracheal intubation using local anesthesia and intravenous sedation:
http:/hml.med.uottawa.ca/Play/103

Assessment & monitoring of neuromuscular function during general anesthesia:
http:/hml.med.uottawa.ca/Play/114

Technique of providing spinal anesthesia:
http:/hml.med.uottawa.ca/Play/115

Thoracic epidural anesthesia and analgesia:
http:/hml.med.uottawa.ca/Play/116

Epidural labour analgesia:
http:/hml.med.uottawa.ca/Play/112

Insertion of a peripheral arterial catheter:
http:/hml.med.uottawa.ca/Play/102

Preoperative Aestiva anesthesia machine checkout procedure:
http:/hml.med.uottawa.ca/Play/101

University of Ottawa central line access self-learning module
http://www.med.uottawa.ca/courses/cvc/e_index.html

University of Toronto 3-D interactive neuraxial anesthesia module
http://pie.med.utoronto.ca/vspine

Anesthesia preoperative assessment sheet
http://www.anesthesiaprimer.com/AP/Ch3PreopEval/PreopSheet.pdf

Ottawa Hospital Preoperative Health Questionnaire
http://www.anesthesiaprimer.com/AP/Ch3PreopEval/PreopQuestionnaire.pdf

Managing pain together: Pathophysiology of pain and self-learning module
www.managingpaintogether.com/pathophysiology

Descriptive explanation of the multiple facets of pain:
http://hml.med.uottawa.ca/Play/119

Optimizing perioperative fluid therapy
http://wwww.anesthesiaprimer.com/AP/Supplement/FluidTherapy.pdf

Optimizing oxygen delivery
http://www.anesthesiaprimer.com/AP/Supplement/Oxygenation.pdf

Echocardiography in the perioperative period
http://www.anesthesiaprimer.com/AP/Ch10Monitoring/EchcardiographyBJA2009.pdf

Echocardiography in the acute trauma patient
http://www.anesthesiaprimer.com/AP/Ch10Monitoring/TraumaEchocardiography.pdf

# CHAPTER 1

# Rotational Learning Objectives

Patrick Sullivan MD, Nikhil Rastogi MD, Marc Doré MD

The learning objectives in the *Ottawa Anesthesia Primer* are designed principally for the anesthesia rotation and are to be tailored to meet the needs of the student. Listed in the knowledge and skills section below are seven traditional objectives designed for medical students during their anesthesia rotation. Students studying in other disciplines may choose to tailor their goals to a limited number of objectives for their rotation. In addition to the general objectives presented here, key learning objectives are listed for the student in each chapter.

Specific attitudes, knowledge, and skills are key elements for a successful rotation in anesthesia. With this in mind, students are encouraged to identify their specific goals and objectives and to discuss these with their supervisor and instructors near the beginning of their anesthesia rotation.

## Attitude:

We hope the time students spend with us will stimulate a thirst for knowledge and understanding of the fascinating physiology and pharmacology that occurs in the patient undergoing surgery. Anesthesia is a somewhat unnatural if not magical state, and it is normal for students to feel technically challenged during their rotation as they acquire vascular access and airway management skills. Each student can expect to experience (as all doctors

have) a humbling but hopefully rewarding technical learning curve. They should remain attentive to their technical challenges and their response to them, as well as the response of their patients and other medical personnel as they meet these challenges. We ask students not to cloud their eyes and senses by technical monitors, but rather, to open their eyes and senses to the overall care of the patient. We expect students to commit to excellence in the care and concern they provide for the well being of the patients and their families. We also insist on punctuality and honesty as a basis of good medicine.

The Royal CanMEDS Physician Competency Framework was created by the Royal College of Physicians and Surgeons of Canada as a competency-based resource to guide students through their individual development as a medical expert in their chosen field. The CanMEDS framework identifies and describes six roles of the medical expert (Fig.1.1): Professional, Scholar, Communicator, Health Advocate, Collaborator, and Manager. Students are encouraged to conduct themselves professionally, to become involved and collaborate with the anesthesia surgical team, to communicate effectively with patients and the surgical team, and to advocate on behalf of the patient. Students should strive to develop a scholarly understanding of the subject matter by reading the required material and by asking questions during their

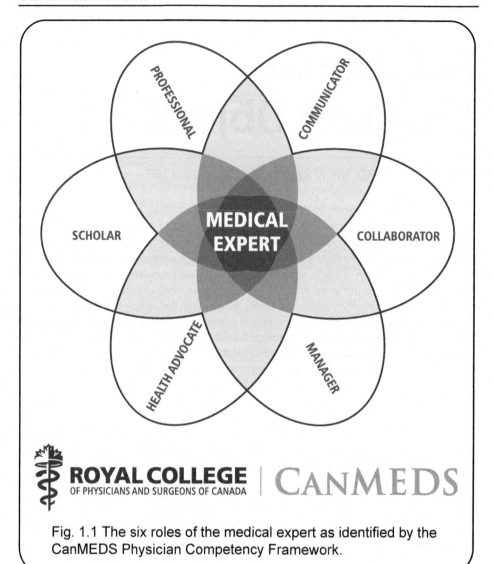

Fig. 1.1 The six roles of the medical expert as identified by the CanMEDS Physician Competency Framework.

anesthesia rotation. Above all, we must always remember that our primary goal is to provide safe and compassionate care for the patient.

While students may view anesthesia as a specialty with limited patient contact, they should ensure that opportunities for communication with the patient and family do not pass by. Fact gathering encounters do not have to be devoid of reassurance, kindness, or a comforting touch. We expect both positive and negative experiences during the anesthesia rotation to be discussed openly with us to ensure the best possible rotation for both current and future students.

# Knowledge and Skills:

### General Objectives
1. To demonstrate an understanding of the anesthetic considerations for a variety of medical conditions and perform the appropriate preoperative assessment and preparation of the patient.
2. To acquire the knowledge necessary to conduct appropriate fluid and blood component therapy.
3. To recognize and describe the main drug classes frequently used in the perioperative period.
4. To acquire knowledge for the safe provision of local anesthesia appropriate for general medical care.
5. To review and describe the principles of acute pain management.
6. To acquire basic skills in airway management.
7. To participate in an emergency resuscitation and, in so doing, to recognize the various roles that health care professionals play in such situations, as assessed by the student's preceptor during a real or simulated emergency.

### Specific Knowledge and Skills Objectives (expanded from general objectives)

**1 To demonstrate an understanding of the anesthetic considerations for a variety of medical conditions and perform the appropriate preoperative assessment and preparation of the patient.**

By the end of the rotation, the medical student will be able to:
a. Obtain and record a pertinent medical history.
b. Perform a focused physical examination, including assessment of the airway, the respiratory and cardiovascular systems, and other systems as indicated by the clinical situation.
c. Interpret basic laboratory data and investigations relevant to the preoperative assessment.
d. Develop a problem list and assign an appropriate American Society of Anesthesiologists' (ASA) physical status based on their patient assessment.
e. Recommend appropriate preoperative medications (e.g., anxiolytics, aspiration prophylaxis) and recognize which medications to refrain from using preoperatively (e.g., anticoagulants, oral hypoglycemic agents).
f. State the recommended preoperative fasting guidelines, list the risk factors for perioperative aspiration, and describe strategies to reduce this risk.

**2 To acquire the knowledge necessary to conduct appropriate fluid and blood component therapy.**

By the end of the rotation, the medical student will be able to:

a. Recognize and describe the physiologic and pathologic routes of fluid losses and be able to estimate these losses.
b. Assess a patient's volume status (i.e., volume of blood in a patient's circulatory system) using history, physical examination, and laboratory investigations.
c. Successfully establish and secure intravenous access using sterile technique with catheters of various sizes.
d. Demonstrate an understanding of the composition of commonly available intravenous fluids by selecting appropriate perioperative fluid and electrolyte replacement while taking into account the patient's deficits, maintenance requirements, and ongoing losses.
e. State the indications and complications of the various blood products, e.g., packed red blood cells (PRBCs), fresh frozen plasma (FFP), and platelets and describe the factors influencing one's decision to administer blood product therapy.

3. **To recognize and describe the main drug classes frequently used in the perioperative period.**

By the end of the rotation, the medical student will be able to describe the main therapeutic effects, side effects, and contraindications of the following classes of medications:
a. Benzodiazepines (midazolam, lorazepam)
b. Opioids (fentanyl, morphine, hydromorphone, codeine, meperidine)
c. Induction agents (propofol)
d. Inhalational agents (desflurane, sevoflurane)
e. Local anesthetics (lidocaine, bupivacaine)
f. Muscle relaxants (succinylcholine, rocuronium)
g. Nonsteriodal anti-inflammatory drugs (NSAIDS; ibuprofen, naproxen, celecoxib)
h. Vasoactive medications (ephedrine, phenylephrine)
i. Antiemetics (dexamethasone, ondansetron, prochlorperazine, haloperidol)

4. **To acquire knowledge for the safe provision of local anesthesia appropriate for general medical care.**

By the end of the rotation, the medical student will be able to:
a. Differentiate the two classes of local anesthetics and state the maximum recommended doses for lidocaine and bupivacaine.
b. List common anesthetic drugs used for topical anesthesia, local infiltration, and peripheral nerve blocks.
c. Describe the signs and symptoms and management of local anesthetic toxicity, including inadvertent intravascular injection of local anesthetics and allergic reactions to local anesthetics.

5. **To review and describe the principles of acute pain management**

By the end of the rotation, the medical student will be able to:
a. Explain the concept of multimodal analgesia.

b.  Identify and describe a variety of modalities commonly used for pain control. Examples of these include patient-controlled analgesia (intravenous PCA), intrathecal (spinal) opioids, epidural infusions, and peripheral nerve blockade.

## 6. To acquire basic skills in airway management

By the end of the rotation, the third-year medical student will be able to demonstrate the ability to manage the airway and ventilation of an unconscious patient.

This will be demonstrated by the ability to:
a.  Label the basic structures of the oropharyngeal and laryngotracheal anatomy.
b.  State the indications and complications of airway management by face mask, laryngeal mask, and intubation.
c.  Identify the appropriate size of face masks, laryngeal masks, oral and nasal airways, laryngoscope blades, and endotracheal tubes.
d.  Recognize upper airway obstruction and independently demonstrate appropriate use of face mask, oral and nasal airways, head positioning, jaw thrust, and chin lift maneuvers.
e.  Independently demonstrate bag-mask ventilation of an unconscious patient.
f.  Successfully prepare appropriate equipment for intubation.
g.  Position and intubate a patient's trachea with minimal supervisory intervention.
h.  Correctly identify within 30 seconds those patients in whom endotracheal intubation was unsuccessful.
i.  Recognize the need for intubation and controlled ventilation using a combination of clinical circumstances, physical signs, and lab results.

## 7. To participate in an emergency resuscitation and, in so doing, to recognize the various roles that health care professionals play in such situations, as assessed by the student's preceptor during a real or simulated emergency.

By the end of the rotation, the medical student will be able to:


a.  Participate in a supportive role in an emergency resuscitative effort and demonstrate knowledge of the ABC approach.
b.  Demonstrate the ability to apply monitoring equipment, including electrocardiogram (ECG) leads and blood pressure (BP) cuff, to a patient with minimal supervisory intervention.

**References:**
1.  Royal College of Physicians and Surgeons of Canada CanMEDS Competencies. http://www.anesthesiaprimer.com/AP/Ch1Objectives/cammeds2005.pdf

# CHAPTER 2

# Anesthesia Overview

Sarah McIsaac MB ChB, Anna Wyand MD

## Learning Objectives

1. To acquire a basic understanding of the history of anesthesia.
2. To gain an appreciation of the different anesthetic modalities.
3. To understand the typical flow of patients to and from the operating room.

## Key Points

1. Anesthesia requires a balance between the role of the surgeon and anesthesiologist and the wishes of the patient as well as a balance between the effects of anesthesia medications and the psychological and physiological stresses of surgery.

2. Anesthesiologists perform a wide variety of roles both inside and outside the operating room.

3. There is a wide spectrum of available anesthetic modalities for patients undergoing surgical procedures.

The word *anesthesia* originates from the Greek prefix *"an"*, which implies without, and *"aesthesia"*, which translates roughly into feeling. In fact, Hippocrates is believed to be the first Greek writer to use the term anesthesia in a medical context.[1] In his collection of writing, Hippocrates refers to *anesthesia* as a loss of consciousness and sedation from a *disease* – not a pharmacological process. It was not until 1846 that the physician and poet, Oliver Wendell Holmes, reintroduced the term in the medical profession with reference to the state of unconsciousness that resulted from the use of the pharmaceutical agent, ether.[2]

In the preanesthesia era, elective surgical procedures were few and far between. The surgical procedures that were performed were often carried out as a last resort given that there was little available to control a patient's pain and agony. To diminish the sensation of pain during an operation, patients were either "knocked" unconscious or given large amounts of opium and alcohol to induce a stupor. In 1897, an elderly Boston physician described surgery in the preanesthetic era as "yells and screams, most horrible in my memory now, after an interval of so many years."[3] There are countless papers describing the efforts of physicians to dull the sensation of pain during surgical procedures prior to anesthesia.

The first successful public administration of inhalational anesthesia is credited to William T.G. Morton, a Boston dentist who demonstrated the use of ether during surgery in the

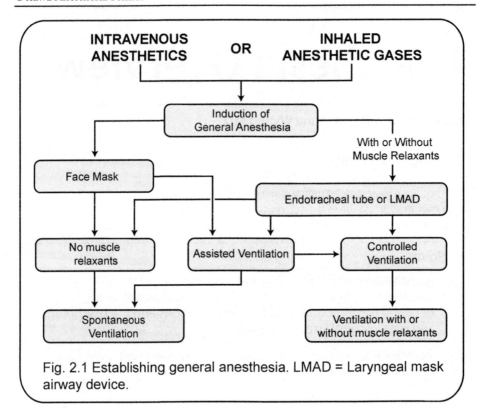

Fig. 2.1 Establishing general anesthesia. LMAD = Laryngeal mask airway device.

famous amphitheater at the Massachusetts General Hospital in Boston. The scripture below the monument honoring William T.G. Morton fittingly reads, "BEFORE WHOM in all time Surgery was Agony..." This remarkable use of inhalational anesthesia propelled a rapid curiosity about "painless surgery". Three months following William T.G. Morton's demonstration, recognition of this technique moved north to Canada, and Canadian physicians embraced this new approach for surgical procedures.[4] In the second half of the 19th century, anesthesia was still very much a craft as practitioners worked tirelessly to understand the basic laws of inhalational anesthesia. The specialty of anesthesia emerged from these seminal procedures, and over the past two centuries, there has been a dramatic increase

in both its depth and knowledge. In concert with the appreciation of anesthetic principles, there has been an equal explosion and growth in the development of surgical procedures and pain management.

Today, modern anesthesia has developed far beyond its rudimentary roots of ether inhalation. Contemporary anesthesia now provides analgesia and/or amnesia to facilitate a multitude of surgical procedures. Three of the most common modalities in the field of anesthesia include general anesthesia, regional anesthesia, and monitored anesthetic care. General anesthesia (GA) can be induced and maintained via a number of different techniques, including the intravenous administration of drugs as well as the administration of an inhaled mixture of anesthetic vapors.

Throughout a general anesthetic, the anesthesiologist attempts to achieve both analgesia and amnesia, with or without muscle relaxation, while maintaining the patient's normal physiological functions.

The delivery of regional anesthesia (RA) refers to the application of a local anesthetic agent to the nerves supplying the anatomical area of surgical interest. Broadly speaking, regional anesthesia is divided into central (neuraxial) and peripheral (nerve block) techniques. These techniques involve the application of a local anesthetic to a specified region to prevent the transmission of pain signals. Finally, monitored anesthetic care refers to anesthetic monitoring with or without the administration of intravenous sedation. Procedures under monitored anesthetic care are commonly performed with intravenous sedation and local anesthesia.

## Anesthetic Modalities Include:

1. **Local anesthesia + monitored anesthetic care**
2. **Sedation + monitored anesthetic care**
3. **General anesthesia (GA)**
   a. Combined intravenous and inhalational anesthesia (e.g., laparotomy)
   b. Inhalational anesthesia (e.g., myringotomy)
   c. Intravenous anesthesia - total intravenous anesthesia (TIVA) (e.g., neurosurgery, malignant hyperthermia)
4. **Regional anesthesia (RA)**
   a. Neuraxial anesthesia (spinal, epidural, and combined spinal/epidural anesthesia)
      Spinal anesthesia: (e.g., total hip arthroplasty, Cesarean delivery)
      Epidural anesthesia: (e.g., epidural analgesia for labour and delivery)
      Combined spinal/epidural anesthesia: (e.g., femoral popliteal bypass surgery)
   b. Major Regional anesthesia:
      Brachial plexus block (e.g., interscalene, infraclavicular, axillary blocks)
      Femoral nerve block
      Popliteal nerve block
      Transversus abdominis plane block (TAP) block
   c. Local Blocks:
      Ankle block
      Bier block
5. **Combined GA + RA**
6. **Combined RA + sedation**

The challenge in anesthesia is to choose the most appropriate modality for a patient undergoing a surgical intervention while maintaining equilibrium between the stress of the surgical procedure and the cardiorespiratory depressant effects of the anesthetic. Thus, modern anesthesia uses a combination of medications in an attempt to minimize the adverse effects and maximize potential benefits of each drug. These medications may include opioids to blunt the pain response to surgery, propofol to induce an anesthetic state, and volatile anesthetic agents to maintain anesthesia. Other common anesthetic medications include benzodiazepines, vasoactive medications, antiemetics, and neuromuscular blocking agents.

In order to formulate an anesthetic plan, the anesthesiologist must consider both the patient's medical condition and the proposed surgical procedure. Patient factors include patient preferences, previous anesthetic experiences, presenting illness, medical history, as well as the patient's medications and allergies. During a physical examination, particular attention is paid to the patient's airway and cardiac and respiratory systems. Each surgical procedure has its own set of anesthetic

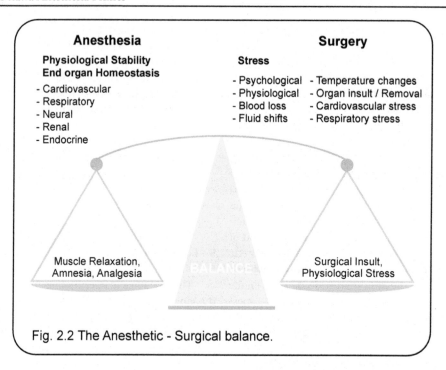

**Anesthesia**

**Physiological Stability**
**End organ Homeostasis**
- Cardiovascular
- Respiratory
- Neural
- Renal
- Endocrine

Muscle Relaxation,
Amnesia, Analgesia

BALANCE

**Surgery**

**Stress**

- Psychological
- Physiological
- Blood loss
- Fluid shifts

- Temperature changes
- Organ insult / Removal
- Cardiovascular stress
- Respiratory stress

Surgical Insult,
Physiological Stress

Fig. 2.2 The Anesthetic - Surgical balance.

considerations that need to be balanced with the patient's physiological status. Procedures may be performed with local anesthesia alone, monitored anesthetic care, regional anesthesia, general anesthesia, or a combination of these choices (e.g., combined epidural and general anesthesia). It is only after considering the patient's preferences and medical condition and the surgical procedure that a reasonable decision can be made regarding the choice of anesthetic modality best suited to the patient's operative procedure.

The scope of anesthesia practice has expanded beyond our primary function in the operating room into a broad spectrum of roles both inside and outside the operating room. The uniqueness of the specialty of anesthesia is the fact that anesthesiologists provide care for all surgical specialties and at all ages of a patient's life twenty-four hours a day.

**The scope of anesthesia practice today may include work in the following areas:**

- Pre-admission unit
- Operating room (OR)
- Obstetrical suites
- Postanesthetic care unit (PACU)
- Intensive care units (ICU)
- Surgical step down units
- Acute pain service
- Chronic pain clinic
- Procedural sedation (endoscopy units, interventional radiology, surgical outpatient clinics)
- Teaching
- Administration
- Research
- Simulation centre (instructor, manager, coordinator, research)
- Surgical/anesthesia care coordinator/facilitator/scheduler

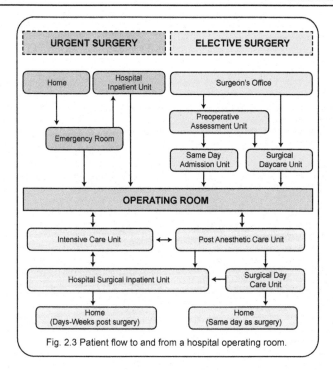

Fig. 2.3 Patient flow to and from a hospital operating room.

Surgical procedures may be performed on an elective, urgent, or emergent basis. Elective procedures are scheduled to permit an assessment of the patient's fitness for the surgery prior to the surgical date (see Chapter 3 Preoperative Assessment). On occasion, time limitations do not permit a complete assessment and optimization of a patient's condition prior to urgent or emergent surgery. Fig. 2.3 is an overview of the typical flow of a patient to and from the operating room.

Anesthesiology is a fascinating specialty where principles of applied pharmacology, physiology, and anatomy are used to provide care for patients of all ages. It has experienced exponential growth from the humble beginnings of Dr. W.G. Morton's experience with inhalational anesthetics to our current practice. Like a painter's brush stroke, no two anesthesiologists have the same practice, and there are subtle nuances that continue to allow for the art as well as the science of medicine. We hope this primer serves as a useful guide during your introduction to our specialty.

**References:**
1. Marcucci, L. (2010). Inside Surgery. Origin of the Word "Anesthesia". From Inside Surgery website http://insidesurgery.com/2010/08/origin-word-anesthesia/.
2. Astyrakaki E, Papioannou A, Askitopoulou H. (2010). References to anesthesia, pain, and analgesia in the Hippocratic Collection. Anesth Analg 2010; 110(1):188-94.
3. Sullivan J. Surgery before anesthesia. Excerpt from the ASA Newsletter 1966;60(9):8-10.
4. Shepard DAE, Turner KE. (2004). Preserving the Heritage of Canadian Anesthesiology: A panorama of People, Ideas, Techniques and Events. From the Canadian Anesthesiology Society web site http://www.cas.ca/English/Archival-Resources

# CHAPTER 3

# Preoperative Evaluation

Raylene Sauvé MD, Gregory Bryson MD

## Learning Objectives

1. To develop an understanding of the anesthetic considerations for patients undergoing surgical procedures.
2. To perform a preoperative assessment and formulate an anesthetic plan.

## Key Points

1 All preoperative visits should include the following steps:
   - Problem identification
   - Perioperative risk assessment
   - Preoperative preparation
   - Proposed plan and technique

2 It is of paramount importance that anesthesiologists perform a final preanesthetic assessment in the immediate preoperative period to formulate their own "patient-specific" assessment and plan.

3 A patient's functional capacity is a powerful predictor of postoperative complications.

4 Laboratory and other diagnostic tests should be ordered only when indicated by the patient's medical comorbidities or drug therapy or the nature of the proposed surgical procedure.

### What is a preoperative assessment, and what is its value to the anesthesiologist?

A preoperative evaluation offers the anesthesiologist an opportunity to define the patient's medical problems and plan an appropriate anesthetic technique. Additional preoperative investigations, consultations, and interventions are used to ensure that the patient is in the best possible condition prior to surgery (i.e., preoperative optimization). Following the optimization process, the anesthesiologist can educate and reassure the patient about the procedure, potentially decreasing the patient's anxiety prior to surgery.

This chapter is intended for care providers who may have little or no exposure to

*◆ In the preoperative evaluation of a patient, the management of certain conditions will be either controversial or require multidisciplinary planning.*

*These "land mines" are identified throughout the text with the symbol◆. If students identify any of these "land mines" in their preoperative evaluation, they should be brought to the attention of the anesthesiologist.*

the specialty of anesthesia. It provides the framework to evaluate a patient's condition, formulate an appropriate anesthetic plan, and communicate this information to colleagues. The preoperative evaluation does not replace the role of the primary care provider and is not meant to address health care issues that are not relevant to the delivery of safe and quality care in the perioperative period.

All preoperative visits should include the following essential steps:
- Problem identification
- Perioperative risk assessment
- Preoperative preparation
- Proposed plan for anesthetic technique

## History of Presenting Illness:

Anesthesiologists must be able to anticipate, avoid, and manage perioperative complications. These complications are specific to the proposed surgery and the patient's coexisting medical problems. This chapter describes how to use an evaluation of the patient's history, physical examination, and laboratory investigations to identify and avoid potential problems, assess the severity of the patient's condition, and optimize the patient's condition prior to surgery. The first step is to ask the patient to explain the reason for the surgery. Ascertain information about the nature of the problem; determine its severity and any therapeutic interventions that have been used. Careful consideration of the surgical procedure will

determine the likelihood of significant blood loss, cardiorespiratory compromise, or unusual positioning requirements (i.e., prone, lateral, lithotomy, etc.). This information can also be useful in planning for venous access, specific monitoring, and choice of anesthetic technique.

## Anesthetic History:

The patient undergoing anesthesia and surgery should be carefully questioned about any reaction to previous anesthetics, and information that the patient considers relevant should be documented. A review of the patient's previous anesthetic records may provide additional information concerning any prior perioperative complications and may offer solutions to avoid similar problems in the future.

The patient should be asked about family history of adverse anesthetic problems. ◆Malignant hyperthermia and plasma cholinesterase deficiency are two such hereditary disorders that manifest under anesthesia (for further information, see Chapter 25: Unusual Anesthetic Complications).

## Problem Identification:

Anesthetic drugs and techniques can have a profound effect on human physiology. The anesthesiologist uses the preoperative evaluation to identify medical conditions that may be adversely affected by the administration of anesthetic medications. Special attention is

⊠ *The American College of Surgeons National Surgical Quality Improvement Program (NSQIP) is a validated, risk-adjusted, program to assess and promote safer and more effective surgical care. NSQIP collects 60 standardized variables for each patient and procedure that influence postoperative outcome. Conditions identified on the preoperative evaluation that are included in NSQIP are indicated with the symbol ⊠.*

paid to symptoms and diseases related to the cardiovascular, respiratory, and neuromuscular systems as they will be directly influenced by the anesthetic medications. A systems-based review can be used to illicit additional relevant information. Ask the patient general screening questions directed at all major body systems, and then narrow the focus if the patient gives positive responses to any of the questions. This information can then be used to develop an appropriate "patient-specific" anesthetic plan.

*When available, a recent preoperative evaluation may be used to guide the assessment.* Even when the patient has been seen in a pre-assessment clinic, it is of paramount importance that anesthesiologists perform a final preanesthetic assessment to formulate their own assessment and plan. The final preoperative evaluation should include a review of the patient's history, physical examination, and most recent investigations.

Optimization prior to surgery requires identifying the patient's medical condition(s) and determining the severity and stability or progression of disease. Patients scheduled for elective surgery who have significant unstable symptoms may need to have their surgery postponed.

## REVIEW OF SYSTEMS

### Functional Capacity

A patient's functional capacity or incapacity is a powerful predictor of postoperative cardiopulmonary[1-3] and neurocognitive[4] complications. Exercise capacity is measured quantitatively in terms of metabolic equivalents (1MET = consumption of 3.5 mL O2·kg$^{-1}$·min$^{-1}$ of body weight). To highlight the possible need for further evaluation, preoperative evaluation guidelines define poor exercise tolerance as ≤ 4 METS. Hence, to evaluate a patient's preoperative functional capacity, one question to ask might be, "Can you climb a flight of stairs without stopping or becoming short of breath?" Table 3.1 provides examples of daily activities and their measured metabolic equivalencies.

## Table 3.1:–Metabolic Equivalency of Activities of Daily Living[5]

| MET | Functional Level of Activity |
|-----|------------------------------|
| 1 | Eating, working at a computer, dressing |
| 2 | Walking down stairs or in your house |
| 3 | Walking 1-2 blocks |
| 4 | Raking leaves, gardening |
| 5 | Climbing 1 flight of stairs, dancing, bicycling |
| 6 | Playing golf, carrying clubs |
| 7 | Playing singles tennis |
| 8 | Rapidly climbing stairs, jogging slowly |
| 9 | Jumping slowly, moderate cycling |
| 10 | Swimming quickly, running or jogging briskly |
| 11 | Skiing cross country, playing full-court basketball |
| 12 | Running rapidly for moderate to long distances |

**The Cardiovascular System:**

Several disease processes can influence the cardiovascular system, and cardiovascular physiology can be altered significantly in the perioperative period.

⊠Patients with coronary artery disease (CAD) are at risk for myocardial ischemia or infarction throughout the perioperative period. The exact mechanism of perioperative myocardial infarction (MI) is complex and involves both thrombus and supply-demand mechanisms. The patients at highest risk are those who have had a recent MI and those with unstable angina.

When assessing a patient at risk for CAD, find out whether the patient previously suffered a MI and, if so, determine the management strategy used. Possible strategies could necessitate treatment with medical therapy alone, ⊠percutaneous coronary intervention (PCI), stenting, or ⊠coronary artery bypass grafting (CABG). ♠※ The patient with a coronary stent placed within the preceding year is at high risk of perioperative cardiac events.[6] The evaluation requires multidisciplinary consultation and careful planning. Cardiology consultation may be required.

⊠Determine the severity and frequency of the patient's ongoing angina pain using standardized reference scales, such as the Canadian Cardiovascular Society Functional Classification of Angina (Table 3.2)[7], and be sure to get a sense of the stability or progression of the patient's disease. Inquire about other coexisting noncardiac diseases, such as hypertension, cerebrovascular disease, diabetes, smoking, and renal insufficiency. The presence of these conditions places the patient at an increased risk of a perioperative cardiac event.

## Table 3.2 CCS Functional Classification of Angina[7]

| Canadian Cardiovascular Society (CCS) Functional Classification of Angina | |
|---|---|
| CLASS I | Ordinary physical activity (walking, climbing stairs) does not cause angina; angina with strenuous, rapid, or prolonged activity |
| CLASS II | Slight limitation of ordinary activity; angina brought on at > 2 blocks on level surface, or climbing ≥ 1 flight of stairs, or by emotional stress |
| CLASS III | Marked limitation of ordinary activity; angina brought on by ≤ 2 blocks on level surface or climbing ≤ 1 flight of stairs |
| CLASS IV | Inability to carry out any physical activity without discomfort; angina may be present at rest |

⊠ The presence of congestive heart failure (CHF) is one of the most important risk factors for perioperative morbidity and mortality. When assessing a patient at risk for cardiac disease, the goal is to identify and minimize the effects of heart failure. Inquire about signs and symptoms of CHF (Table 3.3), including fatigue, syncope, dyspnea, orthopnea, paroxysmal nocturnal dyspnea (PND), and cough.[8] Patients exhibiting signs and symptoms of decompensated or unstable CHF have an increased postoperative risk and should be optimized prior to elective surgery.

## Table 3.3: NYHA Functional Classification of Heart Failure[8]

| New York Heart Association (NYHA) Functional Classification of Heart Failure | |
|---|---|
| CLASS I | Ordinary physical activity does not cause symptoms of heart failure |
| CLASS II | Comfortable at rest; ordinary physical activity results in symptoms |
| CLASS III | Marked limitation of ordinary activity; less than ordinary physical activity results in symptoms |
| CLASS IV | Inability to carry out any physical activity without discomfort; symptoms may be present at rest. |

Valvular heart disease presents a special set of concerns to the anesthesiologist, including unfavorable and even dangerous alterations in hemodynamics with general and major regional anesthetic techniques. Significant valvular disease may present with

17

a murmur, arrhythmia, or poor functional capacity. When a murmur is heard, an attempt should be made to characterize it in terms of intensity, location, timing (within the cardiac cycle), and radiation. ♦A systolic murmur heard over the right clavicle in an elderly patient would be considered highly suspicious of aortic stenosis and require further evaluation if accompanied by left-ventricular hypertrophy (LVH) that has been substantiated by (echocardiography) ECG.[9]

The preoperative assessment may identify a history of arrhythmia, previous pacemaker insertion, or symptoms suggesting the need for a pacemaker. ♦Electrosurgical cautery units as well as other electrical devices in the operating room can interfere with the normal functioning of a pacemaker or implantable cardioverter-defibrillator (ICD). If the patient has a pacemaker or ICD, students should ask the anesthesiologists for their recommendations concerning perioperative management, as a cardiology assessment and intervention may be required prior to the surgery.[10]

## The Respiratory System:

There is wide spectrum of illness associated with the "common cold". ⊠Patients with signs of severe systemic infection or pneumonia (fever, cough, purulent rhinitis, and rhonchi) are at an increased risk for adverse airway events during surgery. Following a complicated upper respiratory tract infection (URTI), hyper-reactive airways may require several weeks to normalize.[11] There is no defined "safe period" to wait, and the decision to postpone anesthetic care should be left to the discretion of the attending anesthesiologist. It is important to ask patients about recent upper respiratory infections.

⊠ Cardiopulmonary pathophysiology associated with smoking includes an increased incidence of hypertension, tachycardia, and peripheral vascular disease (PVD). Cigarette smoke has been shown to decrease the clearance of pulmonary secretions and cause narrowing of the distal airways, leading to an increased frequency of bronchitis, asthma, and chronic obstructive pulmonary disease (COPD) (see below). Carbon monoxide forms a stronger bond with hemoglobin than oxygen, limiting oxygen delivery to the tissues. Patients who continue to smoke immediately prior to surgery will have an increased carboxyhemoglobin (COHb) level and are more prone to hypoxia during the postoperative period. Smoking also impairs wound healing and the immune response.[12]

⊠ It is important to quantitate the patient's smoking history (number of packs/day multiplied by the number of years). A significant smoking history predisposes the patient to perioperative pulmonary complications.[1;13] A systematic review showed that the best postoperative outcomes were achieved when an intensive cessation program was started 4 - 8 wk prior to surgery.[14] This, however, should not discourage clinicians from encouraging smoking cessation when surgery is scheduled in less than four weeks. If the patient is unwilling to quit, stopping for at least 12 - 24 hr prior to surgery should abate the deleterious effects of nicotine and carbon monoxide within the body.

⊠Patients with COPD are at an increased risk of perioperative respiratory complications.[15] Anesthesia, surgery, and postoperative analgesia all predispose the patient with COPD to respiratory depression, atelectasis, retained secretions, pneumonia, and respiratory insufficiency or failure.

Symptoms of COPD may include a decreased exercise tolerance, chronic productive cough, and dyspnea. Respiratory examination may reveal decreased breath sounds, prolonged expiration, and active use of the accessory muscles of respiration. Expiratory wheezing, clubbing, and cyanosis may also be noted. Clinical assessment is generally as good or even better at predicting postoperative respiratory complications when compared with formal testing using pulmonary function tests and arterial blood gases.[17]

The cornerstones of preoperative optimization for patients with COPD include smoking cessation, avoidance of bronchospasm (e.g., preoperative bronchodilation with salbutamol), and treatment of acute COPD exacerbation (e.g., antibiotics for bacterial infections).

Asthmatic patients are prone to bronchospasm with tracheal intubation and exposure to cold, dry anesthetic gases. These patients should be asked about their use of bronchodilator therapy as well as inhalational and oral corticosteroid therapy. The patient's medical history should also determine the frequency and severity of previous asthmatic attacks as well as the need for emergency care, hospitalization, intensive care admission, or tracheal intubation to manage asthma.[18]

Respiratory function in patients with restrictive lung disease, emphysema, and COPD will deteriorate following upper abdominal or thoracic surgery. This deterioration will increase the risk of postoperative respiratory complications. Prior to surgery, patients with limited respiratory reserve undergoing major surgery may benefit from investigations, including chest imaging, pulmonary function testing, and arterial blood gas analysis (assessment of pH, PaO2, PaCO2, and HCO3) to further gauge the severity of their disease and allow for proper anesthetic planning.

♠ It may be difficult to provide positive pressure bag-mask ventilation (BMV) to patients with obstructive sleep apnea (OSA), and it may also be difficult to perform tracheal intubation in these patients using direct laryngoscopy. These difficulties may be due to an abundance of lax soft tissues in the upper airway.[19] These patients also have an increased sensitivity to opioids, benzodiazepines, and volatile anesthetics, which can result in profound respiratory depression, hypoxia, and cardiorespiratory arrest in the postoperative period. Patients with OSA may require alternate or adjusted postoperative analgesic techniques, supplemental oxygen, and prolonged postoperative monitoring.[20] Continuous positive airway pressure (CPAP) ventilation or bilevel positive airway pressure (BiPAP) delivered by a facemask is frequently used in the treatment of patients with OSA. Information concerning the severity of OSA in these patients can be obtained from the findings of previous sleep studies and inferred from the level of pressure prescribed for their device. Patients should be questioned as to the set pressure on their device, and they should be instructed to bring their device on the day of their operation.

Patients with OSA frequently have symptoms of snoring, observed periods of apnea while sleeping, excessive daytime somnolence, and hypertension. A useful mnemonic to identify patients at risk for OSA is "STOP BANG".[21] A positive response to three of the eight criteria is 86% sensitive and 56% specific for the presence of OSA.

## Table 3.4 STOP BANG Mnemonic for Obstructive Sleep Apnea

| | |
|---|---|
| S | Snoring (loud enough to be heard behind a closed door) |
| T | Tired (daytime somnolence) |
| O | Observed periods of apnea |
| P | Pressure (hypertension) |
| B | Body mass index (BMI) > 35 |
| A | Age > 50 years |
| N | Neck circumference > 40 cm |
| G | Sex (males) |

### The Central Nervous and Musculoskeletal Systems:

Patients with cerebrovascular disease may have a history of a ⊠transient ischemic attack (TIA) or previous ⊠cerebral vascular accident (CVA). Important historical features to illicit from the patient include the timing and frequency of events and whether or not there are persistent sensory and motor deficits.[22]

Raised intracranial pressure (ICP) can be life-threatening.[23] At its extreme, raised ICP can result in herniation of cerebral contents causing medullary dysfunction, cardiorespiratory instability, and ultimately death. In patients with central nervous system (CNS) pathology, signs and symptoms of increased ICP may include headache, nausea, vomiting, and papilledema.

Patients with CNS pathology should be questioned about a history of seizures, and if an episode(s) occurred, an attempt should be made to determine the type, frequency, and time of last occurrence. In addition, all anticonvulsant medications should be noted and continued in the perioperative period.[24]

Patients who have a history of ⊠spinal cord injury are at risk for a number of perioperative complications, including respiratory failure, arrhythmias, autonomic hyperreflexia, hyperkalemia, pathologic fractures, and pressure sores.[25] It is important to document both the date and level of neurological injury, as many of these complications are dependent on such variables.

Regional anesthesia may be contraindicated in the presence of certain neurological injuries. Extreme caution should be taken with ♦disorders of the neuromuscular junction (NMJ), such as myasthenia gravis, as they will often result in unpredictable responses to neuromuscular blocking drugs. Lastly, beware that patients with muscular dystrophies and underlying myopathies are known to yield both an increased association with malignant hyperthermia (see Chapter 25) and an increased risk of postoperative respiratory failure.

### The Endocrine System:

Patients with ⊠ diabetes mellitus are prone to a number of vascular complications associated with elevated levels of blood glucose.[26] In particular, chronic hyperglycemia increases the risk of developing coronary artery disease (CAD), myocardial ischemia and infarction (MI), hypertension, neuropathy, and chronic renal failure.

Throughout the perioperative period, the stress of surgery and preoperative fasting can result in marked swings in blood glucose, volume depletion, thrombogenesis, arrhythmias, and silent MIs. Perioperative hyperglycemia also impairs wound healing, and increases the risk of infection. It is important to ask patients about their glucose control, and inquire about their usual blood glucose level and compliance with therapy (diet/ oral hypoglycemic agents/insulin/combination therapy). The presence of comorbidities should be verified, including cardiac ischemia, neuropathy, and nephropathy. If patients are on insulin, it is important to ensure they have followed the preoperative fasting instructions and insulin orders. Typically, patients are instructed to take half of their morning dose of insulin and omit any oral hypoglycemic agents on the day of surgery. At the time of admission to hospital, a glucometer measurement is obtained and an intravenous infusion containing glucose (e.g., 5% dextrose in water [D5W] at 100 mL·hr$^{-1}$) is initiated. Continued management is typically achieved using a "sliding scale" basing additional insulin administration on the results of glucometer measurements repeated at regular intervals. Alternatively, tighter control of blood glucose levels may be desired in the perioperative period. This is generally achieved using a glucose – insulin intravenous infusion protocol.

Patients with thyroid disease may experience difficulties under anesthesia.[27] Profound hypothyroidism is associated with myocardial depression and exaggerated responses to sedative medications. Hyperthyroid patients are at risk for perioperative thyroid storm. Thyroid goiters may either directly compress the airway or involve the recurrent laryngeal nerve, leading to vocal cord palsy and placing the patient at risk for airway obstruction.

Patients with pheochromocytoma can be particularly challenging for the anesthesiologist, surgeon, and internist involved in their care. These patients are at risk for extreme swings in blood pressure and heart rate throughout the perioperative period. They also require intensive preoperative therapy with adrenergic blocking drugs prior to surgery.[28]

Adrenal corticosteroid production increases postoperatively in response to the stress of surgery. Chronic intake of oral steroids may suppress production of adrenal corticosteroids. Patients who are on corticosteroid therapy are at risk of developing postoperative adrenal insufficiency due to their inability to increase endogenous corticosteroid production to match the imposed stress of surgery. The incidence of adrenal suppression is not predictable and depends on the potency and frequency of steroid use as well as the length of steroid therapy.[29] Patients who have received a dose of prednisone > 20 mg per day for more than 5 days in the past 12 months may be at an increased risk of developing postoperative adrenal insufficiency. Supplementation with parenteral corticosteroids may be required to prevent adrenal insufficiency in the perioperative period.

## The Gastrointestinal and Hepatic Systems:

Patients with gastroesophageal reflux disease (GERD) are prone to regurgitation of acidic gastric contents, which could result in aspiration pneumonitis during the perioperative period. Aspiration of an acidic fluid worsens the severity of pneumonitis compared with a fluid with neutral pH. In patients with symptomatic reflux, consider premedication with an H$_2$ blocker, a proton pump inhibitor, or a non-particulate antacid (e.g., 0.3M sodium citrate 30 mL) preoperatively to reduce gastric acidity (see Chapter 4).

Patients with hepatic disease often have issues with fluid and electrolyte imbalance, coagulopathies, and altered drug metabolism.[30] Perioperative complications, including jaundice, hypoalbuminemia, coagulopathy, and renal dysfunction, are increased in patients with advanced liver disease, ⊠ ascites, ⊠ esophageal varices, or acute liver failure. Preoperative workup may warrant investigations, including complete blood count (CBC), electrolytes, international normalized ratio (INR)/activated partial thromboplastin time (aPTT), renal and liver function testing, and correction of these abnormalities may be required.

## The Renal System:

Disorders of fluid and electrolytes are common and may require correction in the perioperative period. Generally, all fluid and electrolyte disorders should be corrected prior to elective surgery.

Patients with⊠ acute and chronic renal failure have abnormal fluid, electrolyte, and drug excretion and may require perioperative dialysis management.[31] Patients should be asked about the relative progression (or stability) of their disease, and particular attention must be paid to fluid and hemodynamic management in order to avoid further renal insult. Patients on ⊠ hemodialysis (HD) should also be asked about their schedule so arrangements can be made to perform HD within the 24-hr period prior to surgery. Potassium levels do not reach a steady state between the intra and extracellular compartments for several hours after HD; hence, measurement of electrolytes (including potassium) immediately following HD is generally not helpful, and it may be misleading, as potassium flux has not reached a steady state.

## The Hematologic System:

Anemia (of various etiologies) is common in surgical patients. The presence of anemia increases the likelihood of a patient receiving blood products in the perioperative period. Perioperative transfusion is associated with an increase in morbidity and mortality.[32] When time permits, therapeutic interventions should be considered to treat and correct the anemia prior to surgery.

There is no defined "transfusion trigger" for patients having surgery, rather, a "patient-specific" decision whether or not to transfuse perioperatively is encouraged. Factors to consider include the chronicity of the anemia, the risk of perioperative blood loss, and the presence of other coexisting diseases. A preoperative blood "type and screen" should be considered, and if transfusion is a possibility, this should be discussed with the patient, and the patient's consent should be obtained for blood product administration prior to commencing surgery. The surgeon should be advised to optimize hemostasis and minimize blood loss. Blood conservation strategies should also be discussed with the patient and operating room (OR) team (see Chapter 21).

Careful management is required for patients with bleeding disorders secondary to clotting factor deficiencies, platelet abnormalities, or medication therapy. Neuraxial anesthesia is generally contraindicated in patients who have a bleeding disorder. Patients with a history of deep vein thrombosis (DVT), pulmonary embolism (PE), cerebral vascular accident (CVA), or atrial fibrillation may be receiving long-term anti-coagulant therapy. These patients require special attention to minimize the risk of bleeding vs the risk of thrombotic complications (DVT, PE, CVA) in the perioperative period. Depending on the nature of the proposed surgery, ♦ anticoagulation therapy (such as acetylsalicylic acid [ASA], coumadin, antiXa inhibitors, and clopidogrel) may need to be stopped. These patients may require "bridging therapy" with low-molecular-weight heparin to "bridge" them in the immediate preoperative period. A preoperative consult (general medicine, hematology, or thrombosis) may be needed for patients requiring bridging therapy.

For further information on management of anticoagulation both before and after surgery, consult the ACCP Guidelines.[16,17]

## Special Populations:

### Pediatrics:

Children are not simply "small adults", they are influenced by a variety of developmental, pharmacological, and physiological changes that influence the delivery of anesthesia (see Chapter 26: Pediatric Anesthesia). In addition to a regular history, ask about the pregnancy and birth history, premature delivery and its complications, and the presence of any known syndromes or organ dysfunction in the child. The preoperative visit is especially important for children as it provides an opportunity to familiarize the child with procedures that will take place in the OR. Consider that the child may benefit from oral premedication with a benzodiazepine as well as the application of a topical local anesthetic applied to potential intravenous access sites. Finally, discuss the potential for parental presence during induction of anesthesia.

### The Elderly:

Physiological changes associated with aging as well as altered drug sensitivity and metabolism place elderly patients at an increased risk of perioperative morbidity and mortality.[33] Bag-mask ventilation may be more difficult in the edentulous patient, and limitations in cervical spine range of motion may make direct laryngoscopy and tracheal intubation more difficult. Elderly patients have an increased incidence of age-related comorbid conditions as well as diminished organ function and reserve. Common comorbidities include CAD, hypertension, diabetes, CHF, and renal failure. Elderly patients are more sensitive to CNS depressants and are at risk of postoperative cognitive dysfunction and delirium.

### Obesity:

The perioperative risk of complications is related to the degree of obesity, which is defined by the body mass index (BMI). Comorbidities commonly associated with morbidly obese patients include CAD, hypertension, OSA, and insulin resistant diabetes mellitus.[34] The World Health Organization (WHO) obesity classification is listed in Table 3.5.

## Table 3.5 WHO Classification of Obesity

| BMI | Classification |
| --- | --- |
| < 18.5 | Underweight |
| > 18.5 to < 25 | Normal |
| > 25 to < 30 | Overweight |
| > 30 to < 35 | Class I obesity |
| > 35 to < 40 | Class II obesity |
| > 45 | Class III obesity (morbid obesity) |

Morbidly obese patients may be difficult to ventilate using positive pressure with bag-mask ventilation (BMV). They are prone to rapid desaturation following induction of general anesthesia (see Fig. 9.1). The rapid desaturation is due to an increase in oxygen consumption as well as a restrictive lung disorder and is accompanied by a reduction in total lung capacity, functional residual capacity (FRC), and expiratory reserve volume. As a result, the FRC can fall below the closing capacity, resulting in small airway collapse even during normal ventilation in an awake obese patient. The onset of general anesthesia results in a further fall in the FRC.

In a small percent of patients with severe obesity, respiratory failure may result from central hypoventilation causing Pickwickian Syndrome. The clinical features of this syndrome include somnolence, hypoxia, hypercapnia, pulmonary hypertension, cor pulmonale, and polycythemia. The risk of aspiration is increased due to low gastric pH, increased abdominal pressures, and increased gastric volume. The obese patient may also face issues with difficult intravenous access, altered drug metabolism, and difficulty with mobilization. Anesthetic techniques, such as epidural analgesia, may be technically challenging to perform. The risk of epidural failure in the postoperative period is increased in obese patients secondary to catheter movement and dislodgement resulting from abundantly mobile and lax soft tissues.

## Patients with Cancer:

Oncology patients commonly present for surgical procedures that may or may not be related to their cancer. In addition to the usual medical history, it is important to discern the type of cancer, staging and presence of metastases, and/or paraneoplastic syndromes. The patient should be asked about treatments received, including chemotherapy and radiation. Certain chemotherapy drugs (anthracyclines, herceptin) can affect cardiac contractility; hence, a review of the patient's functional capacity and available cardiac investigations would be appropriate. If radiation is administered to the patient's neck or chest, be sure to conduct a thorough airway examination as radiation fibrosis of the airway tissues is associated with an unanticipated difficult tracheal intubation (see Chapter 7).

## Other Key Information to Elicit:

In addition to the review of systems, there are several other basic elements of the patient's medical history that should be addressed:

### Current Medications and Allergies:

It is important to obtain a detailed list of the patient's current and recent medications (including all herbal medications) and to note all allergies to drugs. The nature of any adverse reaction should be documented, including the circumstances under which it occurred (e.g., rash, hives, anaphylaxis). Many "allergies" are simply drug side effects, such as nausea and vomiting or pruritus. True allergies to "anesthetic medications" are unusual. Document a careful history of the reaction, and if available, review past medical and anesthetic records.

Particular attention should be paid to cardiovascular and respiratory medications, narcotic analgesics, steroids, and anticoagulants. As a general rule, all medication should be taken with sips of water up to and including the day of surgery. Exceptions to this may include anticoagulants (coumadin, ASA, antiXa inhibitors, and many herbal medications), oral hypoglycemics, insulin (adjustment of the dose is needed on the day of surgery), angiotensin-converting enzyme (ACE) inhibitors, and older generation antidepressants (monoamine oxidase inhibitors, [MAOIs]). Review your local institutional preoperative medication policy.

## Physical Examination:

The physical exam should focus on evaluation of the airway as well as the cardiovascular and respiratory systems. Specific attention should be directed to other systems based on comorbidities identified in the preoperative evaluation.

## General Inspection:

A general assessment of the patient's physical and mental status should be performed, and note should be taken of the patient's vital signs (heart rate, respiratory rate, blood pressure, and oxygen saturation) and biometric measurements (height and weight for calculation of BMI). It is important to check whether the patient is alert, calm, and cooperative, or unusually anxious about the scheduled procedure. Also, does the patient appear young and fit, or elderly, incoherent, emaciated, and bed-ridden? Such obvious differences will dictate the extent and intensity of the examination and the time required to address the patient's concerns and provide reassurance. The patient's mental status may also determine the type and amount of premedication required (if any) and may influence the type of anesthetic technique used (general vs regional).

## Airway Examination:

Examination of the upper airway should be performed on all patients regardless of their planned anesthetic, as this assessment is used as an indicator of potential difficulty with bag-mask ventilation as well as laryngoscopy and tracheal intubation. Identification of abnormalities in the airway exam will assist in the formulation of a rational plan for airway management. Difficulty in securing the airway is associated with significant patient harm that may be avoided with careful assessment and planning. A detailed discussion on the preoperative airway examination can be found in Chapter 6: Intubation and Anatomy of the Airway.

## Cardiovascular Examination:

Assess the patient's heart rate, rhythm, and blood pressure. Auscultate and identify the first and second heart sounds, and listen for the presence of heart murmurs or a third or fourth heart sound. Identify the location of the apical pulse, and note whether it is abnormally displaced. If indicated (i.e., history of CHF), assess the level of the jugular venous pressure (JVP) and look for the presence of peripheral edema.

## Respiratory Examination:

Assess the respiratory rate and work of breathing (i.e., easy and relaxed vs using accessory muscles), and look for the presence or absence of cyanosis or clubbing. Changes in the shape of the thoracic cage may be observed in patients with chronic respiratory disease. The COPD patient with obstructive disease (often referred to as a "blue-bloater") may have a "barrel"-shaped chest that is quite different from a patient with emphysema (commonly referred to as a "pink-puffer") or the restrictive lung defect associated with kyphoscoliosis. Auscultate the patient's chest during quiet and forced respiration, listening for bilateral air entry and noting the presence of crackles or wheezes.

## Neurological Examination:

A basic neurological assessment should be performed and documented in patients with a history of preexisting motor or sensory weakness as well as in patients about to have a regional nerve block. On general inspection, assess for symmetry, look for the presence of muscular tone, and note any abnormal movements or posturing. Assess sensation in the upper and lower extremities in response to light touch and pain (or temperature). Record any gross motor deficits present prior to the proposed procedure.

If neuraxial anesthesia is planned, assess the patient's back, specifically noting the alignment (examining for scoliosis, kyphosis, or lordosis) and the ability to palpate external landmarks, such as the spinous processes and the anterior superior iliac crests.

Anticipate the need for special invasive monitors, and assess the anatomy for arterial line insertion, central vein cannulation, intravenous access, and major regional anesthetic techniques.

## Investigations

Laboratory investigations should not be ordered routinely as part of the preoperative evaluation. Laboratory and diagnostic investigations should be ordered only when indicated by the patient's medical comorbidities, drug therapy, or nature of the proposed procedure. The 2011 Canadian Anesthesiologists' Society (CAS) Guidelines to the Practice of Anesthesia offers suggestions to guide preoperative testing (Table 3.6).

## Table 3.6: Indications for Preoperative Testing[34]

| Test | Indication |
|---|---|
| CBC | Major surgery requiring blood type and screen or crossmatch<br>Chronic cardiovascular, pulmonary, renal, or hepatic disease<br>Malignancy<br>Known or suspected anemia, bleeding diathesis, or myelosuppression<br>Patients < 1 yr of age |
| HbS | Genetically predisposed patient (hemoglobin electrophoresis, if screen is positive) |
| INR<br>aPTT | Anticoagulant therapy<br>Bleeding diathesis<br>Liver disease |
| Electrolytes<br>Cr | Hypertension, renal disease, diabetes<br>Pituitary or adrenal disease<br>Digoxin, diuretic therapy, or other drug therapies affecting electrolytes |
| Fasting Glucose Level | Diabetes (should be repeated on the day of surgery) |
| Pregnancy (β-HCG) | Woman who may be pregnant |
| (ECG) | Heart disease, hypertension, diabetes<br>Subarachnoid or intracranial hemorrhage, cerebrovascular accident, head trauma<br>Other risk factors for cardiac disease (may include age) |

| Chest radiograph (CXR) | Cardiac or pulmonary disease Malignancy |
|---|---|

CBC = complete blood count; HBS = sickle cell screen; INR = international normalized ratio; aPTT = activated partial thromboplastin time; Cr = creatinine; ECG = electrocardiograph; CXR = chest *x-ray*.

In 2007, the American College of Cardiology and the American Heart Association (ACC/AHA) revised their guidelines on perioperative cardiovascular evaluation and care for patients undergoing noncardiac surgery.[1] The following algorithm (Fig. 3.1) can be used to guide investigation and management of patients with cardiovascular disease undergoing noncardiac surgery.

## Summative Risk Assessment

### The Risk of Anesthesia:

Understanding the extent of a patient's disease is of paramount importance as many organ systems are directly affected by the delivery of anesthesia. Evaluation of a patient's overall perioperative risk must consider the patient's preoperative medical condition, the nature of the proposed surgical procedure, and the risks associated with anesthesia. Fortunately, anesthesia-related morbidity and mortality are rare.

It is difficult to make generalized statements about risk due to the wide variety of surgical procedures and anesthetic techniques combined with the diversity of a patient's comorbid conditions. It is rare for patients to receive an anesthetic without undergoing a surgical procedure, which makes it a challenge to separate the relative contributions of anesthesia and surgery from the adverse outcomes.

Generalized estimates of all-cause perioperative mortality of 1:500 and anesthesia-related mortality of 1:13,000 have been relatively consistent over the past forty years.[35]

The question that needs to be answered is "What is the risk of this particular procedure in this particular patient who has these medical conditions and is receiving this specific anesthetic technique?" Numerous investigators have attempted to address this very complex question. Most of the work, however, addresses the operative risk according to the patient's preoperative medical status.

### Perioperative Risk Assessment:

Perhaps the oldest and simplest method of risk assessment is the American Society of Anesthesiologists (ASA) physical status classification system (Table 3.7). The ASA physical status classification originally proposed in 1941 and revised by Dripps in 1961[36] provides a simple clinical assessment of a patient's preoperative physical condition. While initially developed as a tool for classifying a patient's physical condition, the ASA physical status has also been used to stratify patient risk. While open to significant criticism because of its vague categories and inconsistencies in its application, the ASA physical status classification has been shown to correlate with perioperative mortality.[35]

## Table 3.7: ASA Physical Status Classification

| Category | Description | Example |
|---|---|---|
| I | Healthy patient | Healthy patient, no medical problems |
| II | Mild systemic disease – no functional limitation | Controlled hypertension |
| III | Severe systemic disease – definite functional limitation | Emphysema |
| IV | Severe systemic disease – a constant threat to life | Unstable angina |
| V | Moribund patient – not expected to survive with or without an operation for 24 hours | Ruptured abdominal aortic aneurysm in shock, undergoing emergency surgery |
| VI | A declared brain-dead patient whose organs are being removed for donor purposes | Brain death, organ donor |
| E | A suffix E is added to denote an emergency procedure | On call / emergency case |

Perioperative cardiac complications contribute significantly to perioperative mortality, morbidity, and costs.[37] As a result, researchers have focused on identifying the patient at risk for major adverse cardiac events. The best risk prediction model, the Revised Cardiac Risk Index,[38] includes six variables:

- High-risk surgery (i.e., intraperitoneal, intrathoracic, or suprainguinal vascular procedures)
- History of ischemic heart disease (i.e., MI, positive exercise test, presence of angina, use of nitrate therapy, or ECG with Q wave changes).
- History of CHF (i.e., pulmonary edema, PND, bilateral rales, S3 gallop rhythm, chest x-ray with vascular redistribution)
- History of cerebrovascular disease (i.e., transient ischemic attack or cerebrovascular accident)
- Preoperative treatment with insulin
- Preoperative creatinine>176 $\mu mol \cdot L^{-1}$

Once assessed, the patient is given one point for the presence of each risk factor and assigned a Revised Cardiac Risk Index (RCRI) class that corresponds to a percentage value representing the potential for perioperative cardiac complications.

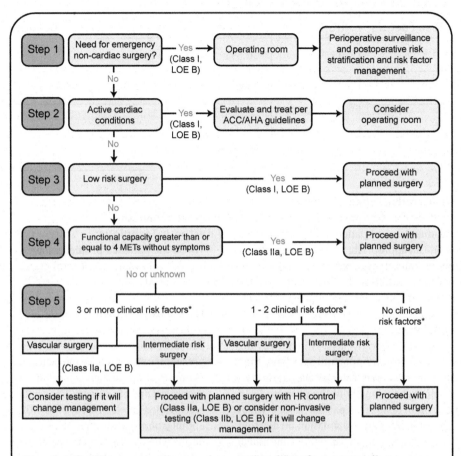

Fig. 3.1 Cardiac evaluation and care algorithm for noncardiac surgery based on active clinical conditions, known cardiovascular disease, or cardiac risk factors for patients 50 years of age or greater. Clinical risk factors* include ischemic heart disease, compensated or prior heart failure, diabetes mellitus, renal insufficiency, and cerebrovascular disease. Consider perioperative beta blockade for populations in which this has been shown to reduce cardiac morbidity/mortality. ACC/AHA indicates American College of Cardiology/American Heart Association; HR, heart rate; LOE, level of evidence; and MET, metabolic equivalent. Adapted from the ACC/AHA.

## Table 3.8:–Revised Cardiac Risk Index

| Risk Factors | RCRI Class | Incidence of Cardiovascular Complications |
|:---:|:---:|:---|
| 0 | I | 0.5% |
| 1 | II | 1% |
| 2 | III | 5% |
| 3 | IV | 10% |

### Preoperative Preparation:

The goal of the preoperative evaluation is to gather relevant patient information to formulate an appropriate anesthetic plan. When time permits, this can be a golden opportunity to arrange additional testing and consultations to optimize the patient prior to surgery (e.g., cardiology, respirology, hematology consultations).

The preoperative assessment provides patients with an opportunity to have their questions answered. This may alleviate anxiety and apprehension about the proposed surgery. On occasion, the patient's anxiety may warrant a preoperative sedation medication. Patients should be instructed to continue or hold existing medications as discussed previously in this Chapter. Preoperative administration of medications for gastroesophageal reflux disease (GERD) or the administration of foundational analgesics, such as acetaminophen and a NSAID, are discussed in Chapter 4: Premedication.

The Preoperative Assessment Summary Sheet (Fig. 3.2) provides a concise reference summary of the salient information that needs to be gathered during a preoperative assessment. This sheet can be downloaded from http://www.anesthesiaprimer.com/AP/Ch3PreopEval/PreopSheet.pdf and used as an aid when performing the preoperative assessment.

### Proposed Plan for Anesthetic Technique:

Once the patient's problems have been identified and evaluated, several questions need to be answered:

1. **Is the patient's condition optimal?**
   Is there sufficient time to optimize the patient? Patients who require emergency procedures may not have the benefit of time to optimize their comorbid conditions prior to surgery. If the patient is scheduled for elective surgery without–optimization, the anesthesiologist must decide whether the surgery can proceed safely despite lack of optimization (low-risk surgery), or whether the surgery should be delayed for further investigations or perhaps cancelled.

2. **Are there any problems that require further consultation or special tests?**
   Patients undergoing major surgical procedures with poorly defined comorbidities may require additional investigations or consultations to assess their perioperative risk and formulate an appropriate plan of management.

## Fig. 3.2      **Preoperative Assessment Sheet**

- Proposed surgery:
  - ☐ Previous Anesthetics
  - ☐ Complications
  - ☐ Previous intubations
  - ☐ Medications
  - ☐ Allergies / Sensitivities

**PMHx**
- **CNS**
  - ☐ Seizures
  - ☐ Stroke
  - ☐ Raised ICP

- **CVS:**
  - ☐ CAD
  - ☐ MI
  - ☐ HTN
  - ☐ CHF
  - ☐ Valvular disease
  - ☐ Dysrhythmias
  - ☐ PVD
  - ☐ Exercise intolerance
  - ☐ NYHA class
- **Respiratory**
  - ☐ Smoking
  - ☐ Asthma
  - ☐ COPD
  - ☐ Recent URTI
  - ☐ Sleep apnea
- **GI**
  - ☐ GERD
  - ☐ Liver disease

- **Renal**
  - ☐ Insufficiency
  - ☐ Dialysis
- **Hematologic**
  - ☐ Anemia
  - ☐ Coagulopathies
  - ☐ Blood dyscrasias
- **MSK**
  - ☐ Conditions associated with difficult intubation
  - ☐ Rheumatoid arthritis
  - ☐ Cervical tumors / infections
  - ☐ Trauma to cervical spine
  - ☐ Trisomy 21
  - ☐ Myasthenia Gravis
- **Endocrine**
  - ☐ DM
  - ☐ Thyroid
  - ☐ Adrenal disorders
  - ☐ Morbid obesity
- **Other**
  - ☐ Pregnancy
  - ☐ ETOH abuse / illicit drug use

**FHx**
- Malignant hyperthermia
- Atypical cholinesterase (pseudocholinesterase)
- Abnormal drug reactions

**PHYSICAL EXAM**
- Oropharynx and airway assessment
  - ☐ Mallampati classificaiton
  - ☐ Mouth opening
  - ☐ Jaw size (thyromental distance)
  - ☐ Tongue size / dentition
  - ☐ C-spine stability, neck flexion / extension
  - ☐ Tracheal deviation
  - ☐ Nasal passage patency
- Bony landmarks and suitable areas for regional anesthetic (if warranted)
- Focused physical exam, including: vital signs, CNS, CVS, respiratory system
- General assessment of nutrition, hydration and mental status
- Pre-existing motor and sensory deficits
- Examine sites for:
  - ☐ Intravenous access
  - ☐ Central line access
  - ☐ Regional anesthesia

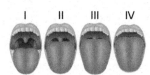

I    II    III    IV

Mallampati Classification

| American Society of Anesthesiology (ASA) Classification ||
| --- | --- |
| ASA 1 | Healthy, fit patient |
| ASA 2 | Mild systemic disease. |
| ASA 3 | Severe systemic disease with functional limitation. |
| ASA 4 | Incapacitating disease, a constant threat to life. |
| ASA 5 | Moribund patient not expected to survive 24 hrs with or without surgery. |
| ASA 6 | Brain dead patient |

### 3. Is there an alternative procedure that may be associated with a lower perioperative risk?

This question is especially important to consider in the high-risk patient. For example, a surgeon may be unaware of significant anesthesia risks for a patient scheduled to undergo major surgery (e.g., radical cystectomy). After discussion with the team, a lower risk procedure may be deemed more appropriate (e.g., insertion of a suprapubic catheter for relief of urinary obstruction). In patients with significant comorbidities undergoing high-risk surgery, the anesthesia and surgical team may explore whether any alternative less-invasive surgical options are available.

### 4. What are the plans for postoperative management of the patient?

The majority of patients will require an initial period of monitoring in the postanesthesia care unit (PACU) following their procedure. They are subsequently returned to a hospital ward or discharged home. Patients with significant underlying diseases or those having major procedures may require postoperative care in a critical care unit. Supplemental oxygen therapy and analgesic plans should also be clearly defined. Analgesic options for the postoperative patient are discussed in Chapters 14 – 17.

### 5. Are blood products likely to be required?

The patient should be informed and consent obtained for possible blood product administration. The availability of blood products should be confirmed, and blood conservation strategies should be discussed with the OR team.

### 6. What premedication (if any) is appropriate? (See Chapter 4: Premedication)

Last but not least, the anesthetic technique must be planned. Options for anesthesia will include:

- Monitored anesthetic care with local anesthesia with or without sedation.
- Regional anesthesia with or without intraoperative sedation.
- General anesthesia with or without tracheal intubation.–If tracheal intubation is required, the anesthesiologist may choose to control ventilation of the lungs or allow the patient to breathe spontaneously.–If controlled ventilation is used, the anesthesiologist may or may not use muscle relaxants.
- Combined regional and general anesthetic.

A well-formulated anesthetic plan includes a plan for induction of anesthesia, maintenance of anesthesia, emergence, transport, and postoperative analgesia.

We encourage students to challenge themselves by performing a preoperative patient-specific assessment and formulating an appropriate anesthetic plan:

- Complete the preoperative assessment
- Develop an anesthetic plan for the patient you have assessed based on the proposed surgery.
- Discuss your plan with the attending anesthesiologist and elicit their thoughts on your management plan and any alternative strategies they would suggest.

## References:

1. Arozullah AM,Khuri SF, Henderson WG, et al. Development and validation of a multifactorial risk index for predicting postoperative pneumonia after major noncardiac surgery. Ann Intern Med 2001 Nov 20;135(10):847-57.
2. Reilly DF, McNeely MJ, Doerner D, et al. Self-reported exercise tolerance and the risk of serious perioperative complications. Arch Intern Med 1999 Oct 11;159(18):2185-92.
3. Fleisher LA, Beckman JA, Brown KA, et al. 2009 ACCF/AHA focused update on perioperative beta blockade incorporated into the ACC/AHA 2007 guidelines on perioperative cardiovascular evaluation and care for noncardiac surgery: a report of the American college of cardiology foundation/American heart association task force on practice guidelines. Circulation 2009 Nov 24;120(21):e169-e276.
4. Marcantonio ER, Goldman L, Mangione CM, et al. A clinical prediction rule for delirium after elective noncardiac surgery. JAMA 1994 Jan 12;271(2):134-9.
5. Jette M, Sidney K, Blumchen G. Metabolic equivalents (METS) in exercise testing, exercise prescription, and evaluation of functional capacity. ClinCardiol 1990 Aug;13(8):555-65.
6. Practice alert for the perioperative management of patients with coronary artery stents: a report by the American Society of Anesthesiologists Committee on Standards and Practice Parameters. Anesthesiology 2009 Jan;110(1):22-3.
7. Campeau L. Letter: Grading of angina pectoris. Circulation 1976 Sep;54(3):522-3.
8. The Criteria Committee of the New York Heart Association. Nomenclature and Criteria for Diagnosis of Diseases of the Heart and Great Vessels.– 9th ed. Boston, Mass: Little, Brown & Co; 1994.
9. Etchells E, Glenns V, Shadowitz S, et al. A bedside clinical prediction rule for detecting moderate or severe aortic stenosis. J Gen Intern Med 1998 Oct;13(10):699-704.
10. Practice advisory for the perioperative management of patients with cardiac implantable electronic devices: pacemakers and implantable cardioverter-defibrillators: an updated report by the American society of anesthesiologists task force on perioperative management of patients with cardiac implantable electronic devices. Anesthesiology 2011 Feb;114(2):247-61.
11. Von Ungern-Sternberg BS, Boda K, Chambers NA, et al. Risk assessment for respiratory complications in paediatric anaesthesia: a prospective cohort study. Lancet 2010 Sep 4;376(9743):773-83.
12. Hawn MT, Houston TK, Campagna EJ, et al. The Attributable Risk of Smoking on Surgical Complications. Ann Surg 2011 Aug 24.
13. Arozullah AM, Daley J, Henderson WG, et al. Multifactorial risk index for predicting postoperative respiratory failure in men after major non cardiac surgery. The National Veterans Administration Surgical Quality Improvement Program. Ann Surg 2000 Aug;232(2):242-53.
14. Thomsen T, Villebro N, Moller AM. Interventions for preoperative smoking cessation. Cochrane Database Syst Rev 2010;(7):CD002294.
15. Smetana GW, Lawrence VA, Cornell JE. Preoperative pulmonary risk stratification for non cardiothoracic surgery: systematic review for the American College of Physicians. Ann Intern Med 2006 Apr 18;144(8):581-95.
16. Douketis JD Berger PB, Dunn AS et al. The perioperative management of antithrombotic therapy: American college of chest physicians evidence-based clinical practice guidelines. Chest 2008; 133;229S-339S.
17. McAlister FA, Bertsch K, Man J, et al. Incidence of and risk factors for pulmonary complications after nonthoracic surgery. Am J Respir Crit Care Med 2005 Mar 1;171(5):514-7.
18. Woods BD, Sladen RN. Perioperative considerations for the patient with asthma and bronchospasm. Br J Anaesth 2009 Dec;103Suppl 1:i57-i65.
19. Siyam MA, Benhamou D. Difficult endotracheal intubation in patients with sleep apnea syndrome. Anesth Analg 2002 Oct;95(4):1098-1102.
20. Gross JB, Bachenberg KL, Benumof JL, et al. Practice guidelines for the perioperative management of patients with obstructive sleep apnea: a report by the American Society of Anesthesiologists Task Force on Perioperative Management of patients with obstructive sleep apnea. Anesthesiology 2006 May;104(5):1081-93.
21. Chung F, Yegneswaran B, Liao P, et al. STOP questionnaire: a tool to screen patients for obstructive sleep apnea. Anesthesiology 2008 May;108(5):812-21.
22. Wong DH. Perioperative stroke. Part I: General surgery, carotid artery disease, and carotid endarterectomy. Can J Anaesth 1991 Apr;38(3):347-73.

23. Steiner LA, Andrews PJ. Monitoring the injured brain: ICP and CBF. Br J Anaesth 2006 Jul;97(1):26-38.
24. Kofke WA. Anesthetic management of the patient with epilepsy or prior seizures.
   Curr Opin Anaesthesiology 2010 Jun;23(3):391-9.
25. Dutton RP. Anesthetic management of spinal cord injury: clinical practice and future initiatives.
   Int Anesthesiology Clin 2002;40(3):103-20.
26. Ahmed Z, Lockhart CH, Weiner M, et al. Advances in diabetic management: implications for anesthesia.
   Anesth Analg 2005 Mar;100(3):666-9.
27. Farling PA. Thyroid disease. Br J Anaesth 2000 Jul;85(1):15-28.
28. Pacak K. Preoperative management of the pheochromocytoma patient.
   J Clin Endocrinol Metab 2007 Nov;92(11):4069-79.
29. Marik PE, Varon J. Requirement of perioperative stress doses of corticosteroids: a systematic review of
   the literature. Arch Surg 2008 Dec;143(12):1222-6.
30. Suman A, Carey WD. Assessing the risk of surgery in patients with liver disease.
   Clev Clin J Med 2006 Apr;73(4):398-404.
31. Craig RG, Hunter JM. Recent developments in the perioperative management of adult patients with
   chronic kidney disease. Br J Anaesth 2008 Sep;101(3):296-310.
32. Beattie WS, Karkouti K, Wijeysundera DN, et al. Risk associated with preoperative anemia in noncardiac
   surgery: a single-center cohort study. Anesthesiology 2009 Mar;110(3):574-81.
33. Preston SD, Southall AR, Nel M, et al. Geriatric surgery is about disease, not age.
   J R Soc Med 2008 Aug;101(8):409-15.
34. Candiotti K, Sharma S, Shankar R. Obesity, obstructive sleep apnoea, and diabetes mellitus:
   anaesthetic implications. Br J Anaesth 2009 Dec;103Suppl 1:i23-i30.
35. Lagasse RS. Anesthesia safety: model or myth? A review of the published literature and analysis of
   current original data. Anesthesiology 2002 Dec;97(6):1609-17.
36. Dripps RD, Lamont A, Eckenhoff JE. The role of anesthesia in surgical mortality.
   JAMA 1961 Oct 21;178:261-6.
37. Fleischmann KE, Goldman L, Young B, et al. Association between cardiac and noncardiac complications
   in patients undergoing noncardiac surgery: outcomes and effects on length of stay.
   Am J Med 2003 Nov;115(7):515-20.
38. Lee TH, Marcantonio ER, Mangione CM, et al. Derivation and prospective validation of a simple index
   for prediction of cardiac risk of major noncardiac surgery. Circulation 1999 Sep 7;100(10):1043-9.

## Additional Resources:

Merchant R, Bosenberg C, Brown K, et al. Guidelines to the Practice of Anesthesia: Revised edition 2011.
Can J Anaesth 2011 Jan;58(1):74-107.
The Ottawa Primer Preoperative Assessment Sheet can be downloaded at
http://www.anesthesiaprimer.com/AP/Ch3PreopEval/PreopSheet.pdf

# CHAPTER 4

# Premedication

Annie Pang MD, Nikhil Rastogi MD

## Learning Objectives

1   To gain an appreciation of the indications and contraindications for prescribing medications prior to an operative procedure.

## Key Points

1.  The majority of adult patients do not require preoperative sedation.

2.  Provided there are no contraindications to their use, acetaminophen and a nonsteroidal anti-inflammatory medication may be used to provide a foundation of analgesia for postoperative pain management (see Chapter 17 Acute Pain Management).

3.  Reasons for prescribing medications prior to an operative procedure can be related to the patient, the procedure, or the patient's coexisting medical condition.

The majority of adult patients do not require sedation prior to their surgical procedure, though a discussion about the procedure and anesthetic in a compassionate way will help reassure the patient. Medications are prescribed preoperatively to avoid potential complications associated with the surgical procedure or to continue the patient's current medications for coexisting medical conditions.

### Reasons for prescribing a preoperative medication include:

**I.   Patient-related reasons:**
1.  Anxiolysis
2.  Amnesia
3.  Analgesia
4.  Antisialagogue effect (to dry oral secretions)
5.  Medications to decrease gastric acidity and gastric volume
   The majority of patients scheduled for surgery experience some degree of apprehension.

The psychological stress patients experience prior to surgery can be more detrimental than the actual physical insult of the surgical procedure. Preoperative anxiety may be caused by many factors. Some of the more common causes include:
1.  The fear of relinquishing control to someone else while under general anesthesia.

2. The fear of experiencing pain postoperatively.
3. The inability to preserve their modesty and dignity during the operation.
4. The fear of separation from family and loved ones.
5. The fear of discovering a serious problem such as cancer.
6. The fear of surgical mutilation and an altered body image.
7. The fear of dying during the operation.

It is important to take time to answer your patients' questions. If you are unable to answer their questions, reassure them that their questions are important to you, and while you may not know the answers, you will speak to the attending staff physician and provide them with answers. Perhaps the most important part of our preoperative visit is to convey a reassuring, honest and caring attitude.

**II. Procedure-related reasons:**
1. Gastric prophylaxis to minimize the risk of gastric aspiration during anesthesia.
2. Corticosteroid coverage in patients who are immunosuppressed (see Chapter 3).
3. Prevention of undesired reflexes arising during a procedure (e.g., vagal reflex during eye surgery).
4. Anticholinergic agents to decrease oral secretions and facilitate a planned awake tracheal intubation with a fiberoptic bronchoscope.

**III.    Coexisting Diseases:**
1. To continue the patient's own medications for coexisting diseases (e.g., beta-blockers, antihypertensive medications, nitrates, antiparkinsonian medications).
2. To optimize the patient's status prior to the procedure (e.g., bronchodilators, nitroglycerine, beta-blockers, antibiotics).

Patients with significant coexisting diseases and those at the extremes of age may be more sensitive to anxiolytics, and the dose should be decreased accordingly. Additional medications can be given intravenously as needed when the patient arrives in the operating room.

Benzodiazepines are the class of drugs most frequently used preoperatively to achieve sedation, relief of anxiety, and amnesia. Diazepam (5 -10 mg *po*) may be given with sips of water 1½ - 2 hr preoperatively. Lorazepam (0.5 - 2 mg) may be given either by the sublingual or oral route. Lorazepam provides excellent amnesia and sedation, but occasionally, patients remain excessively drowsy after the surgery.

Oral midazolam may be used for pediatric patients or developmentally delayed adults 30 min preoperatively in a dose of 0.25 - 0.5 mg·kg$^{-1}$. To enhance acceptance, a flavored suspension of acetaminophen, in a dose appropriate to the patient's age, is frequently used as a base to which the midazolam is added. To prevent a fall or injury after the administration of midazolam, the patient should be watched closely and, in the case of a child, the patient may be held in the parent's arms.

Melatonin is a naturally occurring hormone found in the pineal gland and is involved in the regulation of circadian rhythms. Exogenous administration facilitates both the onset and quality of sleep and does not suppress rapid eye movement (REM) sleep. In contrast, benzodiazepines impair sleep quality and reduce the duration of REM sleep. Unlike benzodiazepines, melatonin is not associated with a "hang over" effect.[1] A single dose of melatonin 5 mg resulted in a reduction in anxiety comparable with  sublingual midazolam 15 mg when administered 100 min prior to surgery.[2] Melatonin 0.25 mg·kg$^{-1}$ was comparable with midazolam 0.5 mg·kg$^{-1}$ in reducing preoperative anxiety in children.[3] In this study, children given melatonin preoperatively experienced a faster recovery, a lower incidence of postoperative excitement, and less sleep disturbance postoperatively compared with children given midazolam. A recent review highlighted the role of melatonin in the perioperative period for its sedative, analgesic, and antioxidant properties.[4] Despite the theoretical advantages of melatonin compared with a benzodiazepine, its use has not been widely adopted as a preoperative sedative.

Opioids, such as hydromorphone, morphine, and meperidine, provide both sedation and analgesia. They are appropriate for patients experiencing pain prior to their surgery (e.g., fractured extremity awaiting surgery). Troublesome side effects of opioids may occur, including nausea, vomiting, biliary spasm, respiratory depression, bradycardia, hypotension, and true allergic reactions. Consider ordering supplemental oxygen for patients requiring an opioid medication.

An anticholinergic agent may also be used if an "awake" fibreoptic-assisted tracheal intubation is planned. The use of an anticholinergic in these patients causes decreased secretions from oral salivary glands, thereby facilitating both absorption of topical anesthetics and visualization of the airway when using a fiberoptic scope. Glycopyrrolate (0.2 - 0.4 mg *im*) is a good drying agent. It does not cross the blood brain barrier and causes less tachycardia than atropine.

Medications may be prescribed to decrease the gastric volume and acidity preoperatively, which, in turn, may decrease both the risk and severity of perioperative aspiration of gastric contents (see Chapter 25 Unusual Anesthetic Complications: Aspiration). A non-particulate antacid, such as 0.3 M sodium citrate 30 mL *po*, may be used to neutralize the gastric acid. A prokinetic drug, such as metochlorpropamide 10 mg intravenously, may be administered to facilitate gastric emptying. Medications, such as an H$_2$ blocker, may be given by mouth 1 hr prior to surgery (e.g., ranitidine 150 mg). Alternatively, patients may be asked to take their own usual medications (e.g., omeprazole or pantoprazole) prior to surgery.

Gabapentin and pregabalin are gabapentinoid compounds with sedative, analgesic, and anticonvulsant properties, and they are commonly prescribed in patients with neuropathic pain (see Chapters 17 & 18). Surgical injury initiates a cascade of effects on both the peripheral and central pain pathways, which may result in a "pathological" mode of processing afferent pain information in the postoperative period. Promising results have arisen from studies using gabapentin and pregabalin for the postoperative management of pain. Clinicians are now using pregabalin as a medication prior to surgery for an off-label indication in an attempt to improve postoperative pain management.

A recent study using pregabalin 75 - 300 mg *po* prior to surgery failed to show any benefit with respect to a reduction in preoperative anxiety, improvements in postoperative pain, or improvements in postoperative recovery following minor elective surgery. In this study, the patients who received pregabalin 300 mg preoperatively experienced more sedation prior to surgery as well as 90 and 120 min after surgery.[5] In another study of a single dose of pregabalin 150 mg administered preoperatively in patients undergoing laparoscopic cholecystectomy, results showed an improvement in postoperative pain at rest and with activity, a reduction in opioid consumption, and no increased side effects.[6] A systematic review showed that preoperative administration of gabapentin and pregabalin reduced postoperative pain, opioid use, and opioid-related adverse effects without major risks.[7] Conclusions about the optimal dose and duration of the treatment could not be determined due to the heterogeneity of the studies. The role of these medications in the preoperative period continues to be studied.

Acetaminophen and a nonsteroidal anti-inflammatory drug (NSAID) may be prescribed preoperatively in an attempt to establish a foundation of analgesia for postoperative pain management (see Chapter 17 Acute Pain Management). A recent meta-analysis found that acetaminophen reduced postoperative morphine requirements significantly, but it had no effect on the incidence of morphine-related adverse side effects.[8] In adults, acetaminophen 975 mg may be prescribed with sips of water on call to the operating room.

In meta-analysis, preoperative NSAIDs were found to decrease postoperative nausea, vomiting, and sedation by 30%.[9] NSAIDs have a 30 – 50% sparing effect on morphine consumption. In this review, morphine consumption was found to correlate with the incidence of nausea and vomiting, and pruritus, urinary retention, and respiratory depression were not significantly decreased by NSAIDs. A systematic review in children undergoing tonsillectomy found no significant increase in bleeding associated with the perioperative use of NSAIDs and a significant reduction in nausea and vomiting with the preoperative use of NSAIDs (odds ratio 0.49; 95% CI 0.29 to 0.83).[10] Provided there is no contraindication to its use, a NSAID (e.g., celecoxib 200 - 400 mg for an adult) may be given at the same time as acetaminophen.

Other special premedications may include: supplemental oxygen, antibiotics, steroids, antihistamines, beta-blockers, bronchodilators, antacids, insulin. Students should ask their staff anesthesiologists when and why they would prescribe these medications.

## General contraindications to the use of a premedication include:

1. Allergy or hypersensitivity to the drug.
2. Upper airway compromise or respiratory failure.
3. Hemodynamic instability or shock.
4. Decreased level of consciousness or increased intracranial pressure.
5. Severe liver, renal, or thyroid disease.
6. Elderly or debilitated patients.

## References:

1. Zhdanova IV, Wurtman RJ, Lynch HJ, et al. Sleep-inducing effects of low doses of melatonin ingested in the evening. Clin Pharmacol Ther 1995; 57: 552-8.
2. Naguib M, Samarkandi AH. Premedication with melatonin: a double-blind, placebo-controlled comparison with midazolam. BJA 1999; 82: 875-80.
3. Samarkandi A, Naguib AM, Riad W, et al. Melatonin vs. midazolam premedication in children: a double-blind, placebo-controlled study. Eur J Anaesth 2005; 22: 189-196.
4. Jarratt J. Review: Perioperative melatonin use. Anaesth Int Care 2011;39:171-181.
5. White PF, Tufanogullari B, Taylor J et al. The Effect of Pregabalin on Preoperative Anxiety and Sedation Levels: A Dose-Ranging Study. Anesth Analg 2009; 108:1140-1145.
6. Agarwal A, Gautam S, Gupta D, et al. Evaluation of a single preoperative dose of pregabalin for attenuation of postoperative pain after laparoscopic cholecystectomy. BJA 2008; 101: 700-4.
7. Tiippana EM, Hamunen K, Kontinen VK, et al. Do surgical patients benefit from perioperative gabapentin/pregabalin? A systematic review of efficacy and safety. Anesth Analg 2007; 104: 1545-1556.
8. Remy C, Marret E, Bonnet F. Effects of acetaminophen on morphine side-effects and consumption after major surgery: meta-analysis of randomized controlled trials. BJA 2005; 94: 505-13.
9. Emmanuel M, Okba K, Paul Z, et al. Effects of nonsteroidal anti-inflammatory drugs on patient-controlled analgesia morphine side effects: meta-analysis of randomized controlled trials. Anesthesiology 2005; 102: 1249-1260.
10. Cardwell ME, Siviter G, Smith AF. Nonsteroidal anti-inflammatory drugs and perioperative bleeding in paediatric tonsillectomy. The Cochrane Library; Oct 8 2008.

### Additional Resources:

Dotson R, Wiener-Kronish JP, Ajayi T: Preoperative evaluation and medication. In Stoelting RK, Miller RD, editors: Basics of anesthesia, 5th edition, Churchill Livingstone, New York 2007; 157 – 177.

Hata TM, Moyers JR: Preoperative Patient Assessment and Management. In Barash PG, et al. editors. Clinical Anesthesia 6th edition, Lippincott Williams & Wilkins, Philadelphia PA 2009; 567 – 597.

The Ottawa Hospital "My Surgery" website:
http://www.ottawahospital.on.ca/mysurgery

The Ottawa Hospital Preoperative Health History Patient Questionnaire
http://www.anesthesiaprimer.com/AP/Ch3/PrepoEval/PreopQuestionnaire.pdf

# CHAPTER 5

# Getting Started

Patti Murphy MD, Jordan Zacny MD

## Learning Objectives

1. To provide a practical overview of the student's role as part of the anesthesia care team.
2. To provide a practical overview for establishing intravenous access and monitoring procedures for patients requiring anesthesia care.

In this chapter, students are presented with a brief introduction to the anesthetic care of patients beginning with step-by-step guidelines for establishing monitoring procedures, intravenous access, and initial airway management. Students rotating through the operating room may find participating in the anesthetic care of patients daunting. As important members of the anesthesia care team, we encourage students to participate actively in operating room (OR) activities to maximize their learning opportunities. Anesthesiologists are uniquely positioned to pass on a wealth of knowledge in pharmacology and applied physiology as well as important skill sets involving airway management and intravenous access. This knowledge base and accompanying basic skills are valuable for all physicians. Few specialties can offer the precious one-on-one teaching that anesthesia provides.

Anesthesiology is a unique and fascinating specialty! We hope all students enjoy their anesthesia rotation!

## Key Points

1. The degree to which students actively participate in the anesthetic care of a patient correlates directly with their knowledge and their acquired technical skill set.

2. The mnemonic 'STATICS' can be used as a memory prompt for preparing equipment.

3. A blood pressure (BP) cuff can be used as a tourniquet in patients with difficult intravenous access. Inflation of the cuff to approximately 60 mmHg results in distension of both the deep and superficial veins.

4. To decrease the chance of a medication error, avoid distractions when preparing medications, and label syringes before drawing up medications.

5. For patient safety, students should not attempt to perform unfamiliar tasks unless under supervision.

# Preparing the OR:

To ensure safe anesthetic care, a number of steps must be completed before the patient is brought into the operating room.

## Anesthesia Machine and Equipment:

The anesthesia machine and equipment must be checked and prepared. A link to the anesthetic machine checkout procedure is provided in the reference section, although the detail extends beyond the expectations and objectives of most students. Students find the mnemonic 'STATICS' helpful as a quick reminder of the equipment required for safe management of a patient's airway (see Chapter 6 for further discussion on this topic). The mnemonic is useful in the operating room and can easily be adapted to any site in the hospital (ward, emergency, postanesthetic care unit [PACU] or intensive care unit [ICU]).

- **S**uction
- **T**ube (endotracheal tube)
- **A**irway (oral and / or nasopharyngeal)
- **T**ape (for securing the endotracheal tube)
- **I**ntroducer (or stylet for the endotracheal tube)
- **C**ircuit (anesthesia machine) or AMBU bag
- **S**cope (laryngoscope)

## Medications:

Intravenous medications must be prepared and labelled. Students should ask the anesthesiologist if they can assist. Some anesthesiologists may prefer not to delegate this task, following the principle that they will not give medications that they did not prepare. Preparing medications that are not used is both wasteful and expensive and should be minimized.

Medication errors can have serious consequences. They arise when:

- A correct medication is given to the wrong patient.
- The wrong medication is given to the right patient.
- Medication allergies are not identified or checked before a medication is administered.
- The medication concentration is miscalculated.
- Look-alike and sound-alike medications are involved.
- Care providers are distracted or hurried (medication errors are more prevalent at this time).
- Infrequently used medications are given (medication concentration calculations are more prevalent at this time, hence, more likelihood of error).

Before administering any medications, confirm the patient's identity and any known allergies. Common identified high-risk medications[1] with potential serious consequences in the critical care setting include opioids, insulin, heparin, protamine, vancomycin, muscle relaxants, and vasoactive medications, such as phenylephrine and epinephrine. Students should ask their staff anesthesiologist why these medications are considered high-risk.

It is absolutely imperative to be cautious and conscientious when preparing medications. Always:

- Give your full attention to this task.
- Avoid distractors (conversation, multi-tasking).
- Label the syringe first. Place the label at the volume that is to be drawn into the syringe. For example, if 5 mL are to be drawn up, place the label at the 5 mL mark. If the drug is to be diluted, ensure the final concentration is written on the label. For example, ephedrine comes in vials of 50 mg·mL$^{-1}$, but it is commonly

diluted to 10 mL, which equates to a concentration of 5 mg·mL$^{-1}$.

$$\frac{50 \text{ mg·mL}^{-1}}{10 \text{ mL saline}} = 5 \text{ mg·mL}^{-1}$$

- Read the label on the vial.
- Draw up the drug.
- Read the label again before you put the vial down.
- Record the concentration on the label.
- Consider having another more experienced health care provider check your calculations for drugs that are unfamiliar or used infrequently.

Medications must always be prepared and labelled in unused clean syringes. Once the syringe comes in contact with the patient's intravenous, it is considered contaminated and must not be used either to draw up medications from a multi-dose vial or to administer to any other patient.

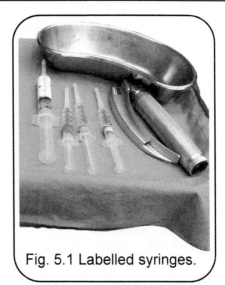

Fig. 5.1 Labelled syringes.

### Intravenous (IV) Access:

Every patient having a surgical procedure will require intravenous access. If available, pre-warmed fluids can be used. For adult patients, a litre of Normal Saline or Ringer's Lactate with standard intravenous tubing

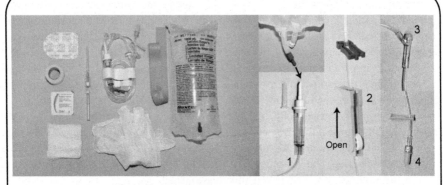

Fig. 5.2 Equipment for intravenous access. Sterile occlusive dressing, tape, alcohol swab, gauze, iv cannula, iv tubing, disposable gloves, tourniquet and intravenous fluid. **1** = iv spike, **2** = roller clamp, **3** = injection port, **4** = luer lock end.

can be prepared. If the patient is having a procedure where a blood transfusion may be required, special tubing with a blood filter and warmer should be prepared.

Preparing a standard intravenous infusion:

- Hang the intravenous bag on an IV pole.
- Close the roller clamp on the tubing to control the flow of fluid. Remove the seal over the IV tubing "spike", and take care not to touch the spike as it is sterile and will come in contact with the intravenous fluid.
- Grasp the IV bag port at the base.
- Insert the tubing spike into the bag port with a pushing and upward twisting motion until the spike is in the port up to its hilt.
- Squeeze and release the drip chamber until it is ½ filled with liquid.
- Open the roller clamp, and flush the air out of the tubing.

## Patient Safety:

To ensure the correct procedure is performed on the correct side and on the correct patient, a number of safety checks must be completed. The patient's identity must be confirmed both verbally and against their identifying arm bracelet. The patient's procedure, consent, and signature must also be confirmed.

Once inside the operating room, a "Preoperative Pause" is conducted by the OR team. The team members verbally identify themselves and their role if this has not been done previously in the day, and the patient's identity is again verified. The indications for antibiotic administration are reviewed and administered, when appropriate, if this has not already been done. This is followed by a discussion of the proposed procedure, sterility of equipment, known allergies, and any problems anticipated by the anesthesia, surgical, and

nursing teams. To communicate this vital information effectively, everyone in the OR must pay close attention to minimize the risk of error. At the completion of surgery, a "Debriefing Pause" is conducted to point out any deviations from the planned procedure that may have occurred.

## Hand Hygiene:

Every year, thousands of Canadians die from infections acquired while being treated in our hospitals.[2] One in nine patients in our hospitals will acquire an infection while being treated for a different medical condition. Proper hand hygiene by health care providers is one of the most effective ways to prevent infections associated with health care. Proper hand hygiene involves the use of an alcohol-based solution or soap and water. The four essential moments for hand hygiene are:

1. Before initial contact with a patient and the patient's environment,
2. Before aseptic techniques,
3. After body fluid exposure, and
4. After contact with a patient and the patient's environment.

Ensure proper hand hygiene before and after interacting with the patient. After proper hand hygiene, the use of disposable gloves is recommended when performing airway and intravenous access tasks. Sterile gloves should be used after proper hand hygiene when performing sterile techniques (e.g., spinal, epidural anesthesia, arterial line insertion).

### Monitoring Procedures:

Once the patient has been safely transferred to the OR table, appropriate monitors should be applied and intravenous access established.

Monitors

- Initial basic monitoring for all patients includes:
- A noninvasive blood pressure (NIBP) cuff,
- An electrocardiogram (ECG), and

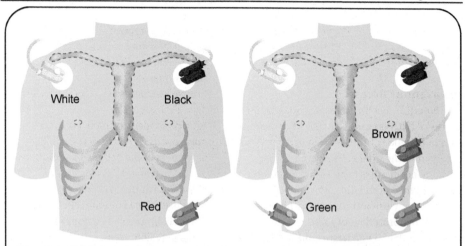

Fig. 5.3 ECG lead placement. Left image: Three lead ECG configuration with white (right arm), black (left arm) and red (left leg) lead placement. Right image: The five lead ECG configuration adds a green lead (right leg), and a brown lead in the V5 chest position.

- A pulse oximeter probe to measure oxygen saturation ($SPO_2$).

The NIBP cuff is typically placed on the patient's upper arm opposite that used for intravenous access. The ECG electrodes are colour-coded and should be placed on flat, hairless sections of the patient's torso far enough away from the surgical prep area.

A three-lead system that includes electrodes for the right arm (RA), left arm (LA), and left leg (LL) is commonly used for healthy patients undergoing minor or moderate-risk surgical procedures. A five-lead system is commonly used for patients who have risk factors for cardiac disease, advanced age, and / or significant comorbid conditions and are undergoing moderate to high-risk surgical procedures. The pulse oximeter probe is typically placed on a digit of the patient's hand on the same side as the intravenous access. See Chapter 10 for a discussion on intraoperative monitors.

## Lead placement and electrode colours

| Lead | 3-lead | 5-lead | Landmarks |
|------|--------|--------|-----------|
| Right arm (RA) | White | White | Right shoulder area |
| Left arm (LA) | Black | Black | Left shoulder area |
| Left leg (LL) | Red | Red | Left chest or flank |
| V5 | | Brown | 5th intercostal space, anterior axillary line |
| Ground | | Green | Right flank |

The saying *"white is right and smoke over fire"* is commonly used to recall the correct position of the white, black and red electrodes.

## Intravenous Access:

Needlestick injuries to health care workers (HCWs) and the risk of transmission of infections to HCWs remains a serious problem in the operative setting.[3,4] The use of safety needles has been shown to decrease the incidence of needlestick injuries. Many hospitals now use intravenous catheters that have incorporated safety features to minimize the risk of a needlestick injury. The BD Insyte™ intravenous catheter safety system uses a spring-loaded mechanism activated by a safety button to retract the needle into a safety chamber once the intravenous catheter is placed in the vein. To further limit needlestick injuries, it is recommended that all needles be disposed of in a designated 'sharps' container, and HCWs should refrain from recapping needles. Newer versions of intravenous insertion cannulas incorporate a membrane in the hub to prevent blood spillage when the needle is retracted (e.g., BD Insyte™ Autoguard™ Blood Control). View the intravenous access video in the additional resources section.

Many operating rooms are configured such that the anesthesiologist is closest to the patients left side. As such, the patient's left hand and forearm are preferentially used for intravenous access. Securing intravenous access closest to the anesthesiologist permits easy access to the site and the ability to monitor the intravenous site should the catheter become interstitial during the procedure. Exceptions to using the left upper extremity for intravenous access include procedures involving the left arm, previous axillary dissection (e.g., mastectomy), the presence of an arteriovenous (AV) fistula for dialysis, and poor venous anatomy. Factors affecting the choice of location for intravenous access include:

- Patient preference
- Venous anatomy
- Short-term use (e.g., day surgery). In this case, dorsal hand veins are suitable.
- Intravenous access is needed for several days. In this case, mid-forearm veins provide an ideal location. Forearm intravenous catheters permit freedom of movement of the patient's arm without occlusion when the arm is flexed.
- Rapid fluid or blood product administration is required. In this case, the cephalic and basilic veins located in the anticubital fossa are larger caliber veins that can be catheterized. Maintenance of an anticubital catheter is more problematic postoperatively as occlusion frequently occurs when the patient's arm is flexed. This can trigger the intravenous infusion pump alarm and disturb the patient's sleep and recovery.

The intravenous catheter gauge refers to the internal diameter of the catheter. A small gauge (G) number indicates the catheter has a larger internal diameter. The larger the diameter the greater the potential flow rate, as flow increases to the fourth power of the catheter radius. Large-bore intravenous catheters (14G and 16G) are used for rapid infusion of large volumes of fluids and blood. A 20-gauge catheter is the most common general purpose catheter used for adults. When venous anatomy is challenging, a smaller 22-gauge intravenous catheter may be used to induce general anesthesia. Under general anesthesia, venous vasodilation occurs as a result of the effects of the volatile anesthetic vapours and the reduction of the patient's emotional stress. With venous vasodilation, an additional larger gauge intravenous catheter can be secured if required.

Local anesthesia may be used to decrease the discomfort associated with intravenous insertion. Either a 25- or 27-gauge needle with 1% or 2% plain lidocaine may be used to raise a skin wheal where the intravenous catheter insertion is planned. Subcutaneous local anesthesia is commonly provided for very anxious patients or in patients requiring a large-bore intravenous catheter. Some clinicians prefer not to use local anesthesia, stating that it involves an additional injection that may be more painful than the intravenous catheter insertion and may obscure the patient's vein. Alternatively, Ametop™, a local topical anesthetic can be applied for 30 – 45 minutes on the dorsum of the patient's hand prior to insertion of the intravenous catheter.

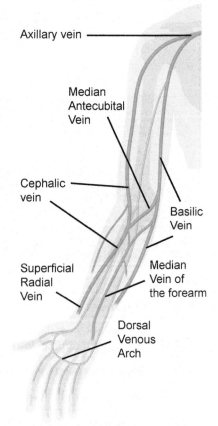

Fig. 5.5 Venous anatomy of the upper limb.

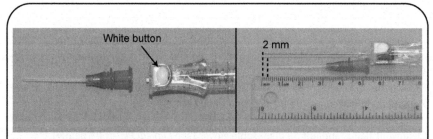

Fig. 5.4 BD Autoguard 20 ga. intravenous safety catheter. Depressing the white button activates the spring loaded needle retraction. Note the needle is approximately 2 mm longer than the catheter.

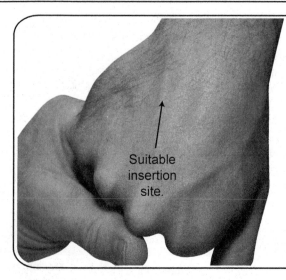

Fig. 5.6 Distal traction is applied to immobilize the dorsal veins of the hand. Note how the operator's thumb is used to apply distal traction on the patient's skin. The thumb is held below the patient's knuckles allowing the intravenous needle to be inserted in the same plane as the vein.

Suitable insertion site.

| Size | Comment |
|------|---------|
| 24G | Infrequently used in adults, used more commonly in pediatrics or adults with difficult intravenous access. |
| 22G | Frequently used for small veins or in pediatric patients. |
| 20G | Most commonly used catheter for adult intravenous access. |
| 18G | Commonly used catheter suitable for moderate fluid requirements. |
| 16G | 16- and 14-gauge catheters are considered "large bore" and are appropriate when significant fluid or blood product administration is anticipated. |
| 14G | "Large bore" catheter used in the setting of significant and rapid blood loss. |

Refer to the addional resourses section to view a brief video demonstrating the necessary steps to secure a peripheral intravenous catheter. Below is a list of the sequential steps required to establish intravenous access.

1. Explain the procedure to the patient and answer any questions the patient may have.
2. Prepare the intravenous tubing and fluid to be used.
3. Place a tourniquet on the patient's upper arm.
4. Clean your hands and put on disposable gloves (see *Clinical Pearls* #4 below).
5. Inspect the patient's hand and forearm for the best site for venous access.
6. Gently tap the vein. This promotes dilation of the vein, increasing its diameter and the chance for success.
7. Clean the site with an alcohol swab.

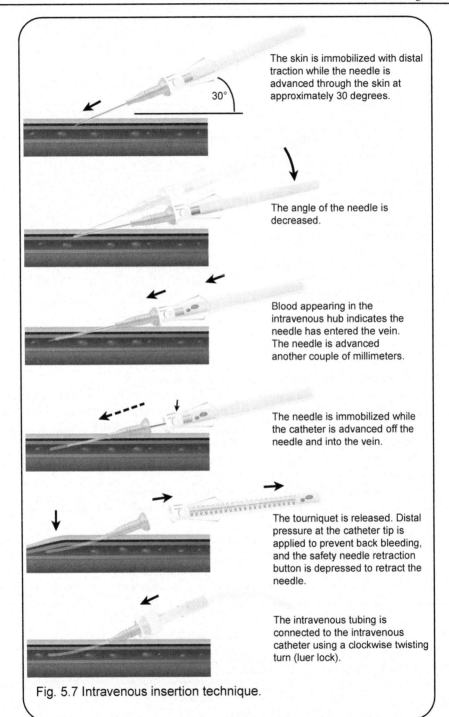

The skin is immobilized with distal traction while the needle is advanced through the skin at approximately 30 degrees.

The angle of the needle is decreased.

Blood appearing in the intravenous hub indicates the needle has entered the vein. The needle is advanced another couple of millimeters.

The needle is immobilized while the catheter is advanced off the needle and into the vein.

The tourniquet is released. Distal pressure at the catheter tip is applied to prevent back bleeding, and the safety needle retraction button is depressed to retract the needle.

The intravenous tubing is connected to the intravenous catheter using a clockwise twisting turn (luer lock).

Fig. 5.7 Intravenous insertion technique.

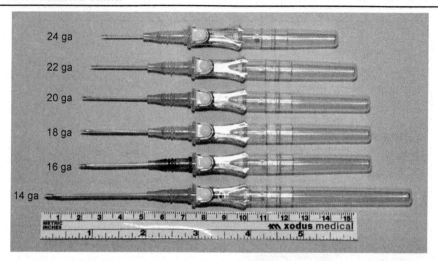

Fig. 5.8 Intravenous catheter sizes. The smaller the gauge number, the larger the diameter of the catheter. The most common sizes are 18, 20 and 22 gauge catheters.

8. If using local anesthesia for intravenous insertion, inject a small amount of local anesthetic at the entry point.
9. Break the seal between the intravenous cannula and needle.
10. Immobilize the vein by applying gentle distal traction on the skin. Distal traction on the skin to is used to immobilize the vein (Fig. 5.6). Once the needle tip pierces through the skin at a 20 – 30 degree angle, decrease the angle of insertion to a shallower 5-degree angle approach to avoid advancing the needle tip beneath the vein. Note that the operator's thumb used to apply distal traction on the veins remains below the patient's knuckles to permit the needle to be advanced at a shallow angle (Fig. 5.6).
11. Insert the needle tip just beneath the skin at a 20 – 30 degree angle.
12. Decrease the angle of entry such that the needle is almost parallel to the skin.
13. Advance the needle towards the vein.
14. Watch for a flashback of blood in the intravenous needle chamber. Some safety needles (e.g., BD Insyte™ 24, 22, and 20G catheters) have incorporated 'Instaflash™' technology. These catheters have a side port in the needle at the distal end such that blood will spill through the port between the needle and catheter as soon as the needle enters the vein. A flash of blood between the needle and catheter immediately confirms that the needle has entered the vascular lumen.
15. Advance the needle another 1 – 2 mm to ensure the catheter is in the vein lumen.
16. Without moving the needle, advance the catheter off the needle and into the vein.
17. Release the tourniquet.
18. Apply pressure over the skin at the tip of the intravenous catheter to prevent back bleeding.
19. For safety needles, deploy the safety needle retraction spring.
20. Attach the intravenous tubing to the catheter.

21. Tighten the luer lock connection between the intravenous tubing and the catheter.
22. Open the intravenous roller clamp and verify that the fluid flow is unrestricted.
23. Place a transparent sterile dressing over the intravenous catheter.
24. Secure the tubing to the patient with tape.
25. Dispose of any needles in an appropriate 'sharps' container.

## The Clinical Pearls of Intravenous Access:

1. The venous tourniquet should be loose enough to permit arterial flow but tight enough to restrict venous flow. It should not be so tight that it causes patient discomfort.
2. Placing the tourniquet on the patient's upper arm permits examination and access to any vein at or below the anticubital fossa.
3. For difficult venous access, a blood pressure cuff can be used as a venous tourniquet. A blood pressure cuff inflated to 60 mmHg will permit arterial inflow while simultaneously obstructing venous outflow. A blood pressure cuff will provide superior occlusion of both the deep and superficial veins compared with a traditional narrow elastic tourniquet. Modern NIBP cuffs often have a 'Venous Stasis Mode' which will maintain a pressure of approximately 60 mmHg while venous access is obtained.
4. The rationale for putting on gloves after applying the tourniquet is to use this time to permit the tourniquet to build up back pressure on the veins. Also, the tourniquet is easier to apply without gloves.
5. Slapping a patient's hand to dilate the veins may result in patient anxiety and discomfort. Gentle tapping of the vein is all that is required to create venous dilation.
6. Use the alcohol swab to wipe the vein in a distal direction. Wiping the alcohol swab towards the heart will tend to empty the vein of blood.
7. Local anesthesia, if used, should be injected only into the superficial dermal skin layer and not into the vein. To be effective, the intravenous catheter should be inserted into the area where the local anesthesia was injected.
8. Gentle distal traction on the vein will immobilize the vein, which is crucial for successful intravenous catheterization.
9. Stabilize the patient's hand with the intravenous catheter by resting the fingers that are not holding the catheter against the patient's hand or forearm.
10. Once the needle tip advances through the skin, avoid downward pressure as this can cause the vein to collapse. Gentle pressure in the direction of the needle will permit the needle to enter the vein without collapsing the vein.
11. Discomfort with intravenous insertion is generally related to sensory feedback from the skin. Intense discomfort can result if the needle is transecting the vein wall or piercing a peripheral nerve. If intense pain occurs with intravenous insertion, remove the needle and reassess.
12. Once the needle tip has advanced through the skin, focus on the position of the needle tip in relation to the vein.
13. A slight 10-15-degree angulation of the needle and catheter unit prior to insertion can be useful to prevent the needle tip from entering too deep into the vein (Fig. 5.9). This is especially helpful for accessing veins in the forearm.

14. With the needle and catheter in the vein, immobilize the needle while the catheter is advanced off the needle. It is important to keep the patient's skin stretched with your non-dominant hand while the catheter is being advanced. If resistance is encountered while advancing the catheter, stop further advancement, as the catheter may be abutting against a valve or exiting the vein lumen. Attach the catheter to the intravenous tubing, open the roller clamp, and if there is no extravasation, attempt to advance the catheter with the intravenous fluid flowing.

15. Difficulties may be encountered in finding a suitable vein for intravenous access. Veins constrict with cold, anxiety, and dehydration. They dilate with gentle tapping, warmth, gravity, and muscle activity. Patients should be kept warm, and preoperative anxiolytics or topical anesthesia should be considered if a patient has a history of difficult venous access and needle phobia. Consider wrapping patients' arms in warm blankets. Apply a tourniquet and ask patients to contract and relax their hand repeatedly and to position their arm (hanging) below the level of their heart.

## General Anesthesia Induction:

With intravenous access secured and appropriate monitoring procedures established, a baseline set of vital signs are recorded. The 'Preoperative Pause' should be completed (if this has not already been done), and the need for antibiotics verified. Oxygen is administered by facemask to maximize the oxygen reserve prior to induction of anesthesia (see Chapter 9 Rationale for Preoxygenation).

Intravenous medications are then administered to the patient to induce a state of general anesthesia. Following induction of anesthesia, loss of consciousness is verified by apnea, loss of response to verbal commands, and loss of the eyelash reflex. Although the patient is asleep, the intravenous medications require an additional period of time to reach their peak effect. During this time, the patient's lungs are supported with a brief period of bag-mask positive pressure ventilation prior to airway management. Airway management may involve the insertion of a laryngeal mask airway device or similar extraglottic device (see Chapter 8) or insertion of an endotracheal tube (see Chapter 6, 7, 9). Now is the student's time to shine! Along with establishing intravenous access, bag-mask ventilation of the lungs is one of the most important skills students will acquire during their anesthesia rotation.

The anesthesia machine can be used to provide bag-mask ventilation in an apneic patient. "The circuit" refers to the clear plastic anesthesia tubing that carries oxygen and anesthetic gases from the anesthesia machine to the patient's airway. It is called a *circle* breathing circuit because the gas flows in a circle directed by one-way valves. The flow of gas (oxygen) into the circuit is controlled by the gas flow meters. The adjustable pressure release valve (APL) valve controls the pressure at which gas leaves the circuit (provided there is a good seal between the patient's face and the mask). Prior to induction of anesthesia, ensure the APL valve is fully open (turned counterclockwise). If the APL valve is closed, the patient will not be able to breathe out with a tightly fitting facemask. Ensure the oxygen flow rate is set at $\geq$ 6 L·min$^{-1}$ before applying the facemask. If there is no oxygen flow, the reservoir bag will be collapsed and the patient will experience difficulty breathing.

After induction of anesthesia, a seal must be created between the patient's face and the anesthesia mask to provide positive pressure ventilation. This is commonly termed 'bag-mask' ventilation. Adjust the APL valve by turning the valve clockwise to 20

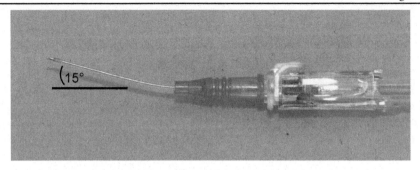

Fig. 5.9 Slight angulation of the intravenous needle and catheter. This simple but useful technique can be used to prevent the needle from going too deep when establishing an intravenous in the forearm.

$cmH_2O$. Airway pressures > 20 $cmH_2O$ may result in gastric insufflation and an increase in nausea, vomiting, and potential aspiration (see Chapters 9, 26). Should the reservoir bag become distended and taut, either lift the facemask from the patient to permit passive exhalation or open the APL valve slightly by turning it counterclockwise.

Squeeze the reservoir bag to deliver positive pressure to the patient. When performed correctly, positive pressure will result in oxygen being delivered to the patient's lungs and the patient's chest wall will rise. As pressure is released from the reservoir bag, the patient's chest wall will fall during exhalation, the capnography will indicate that $CO_2$ is being exhaled, and the ventilator spirometer will record the volume of gas exhaled by the patient. Common causes of failure of the patient's chest wall to rise with positive pressure ventilation include a poor facemask seal and / or an upper airway obstruction. Ask your staff anesthesiologist what they do to problem solve when ventilation by facemask fails (see Chapter 6, 8 for maneuvers used to overcome difficulties with facemask ventilation). After insertion of an endotracheal tube or laryngeal mask airway device, ventilation may be controlled using the anesthesia ventilator. The APL valve is only functional during 'bag-mask' ventilation and becomes inactive once the ventilator is activated.

**References:**
1. Kothari D, Gupta S, Sharma C, et al. Medication error in anaesthesia and critical care: A cause for concern. Ind J Anaesth 2010; 54:187-192.
2. Ontario Ministry of Health and Long Term Care Four Moments of Hand Hygiene.
3. Wilburn SQ, Eijkemans G. Preventing needlestick injuries among healthcare workers. A WHO-ICN Collaboration.
4. Berguer R, Heller PJ. Preventing sharps injuries in the operating room. J Am Coll Surg 2004; 199: 462-467.

# Intubation and Anatomy of the Airway

Patrick Sullivan MD, Ashleigh Farrell MD

## Learning Objectives

1. To identify indicators that would predict difficulty with bag-mask ventilation (BMV).
2. To identify indicators that would lead to difficult direct laryngoscopy.
3. To describe practical clinical maneuvers to resolve an upper airway obstruction in a patient whose trachea is not intubated.

## Key Points

| | |
|---|---|
| 1 | The patient's medical history and clinical exam can help predict difficult bag-mask ventilation as well as difficult tracheal intubation. |
| 2 | Bag-mask ventilation and tracheal intubation will be difficult in a small percentage of patients. These patients require special planning. |
| 3 | Insertion of an extraglottic airway, such as a laryngeal mask airway device (e.g., LMA™) may be life saving in the "cannot intubate, cannot ventilate" scenario. |
| 4 | There are two immediate clinical tools to confirm tracheal intubation: end-tidal carbon dioxide ($ETCO_2$) measurement and visualization of the endotracheal tube (ETT) passing through the glottis. |
| 5 | Clinical experience is correlated directly with successful intubation at first attempt. Enlist expert assistance for anticipated difficult intubations. |
| 6 | Always have a backup airway plan. |

Over 25% of anesthetic-related morbidity and mortality arises from complications related to inadequate ventilation resulting from either difficult BMV or difficult tracheal intubation. The goal of the airway assessment is to identify potential problems with the provision, maintenance, and protection of a patent airway and the provision of adequate ventilation following tracheal intubation. Patient assessment requires a specific history and a directed physical examination (described below).

### History

Patients may be aware of past difficulties with anesthesia pertaining to tracheal intubation, and a review of their previous anesthetic records may provide valuable information concerning prior airway management techniques that were either successful or unsuccessful. A history of restricted neck mobility (e.g., cervical spine (C-spine) fusion, degenerative disc disease [DDD]), restricted mouth opening (e.g., temporal mandibular joint disease), cancer of the oropharynx, or radiation to the head and neck are important predictors of a potentially difficult airway.

Factors predicting difficult BMV include elderly, edentulous patients, obesity, history of obstructive sleep apnea, and the presence of a beard. Patients with predictors of difficult BMV may or may not also have predictors of a difficult intubation. Patients with predictors of both a difficult BMV and difficult intubation require special attention and careful planning to avoid a "cannot intubate, cannot ventilate" crisis. Planning would involve having a difficult airway cart immediately available, enlisting experienced assistance for intubation, use of advanced airway equipment tools, and/or consideration for an "awake" intubation with a fiberoptic scope using topical anesthesia and judicious intravenous sedation. See Chapter 7 for a further discussion on advanced airway options for managing a difficult airway.

In a recent review of 50,000 anesthesia cases, the combined frequency of difficult BMV and tracheal intubation was 0.38% or 1 in 266 patients.[1] Predictors included the presence of sleep apnea, body mass index (BMI) > 31, Mallampati 3 or 4 view, male, beard, edentulous, restricted thyromental distance, and restricted neck extension. A focused preoperative examination can be used to look for these predictors and identify patients at risk for a "failed airway". Either "awake" intubation or use of a regional or local anesthetic technique might then be considered.

## Physical Examination

A focused examination of the airway is used to identify patients who are predicted to experience difficulties with traditional airway management procedures. These procedures commonly include BMV, placement of an extraglottic airway device (e.g., LMA™), or direct laryngoscopy and intubation.

Several clinical predictors of a difficult airway are described below. There is no single test that is both highly sensitive and specific in predicting difficulties. Based on the patient's medical history and using a combination of clinical examinations, we are able to improve our ability to identify patients who will require special attention and equipment so as to provide them with safe airway management.

Difficult BMV is defined as the inability to provide adequate bag-mask ventilation and maintain an oxygen saturation > 90%. The mnemonic "BONES" summarizes the common predictors of difficulty with BMV.

### Clinical Pearl:

*Difficult BMV: Remember the mnemonic* **"BONES"**

**B**eard: A seal between the mask and the patient's face is essential for effective BMV. Assuming the facemask is positioned properly, the most common reason for an incomplete mask seal is the presence of a beard. Less commonly, trauma, secretions, or facial abnormalities prevent an effective seal. If a seal cannot be created, positive pressure will result in oxygen leaking between the patient's face and mask, and ventilation attempts will be ineffective.

**O**besity: Obesity is associated with redundant oropharyngeal tissue. This may result in upper airway obstruction and difficulty with BMV in the unconscious patient.

## BONES

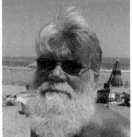

**Beard**

**Obesity**

**No teeth**

**Elderly**

**Snores**

The mnemonic 'BONES' has been used as an aid to identify patients that may be difficult to ventilate using a bag and mask.

No Teeth: Teeth provide a framework by creating a space between the tongue and palate. Without teeth, the tongue collapses against the palate when the mouth is closed, resulting in obstruction of oxygen flow with BMV. The use of an oropharyngeal airway, nasopharyngeal airway, or the patient's dentures may be useful for BMV in the edentulous patient.

Elderly: Increased difficulty with BMV has been observed in patients > 55 years of age. This is thought to be due to a generalized decrease in the elasticity of the tissues and an increased incidence in obstructive and restrictive pulmonary disease.

Snoring & Stiffness: Snoring is a symptom of upper airway obstruction and is associated with obstructive sleep apnea (OSA) as well as difficulties with BMV. Diseases that reduce lung compliance (asthma, pulmonary edema, and fibrosis) are also associated with difficult BMV.

*Clinical Pearl:*

*Difficulty with bag-mask ventilation is not always associated with difficulties in placement of an extraglottic device (e.g., LMA™) or ETT. If difficulties with BMV occur, simple maneuvers, such as placement of an oropharyngeal airway, nasopharyngeal airway, or jaw thrust, may solve the problem. If difficulties persist, consider immediate placement of an extraglottic device or ETT.*

### The Four Step Upper Airway Examination:

The Four Step Upper Airway Examination is used to assess several factors that may affect decisions concerning the patient's airway management. This examination can usually be completed in less than a minute in the elective, awake, and cooperative patient. Modifications of the examination will be dictated by the patient's condition (e.g., unconscious patient, C-spine collar).

### 1st Step:     Assess Temporomandibular Joint Mobility

The first step of the test is to identify any restricted mobility of the temporomandibular joint (TMJ). Ask patients to sit up with their head in the neutral position and their mouth open as wide as possible. Note the mobility of the mandibular condyle at the TM joint. The condyle should rotate forward freely so that the width of the space created between the tragus of the ear and the mandibular condyle is approximately the breadth of one finger.

### 2nd Step:     Assess Mouth Opening and Assign the Mallampati Classification

The aperture of an adult patient's mouth should admit three fingers between the teeth. This corresponds to a distance of

57

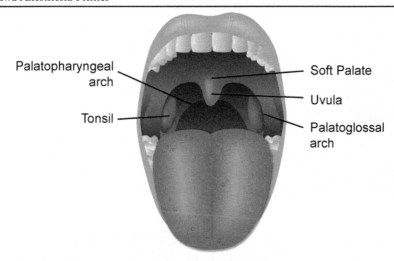

Fig. 6.1 Oropharyngeal Anatomy.

approximately 5 – 6 cm in an adult. If the opening is < 2 fingerbreadths (< 2.5 cm), it will be difficult to insert the laryngoscope blade, let alone visualize the larynx. Note any loose, capped, prominent, or missing teeth as well as any dentures or dental bridge appliances.

**Mallampati Classification:** Mallampati *et al.* first correlated the ability to visualize the oropharyngeal structures with the ease of tracheal intubation with a direct laryngoscope. Their classification was later modified by Samsoon and Young to include four classes. To assign a "modified" Mallampati classification, the examiner should face the patient at eye level. The oropharyngeal structures are classified with the patient sitting upright, head in the neutral position, mouth opened as wide as possible, and tongue maximally protruded without phonating (Fig. 6.1). The structures to visualize include: the pharyngeal arches, uvula, soft palate, hard palate, tonsillar beds, and posterior pharyngeal wall. Technical difficulties with tracheal intubation may be anticipated when only the tongue and soft palate are visualized in a patient during this maneuver. The anticipated difficulty of intubation with direct laryngoscopy increases in relation to the increase in the oropharyngeal class number. For patients with a class I oropharyngeal view, adequate exposure of the glottis during direct laryngoscopy should be easily achieved.

Using this classification, we can predict that the trachea of a patient with a class 4 hypopharynx, a full set of teeth, a restricted thyromental distance, and restricted atlantoocipital extension will be difficult to intubate using direct laryngoscopy. Patients who have a restricted airway may require techniques other than direct laryngoscopy to secure an airway. Choosing regional or local anesthesia rather than general anesthesia is one way to avoid the need for tracheal intubation. Other airway management options include "awake" intubation with topical anesthesia, intravenous conscious sedation, or the use of a laryngeal mask rather than an endotracheal tube.

### 3rd Step: Assess the Thyromental Distance and Mandibular Protrusion

The third step of this test is to assess the characteristics of the patient's mandible, which

Class I    Class II    Class III    Class IV

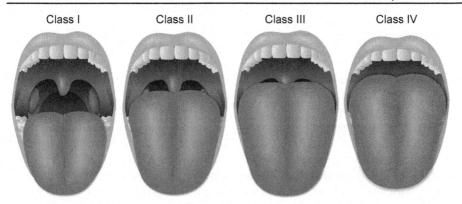

Fig. 6.2 Modified Mallampati classification of pharyngeal structures. Note that the soft palate is visible in Class III but not class IV. (From Samsoon G, Young J. Anaesthesia 1987;42:487 - 490).

involves evaluating the thyromental distance (TMD) and the patient's ability to protrude the mandible.

The TMD is measured with the neck (atlantooccipital junction) in full extension. In adults, the distance from the lower border of the chin (mentum) to the thyroid cartilage notch should be ≥ 3 fingerbreadths (or > 6.5 cm). Distances of < 6.5 cm may be associated with an anterior larynx or a small mandible. A TMD < 6.5 cm would predict difficulty in

exposing the larynx with a classic Macintosh laryngoscope.

Mandibular protrusion is evaluated by asking patients to bring their lower jaw as far forward as possible or to try to bite their upper lip with their bottom teeth. With Class I, the patient is able to protrude the lower incisors anterior to the upper lip. With Class II, the patient's lower incisors can just reach the margin of the upper lip. In Class III, the lower incisors cannot protrude to the upper lip. Class

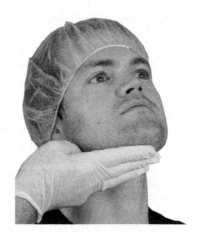

Fig. 6.3 Thyromental distance.

II and III are associated with increased risk of difficult direct laryngoscopy.

### 4th Step: Assess the Range of Motion of the Cervical Spine

The fourth step of the test is to evaluate the mobility of the cervical spine. This is accomplished by asking the patient to flex and extend the neck. Patients should be able to perform this without discomfort. Disease of the C-spine (rheumatoid arthritis [RA], osteoarthritis [OA]), previous injury, or surgical fusion may limit neck extension, which may create difficulties during intubation attempts. This is certainly true if the atlantooccipital joint is involved, as restriction of this joint's mobility may impair the ability to visualize the larynx.

### "Non-reassuring airway" findings:

A number of clinical findings can be used to predict difficulty with direct laryngoscopy and intubation (Table 6.1). When these findings are present, clinicians often describe the patient as having a "non-reassuring" airway. These findings may be used to plan alternate techniques to direct laryngoscopy for intubation.

### Table 6.1 Non-Reassuring Airway

| Non–Reassuring Airway Findings |
| --- |
| Long upper incisors |
| Maxillary overbite |
| Mallampati 3 & 4 |
| Stiff mandibular space |
| Short thyromental space |
| Limited neck extension |
| Limited mouth opening |
| Short thick neck |

### Evaluation of the Lower Airway:

Lastly, an attempt should be made to ascertain any difficulty with the lower airway (glottis, larynx, and trachea). This is particularly important in patients who have experienced a previous airway injury or surgery on their airway, such as a tracheostomy. Observe the patient for hoarseness, stridor, or a previous tracheostomy scar that would suggest a potential underlying tracheal stenosis.

Fig. 6.5 shows visualization of the laryngeal structures at the time of laryngoscopy. Just as the view of the oropharyngeal structures has been classified, the view of the laryngeal

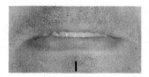 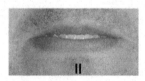 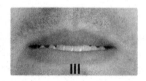

Fig. 6.4 Upper lip bite test. Class I: Lower incisors bite vermilion line. Class II: Lower incisors bite below vermilion line. Class III: Lower incisors cannot bite upper lip.

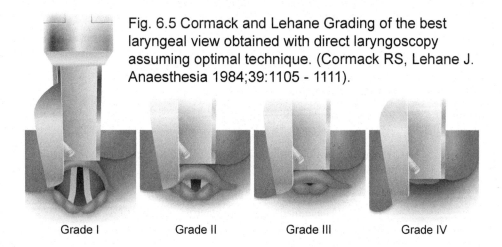

Fig. 6.5 Cormack and Lehane Grading of the best laryngeal view obtained with direct laryngoscopy assuming optimal technique. (Cormack RS, Lehane J. Anaesthesia 1984;39:1105 - 1111).

|  |  |  |  |
|---|---|---|---|
| Grade I | Grade II | Grade III | Grade IV |

structures has been graded from 1 to 4. While there is not a perfect correlation between the oropharyngeal class and the laryngeal grade, we anticipate that a patient with a class 1 oropharyngeal view and no other identified airway abnormalities will have a grade I laryngeal view. Similarly, a class 4 oropharyngeal view predicts difficulty in visualizing laryngeal anatomy.

Before proceeding with intubation **prepare for success** with the mnemonic "**A BASIC MAD POSTER**"

| A BASIC | MAD | POSTER |
|---|---|---|
| **A**ssessment<br>**B**ag, mask<br>**A**irway<br>**S**uction<br>**I**ntravenous<br>**C**apnometry | **M**onitors<br>**A**udible tone<br>**D**rugs | **P**ositioning<br>**O**xygen<br>**S**tylet<br>**T**ape<br>**E**TT, laryngoscope<br>**R**escue – back up airway plans, resuscitation drugs |

"**A BASIC MAD POSTER**" preparation for intubation explained.

**A**ssessment: The preparation for intubation begins with an *assessment* of the airway.

**B**ag-mask: A *bag*-mask system should be checked and capable of delivering oxygen with positive pressure.

**A**irways: Oropharyngeal and nasopharyngeal *airways* should be immediately available.

**S**uction: A tonsillar Yankauer *suction* device with a tapered tip should be immediately available next to the patient's head.

**I**ntravenous: *Intravenous* access should be established.

Capnometry:      *Capnometry* (ETCO$_2$ monitoring) should be immediately available to confirm correct endotracheal placement.

Monitors:      *Monitors,* including pulse oximetry, ECG, and blood pressure (BP), should be attached.

Audible:      The saturation monitor should be configured to provide an *audible* tone during the procedure.

Drugs:      *Drugs* should be prepared and labelled.

Position:      The patient should be in an optimal *position* for tracheal intubation.

Oxygen:      *Oxygen* should be administered to preoxygenate the patient prior to the procedure.

Stylet:      A *stylet* should be positioned in the ETT.

Tape:      *Tape* should be immediately available to secure the ETT.

ETT:      An appropriate sized *endotracheal* tube and functioning laryngoscope should be prepared and checked.

Rescue:      *Rescue* medications and backup airway plans should be considered before intubation.

Common rescue medications include midazolam, fentanyl, and propofol for sedation. Ephedrine and phenylephrine may be required to treat hypotension after intubation. Prior to proceeding with intubation, there should be clearly thought out airway backup plans. Plans may include having special equipment present (e.g., Glidescope or LMA™).

### Clinical Pearl:

*Always ensure that the saturation monitor emits an audible tone when performing tracheal intubation. The audible tone provides immediate information to the operating room team about the patients' heart rate, saturation, and well being that may otherwise go unnoticed during the procedure.*

## Tracheal Intubation:

The technique of tracheal intubation involves five steps.

I.    Position the patient
II.    Open the patient's mouth
III.    Perform laryngoscopy
IV.    Insert the ETT through the vocal cords and remove the laryngoscope
V.    Confirm correct ETT placement and secure the ETT

## I.    Position the patient

Ensure the bed is elevated to a level that is comfortable for the clinician. A rough guide is to position the patient's head at the level of the clinician's umbilicus. When preparing to intubate the patient's trachea, the head and neck should be positioned using a combination of both cervical flexion and atlantooccipital (AO) extension. We describe this as the sniffing position. This enables the clinician to align the axes of the patient's mouth, pharynx, and larynx during laryngoscopy (Fig. 6.6). In addition to the sniffing position, "ramping" up the upper thoracic spine using blankets or specially designed pillows (Troop Pillow) can be very useful to optimize the patient's position prior to tracheal intubation.

*Ideal positioning of the patient for direct laryngoscopy and tracheal intubation occurs when the external auditory meatus aligns in the same horizontal plane as the sternal notch when the patient is examined from the side (see Fig. 6.7, 6.8).*

Atlantooccipital extension alone increases the angle between the axis of the pharynx and the larynx. By contrast, the combination of cervical flexion of the neck with AO extension results in the alignment of the axes of the pharynx and larynx.

Optimizing the position of the patient's head, neck, and thoracic spine before attempting laryngoscopy is an important initial step to ensure a successful tracheal intubation. This is especially true in obese or pregnant patients (Fig. 6.8) or in cases of an anticipated difficult intubation. It is good practice to ensure that your first intubation attempt is your best attempt.

*Clinical Pearl:*

*In addition to placing the patient in the sniffing position, ramping up the thoracic spine is an important maneuver to optimize the patient's position prior to tracheal intubation.*

## II.     Open the patient's mouth

The second step involves opening the patient's mouth. First, the clinician stands directly behind the patient's head and takes the laryngoscope in their left hand. The right hand is used to open the patient's mouth and later to advance the ETT. Mouth opening can be accomplished by using the right hand to open the patient's teeth (e.g., the scissors technique, as illustrated in Fig. 6.10) or by placing the right hand on the patient's occiput and rotating the occiput backward to create an AO

extension (Fig. 6.9). Using the scissors maneuver, the clinician uses the index finger to pull up on the patient's upper right incisors, which serves to open the patient's mouth, extend the AO joint, and protect the teeth and lips. At the same time, the clinician uses the thumb to push down on the lower mandible and further open the patient's mouth. This technique can be modified by opening the patient's mouth using the right middle finger to depress the lower teeth (Fig. 6.10). If the clinician chooses the extraoral technique of mouth opening, the right hand is placed on the patient's occiput and the patients' head is rotated into the sniffing position. With this movement, the mandible drops and the patient's mouth opens. This method of mouth opening is more suitable for the edentulous patient than the scissors technique.

## III.     Laryngoscopy

The third step involves insertion of the laryngoscope into the patient's mouth (Fig. 6.9, 6.10). The tip of the laryngoscope blade is advanced to the base of the patient's tongue by rotating its tip around the tongue (Fig. 6.9). The laryngoscope blade should follow the natural curve of the oropharynx and tongue. The blade should then be inserted to the right of the tongue's midline so that the tongue moves toward the left and out of the line of vision. The patient's tongue should not be pushed into the back of the oropharynx, as visualization will be obscured. Once the tip of the blade lies at the base of the patient's tongue (just above the epiglottis), firm, steady, upward and forward traction should be applied to the laryngoscope. The direction of force should be at 30° from the horizontal. Once the laryngoscope is properly positioned at the base of the tongue, avoid rotating it, as this action might exert pressure on the upper teeth and damage them. Damage is more common to the immobile upper maxillary teeth than to the lower mandibular teeth,

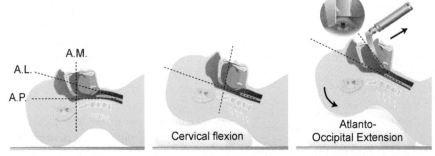

Fig. 6.6 Axes of the airway. A combination of cervical flexion and atlanto-occipital extension aligns the axis of the pharynx (A.P.), larynx (A.L.) and mouth (A.M.). Forward displacement of the mandible then facilitates visualization of the glottis during direct laryngoscopy.

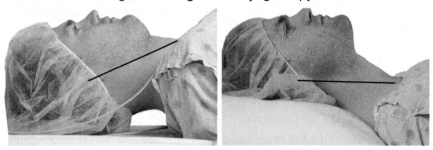

Fig. 6.7 Left image: poor positioning for direct laryngoscopy.
Right image: optimized positioning for direct laryngoscopy. Note the horizontal alignment of the middle ear with the sternum.

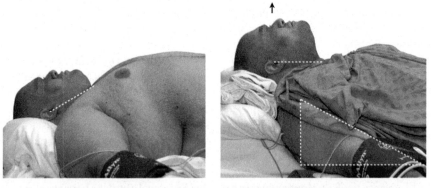

Fig. 6.8 Ramping the thoracic spine to optimize the patients position for direct laryngoscopy and intubation. In addition to pillows under the shoulders and head, a special pillow (e.g., Troop™ pillow) can be used to ramp the thoracic spine (right image). The position is optimized when the tragus of the ear is in the same horizontal plane as the sternal notch.

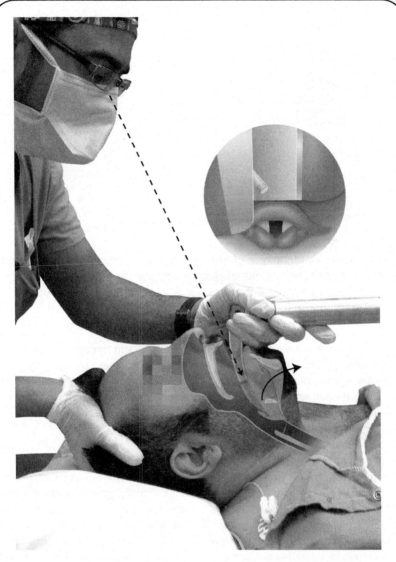

Fig. 6.9 Direct laryngoscopy. A patient pillow provides cervical flexion. The right hand controls atlanto-occipital extension and facilitates mouth opening. The curved laryngoscope has been inserted into the right side of the mouth displacing the tongue to the left. The tip of the curved laryngoscope blade is at the base of the tongue and epiglottis. An upward and forward (30 - 45 degrees) lifting force is used to expose the glottis. Note the operator's proper stance, avoiding a stooped posture.

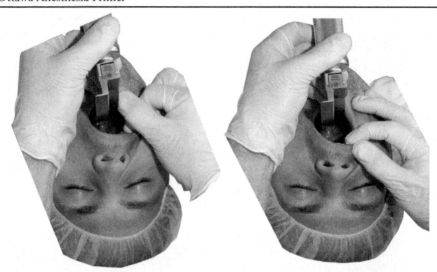

Fig. 6.10 Scissors technique of mouth opening for insertion of a laryngo-scope. Left image: traditional scissors technique. The thumb pushes the mandible forward while the index finger is used to pull back on upper incisor. Right image: modified scissors technique.

which are free to move forward with the jaw during laryngoscopy. Fig. 6.12 shows how the larynx is more visible if the blade of the laryngoscope moves the patient's tongue to the left of the mouth and out of the line of vision.

Students learning the technique of laryngoscopy universally adopt a stooped posture, placing their face within inches of the patient in an attempt to visualize the larynx. A stooped posture limits the power that can be exerted by their arm, making laryngoscopy technically more difficult to perform. In the stooped position, vision becomes monocular. The laryngoscope is typically rotated in an attempt to improve the view resulting in pressure being applied on the patient's upper front teeth. With a stooped posture, it is difficult to visualize the upper teeth and larynx simultaneously while being aware of the pressure being placed on the upper teeth. By maintaining a more erect posture during laryngoscopy, an improved binocular view of both the teeth and larynx is possible. With a more erect posture the muscles

of the arm and forearm can then be used to lift the soft tissues upward and forward with the left hand in the direction of the laryngoscope handle avoiding the need to rotate the laryngoscope with the wrist to improve the laryngeal view.

**Laryngeal Anatomy:**

In adults, the larynx is located at the level of the 4th to 6th cervical vertebrae. It consists of numerous muscles, cartilages, and ligaments. The large thyroid cartilage shields the larynx and articulates inferiorly with the cricoid cartilage. Two pyramidal-shaped arytenoid cartilages sit on the upper lateral borders of the cricoid cartilage. The aryepiglottic fold is a mucosal fold running from the epiglottis posteriorly to the arytenoid cartilages. The cuneiform cartilages appear as small flakes within the margin of the aryepiglottic folds.

The adult epiglottis resembles the shape of a leaf and functions like a trap door for the glottis. In Fig. 6.13, the "trap door" is shown

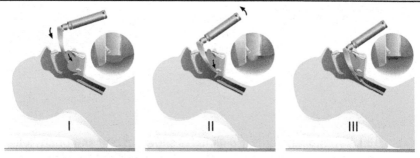

Fig. 6.11 Common problems with direct laryngoscopy. I: Lifting the larygoscope too early results in downfolding of the tongue, obscuring visualization of the glottis. II: Pushing the larygoscope downward may cause the epiglottis to move posterior, obscuring the larygeal view. III: Insertion of the laryngoscope blade too deeply (esophageal inlet) bypasses the glottic aperature.

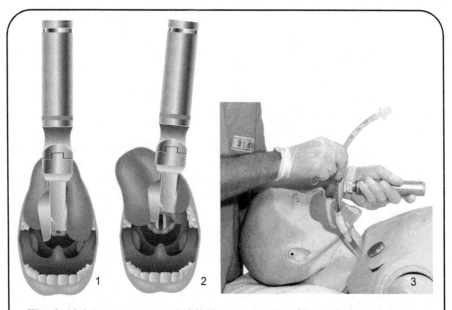

Fig. 6.12 Laryngoscopy. 1. Midline insertion of laryngoscope blade may result in the tongue obscuring the glottis. 2. The laryngoscope blade is inserted on the right side of the patient's mouth, displacing the tongue to the left and exposing the glottis. 3. The patient's head is at the level of the operator's umbilicus. The endotracheal tube is directed immediately behind the epiglottis and anterior to the upper esophageal inlet.

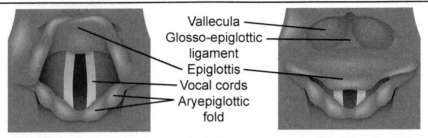

Fig. 6.13 Laryngeal anatomy. Epiglottis is shown in both the open (left image) and closed (right image) position. The cuneiform (medial) and corniculate (lateral) cartilages form the aryepiglottic fold.

in both its open and closed positions. The epiglottis is attached to the back of the thyroid cartilage by the thyroepiglottic ligament and to the base of the tongue by the glossoepiglottic ligament. The covering membrane is termed the glossoepiglottic fold, and the valleys on either side of this fold are called valleculae. When performing laryngoscopy, the tip of the curved laryngoscope blade should be advanced to the base of the tongue at its union with the epiglottis. It helps to try to visualize this anatomy as well as possible when performing laryngoscopy.

## IV.     Insertion of the ETT

Intubation is performed with the left hand controlling the laryngoscope blade while the right hand opens the patient's mouth and then passes the ETT tip through the laryngeal inlet under direct visualization. When a limited laryngeal view is encountered, the epiglottis can be used as a landmark for guiding the ETT through the hidden vocal cords. The tip of the ETT is passed underneath the epiglottis and anterior to the esophageal inlet. Note that the glottis lies anterior to the esophagus (or above the esophagus during laryngoscopy). When the epiglottis partially obscures the view of the glottis, an assistant can be asked to apply pressure to the thyroid cartilage by displacing it in a direction that is backwards, upward, and towards the right side of the patient. This

maneuver is called the "BURP" maneuver. It is used to move the larynx in a manner that improves the clinician's view of the glottis. The BURP maneuver should not be confused with the application of cricoid pressure. Cricoid pressure is discussed in Chapter 9: Rapid Sequence Induction.

A malleable stylet that is shaped to form a distal anterior curve of approximately 35° can be helpful to guide the ETT tip through the laryngeal inlet and should be used for all difficult and/or emergency intubations. Use of an endotracheal stylet that is configured with a more acute 90° "hockey stick" configuration is discouraged as this may result in trauma to the anterior trachea on insertion as well as ETT displacement when the stylet is removed.

When there is a limited view of the ETT passing through the vocal cords, the Ford Maneuver can help with visual confirmation of its correct placement in the glottis immediately after intubation. The maneuver is performed by displacing the glottis posteriorly using downward pressure on the ETT while lifting with the laryngoscope to expose the glottis and ETT. This maneuver is useful in the patient with a grade 3 or 4 larynx when difficulty is encountered visualizing the glottic structures.

The cuff of the ETT should be observed to pass between the vocal cords and should be positioned just inferior (approximately 2 cm) to the vocal cords. Before withdrawing the

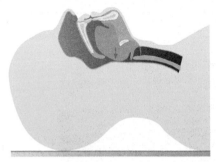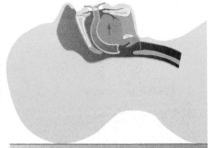

Fig. 6.14 Left image: Upper airway obstruction caused by the tongue falling posterior in the supine unconscious patient. Rght image: Insertion of an oropharyngeal airway restores airway patency.

laryngoscope blade from the patient's mouth, it is helpful to note the length of the ETT at the patient's lips using the cm markers on the ETT. This will be useful information should the ETT move before it can be secured. The usual distance from the tip of the ETT to the patient's mouth is approximately 21 - 24 cm in adult males and 18 – 22 cm in adult females. The ETT cuff is inflated with just enough air to create a seal around the ETT during positive pressure ventilation. A cuff leak may be detected by listening at the patient's mouth or over the larynx.

Bimanual laryngoscopy is an essential maneuver to improve the glottic view when an inadequate view is obtained on first attempt. The maneuver is performed by the clinician using the left hand to lift the laryngoscope blade while the right thumb and forefinger are used to manipulate the thyroid cartilage externally by pushing it posteriorly or to the right to obtain a better view of the glottis. Once an optimal view is obtained, an assistant's hand replaces the clinician's right hand to maintain the thyroid manipulation. The clinician then uses the right hand to direct the ETT into the glottis.

## V. Confirmation of correct ETT placement.

Immediate absolute proof that the ETT is in the tracheal lumen can be obtained by observing the ETT pass between the vocal cords, by observing $ETCO_2$ returning with each respiration, or by visualizing the tracheal lumen through the ETT using a fiberoptic scope. Indirect confirmation that the trachea is intubated with a tracheal tube includes: listening over the epigastrium for the absence of breath sounds with ventilation, observing the chest rise and fall with positive pressure ventilation, observing condensation on the ETT, balloting the endotracheal cuff in the neck, and listening to the apex of each lung field for breath sounds with ventilation. There are reports of physicians auscultating "distant breath sounds" in each lung field when in fact the ETT was incorrectly placed in the esophagus. Hence, listening to the lung fields may reveal bronchospasm or evidence of an endobronchial intubation, but it cannot be relied on as absolute proof that the ETT is correctly positioned in the trachea.

If the ETT is positioned in the tracheal lumen and the patient is breathing spontaneously, the reservoir bag will fill and empty with respiration. An awake patient will not be able to vocalize with an ETT positioned in

69

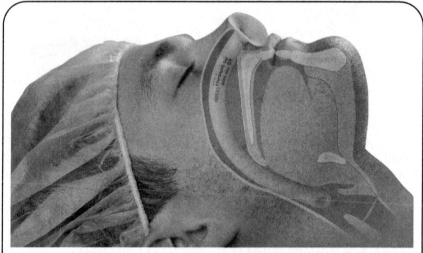

Fig. 6.15 Nasopharyngeal airway relieving dynamic obstruction caused by the tongue falling back in the unconscious patient.

the tracheal lumen. On an anterior-posterior chest *x-ray*, the tip of the ETT should be located between the midpoint of the thoracic inlet and the carina.

Decreased air entry to one lung field may indicate that the ETT is in a mainstem bronchus (usually the right mainstem bronchus). In this situation, the patient may become increasingly hypoxic or continue to cough. An endobronchial intubation may be suspected when one side of the chest is observed moving more than the other with ventilation. In this situation, the airway pressures may be higher than normal (> 25 cm H$_2$O), and an abnormally distant ETT position at the patient's lips will be noted.

**Clinical Pearl:**

"If in doubt, take it out"

*This is prudent advice for anyone who has just attempted tracheal intubation and is unsure and unable to confirm tracheal placement. In this case, rather than risk hypoxic injury and gastric aspiration, it is better to remove the ETT, resume mask ventilation with 100% oxygen, stabilize the patient, and call for help.*

**Clinical Pearl:**

"If in doubt, leave it in"

*This advice applies to the clinician who is considering tracheal extubation in a patient whose trachea has been intubated for a prolonged period of time. When the clinician questions whether the patient's trachea can be safely extubated (see Chapter 7: extubation criteria), it is generally safer to delay extubation, continue to support ventilation, and ensure hemodynamic stability, analgesia, sedation, and oxygenation rather than perform premature tracheal extubation.*

## Potential Problems

### I. Difficulty with Intubation

Repeat intubation attempts should be avoided unless there is a different tactic to improve the chance of success. Persistent repeat attempts at intubation traumatize the patient's airway, interrupts and delays oxygenation and ventilation, and places the patient at risk of significant morbidity and mortality.

If difficulty is encountered, retreat, regroup, and resume manual mask ventilation and oxygenation. Call for help and allow the patient to recover from any sedative or relaxant medications that have been given. No more than three intubation attempts should be made. Discuss with your staff anesthesiologist management option for the patient with an anticipated of unanticipated difficult tracheal intubation.

### II. Upper Airway Obstruction

The most common cause of an upper airway obstruction in an unconscious supine patient is the tongue falling back into the hypopharynx (Fig. 6.14). In the unconscious state, there is a decrease in the tone of muscles attaching the tongue to the mandible, hyoid bone, and epiglottis. The respiratory efforts of the unconscious patient tend to pull the tongue backward causing further airway obstruction, and ultimately, the epiglottis tends to fall downward, also increasing upper airway obstruction. Apart from intubation, simple maneuvers to overcome upper airway obstruction in the unconscious supine patient include:

1. Clear the airway of any foreign material
2. Use a chin lift maneuver
3. Use a jaw thrust maneuver
4. Insert an oral and/or nasal airway
5. Position the patient on the side in the semi-prone recovery position

## Complications of Laryngoscopy and Intubation

Laryngoscopy and intubation result in physiologic stimulation that can lead to hypercarbia and/or hypoxia. Dental damage is always a risk during direct laryngoscopy, and patients should be made aware of this possibility during the preoperative assessment. Other potential complications include airway trauma, recurrent laryngeal nerve damage, vocal cord injury, arytenoid dislocation, or edema of the hypopharyngeal and glottic tissues. ETT malfunction (obstruction, cuff rupture) or malposition can result in adverse events, such as inadequate ventilation, barotrauma, hypoxia, and hypercarbia.

## Laryngospasm

Laryngospasm results from stimulation of the superior laryngeal nerve and causes involuntary muscle spasm resulting in closure of the vocal cords. This can be caused by secretions or by direct stimulation of the cords. Management of laryngospasm includes gentle positive pressure and suction of secretions if the patient is not hypoxemic. Other maneuvers to assist in relieving laryngospasm include a forceful jaw thrust or pressure on the mandible just anterior to the mastoid. Pharmaceutical options include deepening anesthesia with propofol or paralysis with succinylcholine.

Negative pressure pulmonary edema is an uncommon complication that can have serious consequences and result in an otherwise healthy patient becoming critically ill. This topic is discussed in more detail in Chapter 25.

## References:

1. Kheterpal S, Martin L, Shanks AM, et al. Prediction and outcomes of impossible mask ventilation: a review of 50,000 anesthetics.–Anesthesiology. 2009; 110:891-7.
2. Mallampati, SR, Gatt SP, Gugino LD, et al: A clinical sign to predict difficult tracheal intubation: A prospective study. Can J Anaesth 1985; 32:429.
3. Samsoon GLT, Young JRB: Difficult tracheal intubation: A retrospective study. Anaesthesia 1987; 42:487.

# CHAPTER 7

# Intubation Decisions and Challenges

Tim O'Connor MD and Ilia Charapov MD

## Learning Objectives

1. To review the subjective and objective criteria for tracheal intubation and extubation.
2. To review a *goal-directed* and *patient-oriented* approach to the pharmacology of medications used for tracheal intubation.
3. To acquire an appreciation of the specific considerations for tracheal intubation with an emphasis on:
   - The patient's presenting medical condition
   - The identification, anticipation, and management of a difficult airway
   - The rational use of various airway devices in specific patient scenarios.
4. To review complications of tracheal intubation and positive pressure ventilation.

## Key Points

| | |
|---|---|
| 1 | Identifying the goals and conflicts for intubation provides the framework to develop a patient-specific goal-oriented plan for tracheal intubation. |
| 2 | When tracheal intubation fails, bag-mask ventilation or placement of a laryngeal mask airway device (LMAD) may be used as a rescue plan. All efforts should focus on ensuring adequate oxygenation. |
| 3 | "Awake" fiberoptic bronchoscopy (FOB) remains the gold standard for elective intubation in patients with a difficult airway. |
| 4 | A wide array of new airway devices provides clinicians with many equally valid ways to manage a difficult airway apart from FOB. |

Chapter 6 presented an overview of the technical skills required to perform tracheal intubation in adults. This chapter uses clinical cases to illustrate the decision process used to:

- Assess a patient's need for tracheal intubation
- Identify pharmacologic goals for intubation
- Choose an appropriate intubation technique
- Develop a plan to manage an identified difficult airway

- Anticipate and manage problems related to positive pressure ventilation.

**Indications for tracheal intubation**

The need to intubate a patient's trachea may be obvious, but it can also be challenging and controversial. Tables 7.1 and 7.2 list common criteria anesthesiologists use to evaluate a patient's need for tracheal intubation. An individual criterion is not an absolute indication. The criteria are to be used together in the context of the patient's clinical presentation to formulate a decision concerning the patient's need for tracheal intubation.

## Table 7.1 Objective Criteria for Intubation

| **Objective Criteria for Intubation (with or without ventilation) Oxygenation / Ventilation / Mechanics** | |
|---|---|
| **Oxygenation** | • **PaO$_2$ < 70 mm Hg** with F$_i$O$_2$ = 70%. When 100% oxygen is administered to a spontaneously breathing patient using high oxygen flow rates with a non-rebreathing mask or a puritan face mask, the maximum inspired oxygen concentration (F$_i$O$_2$) is generally limited to 70% due to entrainment of room air (see Chapter 24).<br><br>• **A-a DO$_2$ gradient > 350 mm Hg**. The normal alveolar – arterial difference of oxygen gradient (A-a DO$_2$) is < 15 mm Hg and more than doubles with increasing age.[1] Using an arterial blood gas sample, the alveolar gas equation is used to calculate the A-a DO$_2$ gradient; where: A-a DO$_2$ = P$_A$O$_2$ – PaO$_2$<br>P$_A$O$_2$ = partial pressure of alveolar oxygen<br>P$_A$O$_2$ = (P$_{ATM}$ – P$_{H2O}$) x FiO2 – (PaCO$_2$/0.8)<br>P$_{ATM}$ = atmospheric pressure = 760 mm Hg; P$_{H2O}$ = water vapor pressure = 47 mm Hg at 37°C<br>P$_a$O$_2$ = partial pressure of arterial oxygen measured from an arterial sample<br>P$_a$CO$_2$ = partial pressure of carbon dioxide measured from an arterial sample. |
| **Ventilation** | • **RR > 35 breaths·min$^{-1}$ in adults.** Muscles fatigue at respiratory rate (RR) > 35 breaths·min$^{-1}$.<br>• **PaCO$_2$ > 60 mm Hg** (in previously normal adults).<br>• **PaCO$_2$ > 45 mm Hg in status asthmaticus** and rising despite maximum medical management (must use additional objective and subjective criteria).<br>• **Respiratory acidosis with pH < 7.20 in chronic obstructive pulmonary disease (COPD) patients.** |
| **Mechanics** | • **VC < 15 mL·kg$^{-1}$.** Normal vital capacity = 70 mL·kg$^{-1}$ or approximately 5 L. A vital capacity (VC) of ≥15 mL·kg$^{-1}$ is required to cough effectively to clear secretions.<br>• **NIF > - 25 cm H2O.** The normal negative inspiratory force (NIF) is approximately - 80 to - 100 cm H$_2$O. |

## Table 7.2 Subjective Criteria for Intubation.

| Subjective Criteria for Intubation (with or without ventilation) Protect / Provide / Maintain / Tracheal Bronchial Toilet | |
|---|---|
| 1 | Protect the airway (e.g., decreased level of consciousness, drug overdose). |
| 2 | Provide an airway (e.g., impending airway obstruction: epiglottitis, thermal burns, anaphylaxis). |
| 3 | Provide positive pressure ventilation during general anesthesia. There are many reasons why endotracheal intubation is chosen to manage an airway under general anesthesia. These include but are not limited to long surgical procedures, difficult mask ventilation, contraindications to use of a LMAD, prone position, operative site near the head and neck, thoracic surgery, and major abdominal surgery. |
| 4 | Provide a tracheal bronchial toilet (TBT). For patients who are unable to clear their secretions, an endotracheal tube (ETT) provides direct access for suctioning secretions (e.g., COPD patient with pneumonitis). |
| 5 | Clinical signs of respiratory failure and fatigue (e.g., diaphoresis, tachypnea, tachycardia, accessory muscle use, pulsus paradoxus, and cyanosis). |
| 6 | Shock is not immediately reversed with medical treatment (i.e., the patient is not responding to medical management in the first 35 – 45 min). Normal respiratory muscles use approximately 2 – 5% of the cardiac output. In shock states, this may increase to 15 – 20%, diverting vital oxygen delivery from other organs, such as the heart and brain. If dogs subjected to septic shock conditions are allowed to breathe on their own, they will die much earlier than dogs with an intubated trachea and ventilated lungs. |

**Tracheal Intubation: A goal-directed patient-oriented approach to the rational use of medications**

Tracheal intubation is frequently performed using a variety of medications. For the student, the rationale behind the choice, dosage, and timing of medications used for tracheal intubation is often obscure. This can be both confusing and daunting for physicians who have limited experience with intubation and are attempting to learn this skill. As a consequence, the temptation is to learn a standard "recipe" and apply it to all patients requiring tracheal intubation. The recipe approach is generally successful in achieving tracheal intubation, but often will fail to meet other important goals specific to the patient.

In formulating a rational plan for tracheal intubation, it is essential to develop specific goals for each patient. The specific goals provide a foundation for the choice of medications used to perform tracheal intubation.

The specific goals may include some or all of the following:

• Amnesia
• Anxiolysis
• Analgesia
• Muscle relaxation

- Hemodynamic stability (avoidance of tachycardia, bradycardia, hypotension, hypertension)
- Minimal changes in intracerebral pressure (ICP)
- Prevention of gastric aspiration
- Tracheal intubation

Identify the important patient-specific goals for intubation. Concentrating on a subgroup of these goals may minimize the use of unnecessary medications and their potential side effects. Prior to proceeding, plan and prepare backup airway plans and rescue medications to manage adverse events. This may include having specialized rescue airway equipment available for use and the preparation of additional sedative medications or vasoactive medications to manage deviations in hemodynamic parameters.

Once the above goals are identified, medications can be selected to achieve these goals. A patient is identified as having a "reassuring airway" when the airway examination and clinical history fail to identify any predictors of difficulty with bag-mask ventilation or intubation (see Chapter 6).

To illustrate a *goal-directed patient-oriented* approach to medication administration for tracheal intubation, consider a healthy fasted adult with a reassuring airway who requires elective tracheal intubation. The identified goals may include general anesthesia (unconsciousness), attenuation of the sympathetic response to intubation (control of heart rate and blood pressure), avoidance of an overdose of medications (avoidance of bradycardia and hypotension), muscle relaxation, rapid recovery from the effects of muscle relaxation, and tracheal intubation. A rational goal-directed plan for this patient can then be formulated and might consist of an intravenous anesthetic agent, such as propofol 1-2 mg·kg⁻¹, an opioid, such as fentanyl 1-3 μg·kg⁻¹, and a muscle relaxant, such as succinylcholine

1 mg·kg⁻¹. The dose of propofol and fentanyl administered to the patient can be titrated over a brief period based on the patient's clinical response. Alternatively, if the clinician wishes to avoid some of the undesirable side effects of succinylcholine (e.g., myalgia) and accept a longer duration of muscle relaxation, a nondepolarizing muscle relaxant, such as rocuronium 0.3 – 0.6 mg·kg⁻¹ may be substituted in place of succinylcholine.

Chapters 11, 12, and 14 provide information about the pharmacologic properties of medications commonly used for tracheal intubation. It is important to have an understanding of the pharmacology of these medications and the synergistic effects these medications have when they are administered together. The effect of medication synergism often mandates a reduction in the amount of one or both medications administered in order to avoid a relative overdose. See Chapter 14 for a discussion of the synergistic effects of propofol and remifentanil. Midazolam, opioids (e.g., fentanyl), intravenous lidocaine, and propofol all exhibit synergism when administered together.

Other adjuvant medications may be used to attenuate the sympathetic response to intubation. Common examples include the intravenous administration of lidocaine and midazolam prior to the induction of anesthesia. Lidocaine in a dose of 1-1.5 mg·kg⁻¹ may be administered 3 - 4 min prior to intubation. The use of lidocaine may limit the hemodynamic response (elevation of blood pressure [BP] and heart rate [HR]), the ICP response (elevation in ICP), and airway responses (bronchospasm) to tracheal intubation. The administration of a benzodiazepine, such as midazolam, in a dose of 20 – 40 μg·kg⁻¹ may be used for both its anxiolytic properties prior to induction of anesthesia as well as its synergistic effect with other anesthetic agents. Administration of these medications may require a reduction in the dose of other anesthetic agents, such as propofol and opioids, to avoid the potential of a relative anesthetic overdose.

It is important to understand the pharmacologic properties of the different medications being used and the time needed for these medications to reach their peak effect. Typically, fentanyl and lidocaine will reach their peak effect approximately 3 – 4 min after administration. Laryngoscopy can then be timed 4 – 5 min after their administration. The effect of opioids, benzodiazepines, and lidocaine may result in a depression in the level of consciousness and respiration, and the patient should be closely monitored during this period, encouraged to breathe, and / or supported with positive pressure ventilation.

In the real world, the majority of patients will have other additional issues to consider when planning tracheal intubation. The patient's condition and the clinical setting will have a major influence on the specific goals for intubation. Some of the considerations influencing the technique of intubation and choice of medications include:
- Urgency of intubation
- Anticipated difficulty with bag-mask ventilation
- Anticipated difficulty with direct laryngoscopy
- Risk of aspiration
- Identified contraindications to medications (e.g., succinylcholine)
- Whether or not a muscle relaxant should be used
- Whether a short or intermediate period of muscle paralysis is desirable
- Hemodynamic stability of the patient
- Medical history and coexisting conditions (e.g., aortic stenosis, opioid tolerance)
- Resources available (e.g., airway equipment, monitoring, personnel)

The patient-specific goals for intubation and the restrictions imposed by the above considerations frequently create conflicts. These conflicts are important to identify. Once identified, each conflict can be approached as a challenge to overcome.

In the context of the identified patient-specific goals and considerations for intubation, additional questions may need to be addressed. Examples include:
- What is the anticipated hemodynamic response using these induction medications?
- Is there a risk of injury with the proposed plan (e.g., exacerbation of raised ICP in a patient with elevated ICP)?
- Is the patient at high risk for gastric aspiration (see Chapters 9 and 25)?
- Are the resources (e.g., location, equipment, monitoring, and personnel) adequate to perform intubation safely? If time permits, consider moving the patient to a location with appropriate resources.
- Are there other investigations required prior to performing intubation (e.g., identification of associated injuries in the trauma patient)?
- Is difficulty with bag-mask ventilation and intubation anticipated? Consider alternative techniques for intubation, such as the use of airway adjuvants or fiberoptic intubation, with appropriate local anesthesia and sedation (see Chapter 6).
- What are the plans for managing the patient after tracheal intubation (e.g., emergency patient requiring admission to the intensive care unit [ICU])?

The following case discussions illustrate how a goal-directed patient-oriented approach can be used in the context of identified patient considerations affecting airway management.

## Case I

A previously healthy 40-yr-old male was involved in a high-speed motor vehicle accident. The paramedics have transported him urgently to the emergency department. Initial assessment reveals a pale middle-aged male in moderate distress and moaning incoherently. His BP is 90/30, HR 140 beats·min$^{-1}$, and he has a Glasgow Coma Scale (GCS) of 12. A non-rebreathing facemask with oxygen is applied, respiration is 30 breaths·min$^{-1}$, and pulse oximetry records 90% saturation. The trauma surgeon requests intubation and transport to the operating room (OR) for an urgent exploratory laparotomy. The patient has a clinically reassuring airway examination for direct laryngoscopy, a distended abdomen, and no evidence of head or spinal trauma. Heart sounds are normal, his trachea is midline, and air entry is present in both lung fields. Two large bore intravenous catheters are secured, a bolus of warmed crystalloid is administered, and blood is sent for laboratory investigations with a stat crossmatch for four units of packed red blood cells (PRBCs).

## The specific goals for intubation include:

1. Amnesia for intubation
2. Avoiding further exacerbation of the shock state (i.e., further depression of the blood pressure or elevation of the heart rate)
3. Hemodynamic support and fluid resuscitation
4. Prevention of gastric aspiration
5. Rapid paralysis to optimize conditions for direct laryngoscopy and tracheal intubation
6. Tracheal intubation
7. Preparation of rescue airway equipment and medications prior to induction of anesthesia.

## The immediate considerations for this patient include:

1. Trauma patient with both identified and unidentified injuries
2. Limited information regarding the patient's medical history, medications, allergies, and anesthetic history
3. Limited time to assess and optimize the patient
4. Full stomach and heightened risk of aspiration
5. A shock state presumed to be secondary to hypovolemic shock
6. Urgent need for tracheal intubation
7. Urgent need for medical (fluid and blood product resuscitation) and surgical control of the bleeding
8. Limited oxygen reserve and potential for rapid desaturation with induction of anesthesia
9. Remote location with limitations in available equipment and personnel

## The identified conflicts between our goals for intubation and immediate considerations include:

1. The need for rapid sequence induction (RSI) with cricoid pressure (CP) using a fixed dose of drugs to decrease the risk of aspiration (see Chapter 9)
2. An increased risk of hemodynamic collapse if a standard RSI dose of medication is administered
3. A heightened risk of aspiration if drugs are titrated slowly
4. A heightened risk of hemodynamic collapse if drugs are not titrated slowly
5. Recognition that drugs used to provide amnesia and decrease awareness may also further depress blood pressure.

Identifying the goals, considerations, and conflicts for tracheal intubation in this patient highlights the importance of developing a patient-specific goal-oriented modification to the induction plan.

Having identified the goals, considerations, and conflicts, an anesthetic plan is developed to proceed with a RSI using CP. The mnemonic "A Basic Mad Poster" (Chapter 6) was used as a memory aid to prepare the equipment and medications for intubation. The patient is administered 100% oxygen using an AMBU® bag and mask unit; a no. 7.5 endotracheal tube with a stylet is prepared, and suction with a rigid Yankauer suction tip is checked and confirmed to be functional. The patient's weight is estimated to be 80 kg. Medications for anesthesia induction as well as rescue medications (i.e., atropine, phenylephrine, ephedrine, midazolam, and fentanyl) are prepared. A rescue video laryngoscope is checked, functional, and available for use if difficulty with direct laryngoscopy and tracheal intubation is encountered. A pillow is placed behind the patient's head to create mild flexion of the cervical spine. The height of the patient's bed is adjusted such that the patient's head is at the level of the clinician's waist. The audible tone on the saturation monitor is enabled and continuous echocardiography (ECG) and noninvasive blood pressure (NIBP) monitoring is confirmed. The laryngoscope is checked, and an assistant instructed in the proper application of cricoid pressure is positioned to the right of the patient's head.

A decision to avoid propofol is made due to its potential to depress blood pressure and perfusion further in the setting of hypovolemic shock. As the assistant applies cricoid pressure, intravenous ketamine 1 mg·kg$^{-1}$ is administered and immediately followed by succinylcholine 1 mg·kg$^{-1}$. The patient's trachea is intubated with direct laryngoscopy, and the position of the endotracheal tube is confirmed by auscultation and end-tidal carbon dioxide (ETCO$_2$). The endotracheal tube position is secured and mechanical ventilation is initiated.

The patient's heat rate and blood pressure continue to be monitored, and small doses of midazolam (20 µg·kg$^{-1}$) and fentanyl (1 µg·kg$^{-1}$) are titrated to effect while attention is directed to further fluid resuscitation and transport the patient to the OR.

Intravenous anesthetic drugs, such as ketamine and etomidate, cause minimal cardiac depression with administration. In hypovolemic shock, these agents may be preferred over thiopentothal and propofol, both of which will accentuate myocardial depression in this setting. In this case, ketamine was chosen as the intravenous induction agent due to its tendency to cause less cardiac depression compared with an induction dose of propofol. Etomidate in a 0.3 mg·kg$^{-1}$ dose could also have been used for anesthetic induction in this patient. If propofol is used for induction, consider reducing the dose and adding a vasoactive agent, such as phenylephrine, norepinephrine or ephedrine, to avoid hypotension with its administration.

In the setting of more severe degrees of shock, a small dose of benzodiazepine to provide amnesia (e.g., midazolam 20-40 µg·kg$^{-1}$) and a muscle relaxant administered in a RSI fashion with cricoid pressure may be all that is required to ensure preservation of sympathetic tone, hemodynamic stability, and optimum muscle relaxation for laryngoscopy and tracheal intubation. In the setting of circulatory collapse or a full cardiac arrest, anesthesia is a luxury that simply cannot be afforded. In this setting, direct laryngoscopy and tracheal intubation are performed with or without the aid of a muscle relaxant.

Following successful intubation of this patient's trachea, the focus is changed to optimize tissue perfusion and oxygenation (see Chapter 23). The patient's vital signs are consistent with class IV hemorrhagic shock and a blood loss equivalent to > 40% of his blood volume (see Chapter 22 hypovolemic shock).

Immediate goals include blood loss replacement and surgical control of the bleeding. Immediate transfusion should be initiated using a fluid warmer for transfusion of both PRBCs and fresh frozen plasma (FFP). In additional to crystalloid and colloid administration, calcium chloride and other blood products, including cryoprecipitate and platelets, may also be required (see Chapter 21).

## Management of the difficult airway

Airway management is the cornerstone of anesthesia practice. Anesthesiologists must have the knowledge and skills to control ventilation safely in any clinical setting. This may be required in the operating room, intensive care unit, emergency department, or outside the hospital environment. In the past 25 years, there has been an exponential growth in our understanding of airway management as well as the available equipment and monitors to perform intubation safely and control ventilation. Despite these advancements, it is impossible to predict all cases where difficulty in airway management will be encountered. With the rapid growth in airway equipment, most clinicians will be unable to acquire expertise with all airway devices. Nevertheless, any clinician involved in airway management must have a clear management plan and appropriate reaction to an airway emergency. Clinicians often have equally valid but different management approaches to the difficult airway. The differences are generally founded in the clinicians past experience and skills acquired with specific airway devices and equipment.

In the patient undergoing an elective surgical procedure, the anesthesiogist has the luxury of time to permit a full assessment of the airway, to predict difficulties with ventilation and intubation (see Chapter 6), to prepare equipment and medications, and to request assistance from other health care personnel. In an emergency setting, when oxygenation is compromised, only a very limited airway assessment may be possible. Additionally, there may be an inadequate amount of time to prepare equipment and medications properly and to seek assistance from other health care personnel. When difficulty in tracheal intubation is encountered, all efforts should focus on oxygenation not intubation. This is the overwhelming lesson learned from case studies involving the management of a failed airway.

Chapter 6 includes a discussion regarding the assessment and evaluation of the airway and preparation of equipment prior to intubation. The use of an LMA™ or other laryngeal mask airway device (LMAD) as both a primary airway tool and rescue airway device is discussed in Chapter 8. The following information pertains to the use of specialized airway equipment and devices used for both elective and emergent intubation of the difficult or failed airway. The investment of learning a rational approach to the difficult airway provides the learner with a platform from which to both understand and approach the patient who requires emergent airway management when time is limited.

The four levels of airway management are:

1. Bag-mask ventilation (BMV)
2. Placement of an LMA™ or LMAD
3. Endotracheal intubation
4. Surgical airway

Spontaneous or controlled ventilation with the use of a bag and mask or the placement of an LMA™ (or LMAD) may provide acceptable oxygenation and ventilation. When difficulty is encountered with tracheal intubation, it is important that efforts are focused on ensuring adequate oxygenation. In this setting, reverting to bag-mask ventilation or placement of a LMAD may be used as a rescue plan. A specialized LMA™, such as the LMA Fastrach™, may be used a conduit for intubation should this be required.

Common strategies to improve success with BMV are discussed in Chapter 6, and strategies to overcome difficulties with placement of a LMAD are discussed in Chapter 8. Advanced airway techniques may be required to achieve tracheal intubation in patients with a difficult airway. When BMV fails and placement of a LMAD or tracheal tube fails, a situation known as a "can't intubate – can't ventilate" (CICV) emergency is declared. This is a rare event with an estimated incidence of 0.01 – 0.07% of all intubations, but it is a potentially life-threatening emergency that requires immediate action to avert a disaster. All efforts are focused on optimizing oxygenation of the patient. An emergency call should go out to notify any available health care provider with airway management skills of the emergency and to enlist their assistance. Should attempts at oxygenation fail, an emergency cricothyroidotomy may be required. As soon as the need of an emergency cricothyroidotomy is considered, preferably before a CICV situation arises, the presence of a surgeon skilled in providing an emergency surgical airway should be requested. Early notification may allow time for the surgeon to prepare mentally, examine the patient's neck, and prepare the necessary equipment. With proper airway evaluation, preparation, and consideration of alternative management strategies, many cases of CICV emergencies can be avoided, but unfortunately not all. The American Society of Anesthesiology have published practice guidelines for management of the difficult airway (see Fig. 7.1 and 7.2)

## Management of a difficult intubation

Visualization of the glottis during direct laryngoscopy may be improved using a "**BURP**" maneuver [2] i.e., **B**ackward, **U**pward, and **R**ightward displacement and **P**ressure on the thyroid cartilage. The purpose of the BURP maneuver is to improve the glottic view during laryngoscopy. To perform the maneuver, an assistant applies pressure to the patient's thyroid cartilage while the clinician performs laryngoscopy. The clinician may use their right hand to guide the assistant's hand into a position that provides the best view of the glottis. The BURP maneuver should not be confused with the application of cricoid pressure (see Chapter 9), which is performed in an effort to prevent aspiration of gastric contents.

The McCoy laryngoscope has a distal articulating tip that can be flexed to lift the tissues at the tip of the blade and improve visualization of the glottis. It has been shown to improve laryngeal grade view compared with a standard laryngoscope blade.

An Eschmann tracheal tube introducer, referred to frequently as a gum elastic bougie (GEB), can be used to guide an endotracheal tube into the trachea. The GEB is particularly useful in situations when the glottic view is restricted (i.e., Cormack-Lehane grade 3 view; see Chapter 6). The GEB is 55 cm long with a distal "J-tip" that has a 35° angulation. To use the GEB, the clinician first performs laryngoscopy and attempts to achieve the best possible view of the glottis. The clinician then passes the soft angulated tip of the GEB just behind the epiglottis towards the trachea. Tracheal placement is confirmed by tactile feedback as the GEB tip is advanced and bumps along the tracheal rings. Alternatively, the GEB can be advanced until gentle resistance is felt (usually at 30 – 35 cm) when it lodges in a small airway. Esophageal placement is likely to have occurred when no tactile clicks are felt and there is no resistance to advancement of the GEB.

Once the GEB is positioned in the trachea, it is pulled back to the 20 cm marking at the teeth. As the clinician maintains laryngoscopy, an assistant advances an ETT, "railroading" it over the GEB into the trachea. Laryngoscopy is continued during this time to facilitate advancement of the ETT over the GEB. Resistance to advancement at the level of the glottis (referred to as ETT "hang-up") can be overcome by ensuring that the patient is paralyzed and / or by using a 90° counterclockwise rotation of the ETT. Rotation of the ETT 90° counterclockwise positions the ETT bevel posteriorly, minimizing the risk of it catching on the glottis structures. Once the ETT is positioned in the trachea, the GEB can be removed and tracheal placement can be confirmed with $ETCO_2$ and clinical examination.

The combined use of a McCoy laryngoscope, BURP maneuver, and GEB can be a very effective way to improve visualization of the glottis in patients whose tracheas are difficult to intubate with direct laryngoscopy (e.g., Cormack-Lehane laryngeal grade 3 – 4).

An LMA™ or other LMAD can be used either as a rescue device or as a conduit for tracheal intubation following a failed attempt at intubation. Elective use of an LMA™ is generally considered to be contraindicated in patients at risk of gastric aspiration (see Chapters 9 and 25). However, in a CICV situation, an LMA™ or other LMAD may be lifesaving, providing oxygenation and ventilation and preventing hypoxic brain injury or death. When such a device is used in a CICV situation where gastric aspiration remains a real risk, a decision must be made either to proceed with surgery or to awake the patient and abandon the procedure. In Chapter 8, there is a review of specialized LMAs, such as the LMA Proseal™ and the LMA Fastrach™, that may be superior to a LMA Classic™ in providing oxygenation and ventilation with positive pressure, decreasing the risk of aspiration and providing a conduit for tracheal intubation.

A number of malleable lighted stylets are available to manage a difficult intubation. The Trachlight® is a small battery powered stylet with a bright light at the distal end. The tip of the Trachlight® stylet is positioned at the end

of the ETT where the distal 5 cm of the ETT is acutely angulated at 90°. The stylet is inserted into the patient's mouth with the jaw lifted forward to unfold the epiglottis, and the tip of the stylet is directed towards the glottis opening. As the trachea is anterior to the esophagus when the stylet is correctly positioned, a bright glow will be visible below the thyroid cartilage. When the tip of the ETT is in the esophagus, the transmitted light will be dim and diffuse. The clinician uses the intensity and location of the transilluminated light to direct the ETT into the trachea without the use of a laryngoscope. Muscle relaxation is recommended with this technique to prevent glottis closure (laryngospasm) when the stylet approaches the glottis. Lighted stylets are particularly useful in patients with restricted mouth opening or neck mobility as well as those with an overbite with prominent upper front teeth. In patients with upper airway pathology (e.g., tumor, infection, trauma, goiter, obesity), light transmission from the stylet through the tissues may be difficult or impossible to visualize.

A number of rigid video laryngoscopes are now available, including the Glidescope®, Storz C-MAC®, Pentax Airway Scope®, McGrath® video laryngoscope, BONFILS® scope, Bullard® scope, Clarus® Video System, and King Vision® video laryngoscope. These video laryngoscopes have provided clinicians with a wide repertoire of tools to manage patients with both anticipated and unanticipated difficult airways. These devices are not dependent on neck mobility or alignment of the axis of the airway to provide an excellent view of the glottis for intubation.

**Fiberoptic bronchoscope (FOB) and the "awake" intubation:** "Awake" bronchoscopy and intubation can be performed with appropriate sedation and topical anesthesia. Local anesthesia of the airway allows advancement of a flexible bronchoscope into the oral or nasal airway past the vocal cords

Fig. 7.1 **_ASA Difficult Airway Algorithm_**

1. Assess the likelihood and clinical impact of basic management problems:
   A. Difficult Ventilation
   B. Difficult Intubation
   C. Difficulty with Patient Cooperation and Consent
   D. Difficult Tracheostomy

2. Actively pursue opportunities to deliver supplemental oxygen throughout the process of difficult airway management.

3. Consider the relative merits and feasibility of basic management choices:

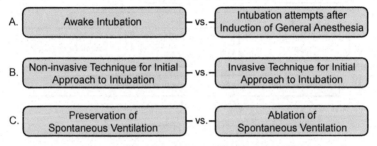

4. Develop primary an alternative strategies: See Figure 7.2 A & B Strategies.

Legend for Fig. 7.2

\* **Confirm ventilation, tracheal intubation, or LMA placement with exhaled $CO_2$**

a. Other options include (but are not limited to): surgery utilizing face mask or LMA anesthesia, local anesthesia infiltration or regional nerve blockade. Pursuit of these options usually implies that mask ventilation will not be problematic. Therefore, these options may be of limited value if this step in the algorithm has been reached via the Emergency Pathway.

b. Invasive airway access includes surgical or percutaneous tracheostomy or cricothyroidotomy.

c. Alternative non-invasive approaches to difficult intubation include (but are not limited to): use of different laryngoscope blades, LMA as an intubation conduit (with or without fiberoptic guidance), fiberoptic intubation, intubating stylet or tube changer, light wand, retrograde intubation, and blind oral or nasal intubation.

d. Consider re-preparation of the patient for awake intubation or cancelling surgery.

e. Options for emergency non-invasive airway ventilation include (but are not limited to): rigid bronchoscope, esophageal-tracheal combitube ventilation, or transtracheal jet ventilation.

*Adapted from Caplan RA, Benumof JL, Berry FA et al. Practice guidelines for management of the difficult airway. An updated report by the American Society of Anesthesiologists Task Force on management of the difficult airway. Anesthesiology 2003; 98:1269-77.*

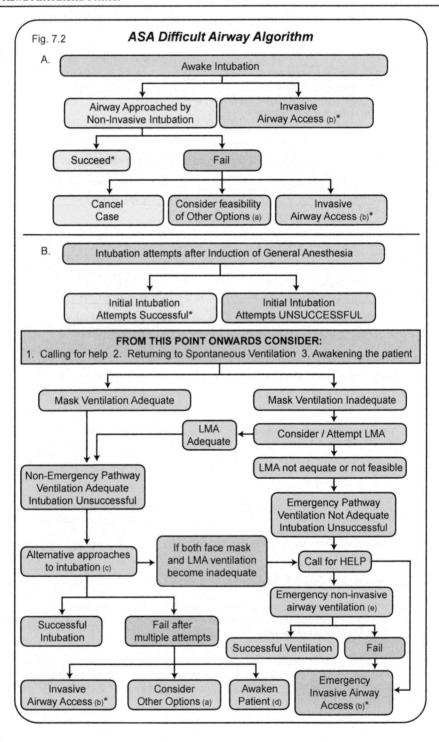

Fig. 7.2 **ASA Difficult Airway Algorithm**

A.
Awake Intubation

Airway Approached by Non-Invasive Intubation
Invasive Airway Access (b)*

Succeed*
Fail

Cancel Case
Consider feasibility of Other Options (a)
Invasive Airway Access (b)*

B.
Intubation attempts after Induction of General Anesthesia

Initial Intubation Attempts Successful*
Initial Intubation Attempts UNSUCCESSFUL

**FROM THIS POINT ONWARDS CONSIDER:**
1. Calling for help  2. Returning to Spontaneous Ventilation  3. Awakening the patient

Mask Ventilation Adequate
Mask Ventilation Inadequate

LMA Adequate
Consider / Attempt LMA

LMA not aequate or not feasible

Non-Emergency Pathway Ventilation Adequate Intubation Unsuccessful

Emergency Pathway Ventilation Not Adequate Intubation Unsuccessful

Alternative approaches to intubation (c)
If both face mask and LMA ventilation become inadequate
Call for HELP

Emergency non-invasive airway ventilation (e)

Successful Intubation
Fail after multiple attempts
Successful Ventilation
Fail

Invasive Airway Access (b)*
Consider Other Options (a)
Awaken Patient (d)
Emergency Invasive Airway Access (b)*

and into the trachea. Prior to bronchoscopy, an endotracheal tube is loaded onto the bronchoscope. Once the bronchoscope is positioned in the mid-trachea, the endotracheal tube is advanced over the bronchoscope and into the trachea. The bronchoscope is then removed. Bronchoscopes today are commonly connected to an LCD viewing screen, which provides excellent imaging of the airway during FOB and intubation. FOB and intubation is ideally performed with the patient breathing spontaneously with appropriate local anesthesia and sedation. This permits intubation to proceed in a safe and controlled manner. "Awake" FOB and intubation may be used in the patient with an identified difficult airway, difficult ventilation, or known upper airway pathology (e.g., tumor or abscess). Once the ETT is positioned correctly, the patient can then be given other medications to induce general anesthesia. FOB and intubation are less suited to emergency situations where there may be insufficient time for application of topical anesthesia and where blood or secretions may obscure the view. The presence of blood or vomitus is generally considered a contraindication to fiberoptic bronchoscopy and intubation.

FOB and tracheal intubation in the unconscious patient can be performed but is considered an advanced skill. The use of a jaw thrust maneuver and a specialized split oral airway (e.g., Berman Airway®) can be useful in guiding the tip of the bronchoscope to a position just above the glottic opening. The Berman Airway® functions as a bite block and intubation guide for the bronchoscope and can be used in both the awake and asleep patient. A short video of an "awake" fiberoptic intubation is available as a URL link in the additional resources.

Clinicians now have a wide array of airway equipment that can be used for safe management of patients with a difficult airway. Awake FOB and intubation is the gold standard for the elective management of patients with a difficult airway. Nonetheless, new developments in airway equipment now provide clinicians with many equally valid ways to manage a difficult airway. The plan of airway management is commonly based on the availability of airway equipment and the skill set of the attending clinician.

## Case II

On the first day of rotation, you are scheduled to assist with anesthesia in the general surgical room. The first patient is a moderately obese 40-yr-old female who is scheduled for a laparoscopic cholecystectomy. What kind of anesthesia should we provide for this patient? You ponder whether you should prepare equipment and medications for tracheal intubation.

Most cholecystectomies today are performed under general anesthesia with tracheal intubation. While it may be possible to provide regional anesthesia (e.g., epidural anesthesia) for this procedure, most anesthesiologists will opt to provide general anesthesia with tracheal intubation. The rationale for this decision includes:

- The need for muscle relaxation
- Abdominal insufflation that will impair spontaneous ventilation
- Carbon dioxide ($CO_2$) insufflation and absorption requiring increased minute ventilation to maintain a normal pH
- A moderately obese patient who will have difficulty breathing spontaneously when lying supine due to procedure-related pain and peritoneal insufflation.

Epidural anesthesia alone would require a high block to provide adequate anesthesia. This could impair the patient's intercostal and abdominal muscles of respiration, resulting in respiratory insufficiency. In the early days of anesthesia, open cholecystectomies were performed using ether or chloroform administered by a facemask with the patient breathing spontaneously during the procedure. Ether produced marked muscle relaxation when used with small doses of muscle relaxants (e.g., curare 6 mg). Respiratory depression was accepted. When the ether was discontinued, the patient's muscle strength recovered and ventilation increased to match the metabolic needs. Pulse oximeters, $ETCO_2$ monitors, nerve stimulators, mechanical ventilators, and antagonists for muscle relaxants were not available to the anesthesiologist during the early years. Today, by contrast, we routinely plan general anesthesia with intubation, muscle relaxation, and controlled mechanical ventilation for patients undergoing a cholecystectomy. This allows the anesthesiologist to provide profound muscle relaxation during the procedure, protect the airway from aspiration of gastric contents, and optimize ventilation and oxygenation. The anesthesiologist can also administer potent anesthetic drugs, such as opioids and volatile anesthetic agents (e.g., sevoflurane, desflurane), to minimize the stress of the surgical procedure. Accordingly, you should plan to assist by preparing the endotracheal tube, checking the anesthesia machine, and preparing the anesthetic medications.

**Case III**

Having recently completed your anesthesia rotation, you are working in the emergency department when a pale diaphoretic 50-yr-old man stumbles through the door and collapses in front of the receptionist. The patient is quickly placed on a bed and taken to the resuscitation room. Unable to find a pulse, a nurse initiates chest compressions while the emergency physician applies chest paddles and delivers a biphasic shock of 150 joules. Unfortunately, despite three consecutive shocks, the patient fails to respond. You are at the head of the bed and have initiated manual ventilation with an Ambu® bag and mask. Chest compressions continue while a nurse attempts, unsuccessfully, to insert an intravenous catheter. Should you proceed to intubate the patient's trachea?

The emergency physician appreciates your help and asks you to proceed with tracheal intubation. After placing the ETT, you confirm its position, secure it, and continue with controlled ventilation. At your suggestion, 10 mL of 1:10,000 epinephrine is injected down the ETT into the patient's lungs and central circulation. The cardiac rhythm subsequently changes to a coarser form of ventricular fibrillation, and repeat defibrillation with 150 joules converts the man's rhythm to a sinus tachycardia with a systolic pressure of 110 mm Hg. Frequent ventricular premature beats (VPBs) are noted, and amiodarone 150 mg is infused slowly over 10 min while arrangements are made for the patient's transfer to the coronary care unit (CCU).

The resuscitation of this patient could have proceeded with mask ventilation and chest compressions. By choosing to intubate this patient's trachea, the clinicians were able to protect the patient's lungs from the risk of gastric aspiration. The ETT also provided a route for the administration of epinephrine, which played an important role in this man's resuscitation.

Later, a classmate asks why medications weren't given to the patient for tracheal intubation. You explain that patients with profound cardiovascular collapse requiring emergent tracheal intubation do not need any anesthetic medications, such as thiopental, propofol or succinylcholine, to perform tracheal intubation. In fact, the administration of these medications could have a detrimental effect by further depression of the patient's already compromised myocardium. If your colleague asks what other medications can be given through the ETT, remind him of the mnemonic

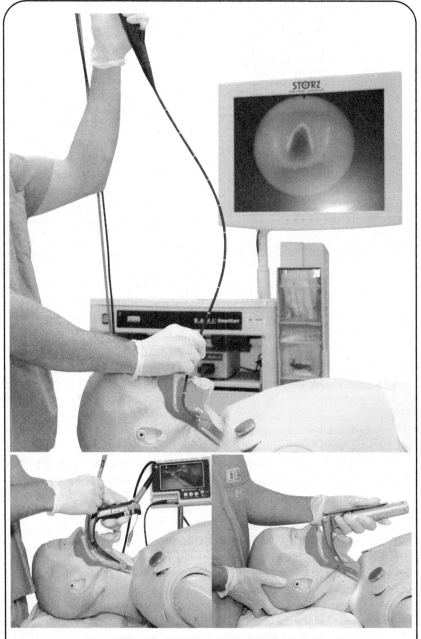

Fig. 7.3 Common advanced airway intubation tools. Fiberoptic bronchoscopy (top image), Glidescope™ video laryngoscopy with intubation stylet (bottom left), McCoy laryngoscope (bottom right).

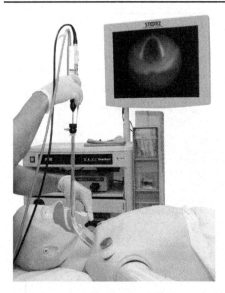

**Fig. 7.4** The Karl Storz Bonfils rigid fiberoptic video stylet has a 40 degree curved tip. It offers an alternative method of performing tracheal intubation using either a midline or retromolar approach in patients with an identified difficult direct laryngoscopy.

"NAVEL" used to remember the drugs that can be administered through an endotracheal tube, i.e., naloxone, atropine, Ventolin®, epinephrine and lidocaine.

### Case IV

Later, another clinical clerk asks for your opinion regarding a 68-yr-old man with known COPD. He is evaluating this patient in the emergency room because the patient is feeling more short of breath than usual. Your colleague was ready to send him home on antibiotics but hesitated after seeing his arterial blood gases (ABGs). He is concerned that this man may need tracheal intubation because his $PaCO_2$ is so high. His ABGs on room air were pH = 7.34, $PaCO_2$ = 65 mm Hg, $PaO_2$ = 54 mm Hg, $HCO_3$ = 34 mEq$\cdot L^{-1}$. How would you assess and treat this patient?

The patient's ABGs demonstrate hypoxemia and an acute on chronic respiratory acidosis with metabolic compensation. You review his old chart and note that his bicarbonate ($HCO_3$) was 33 mEq$\cdot L^{-1}$and his $PaO_2$ was 59 mm Hg at the time of discharge four months previously. This, you suggest, probably represents his optimal blood gas values. You complete your evaluation by examining the patient noting a RR = 22 breaths$\cdot min^{-1}$, HR = 90 beats$\cdot min^{-1}$, BP = 160/85, and diffuse mild rhonchi throughout the chest with no significant pulsus paradoxus (i.e. < 10 mm Hg). You also note that the patient is able to talk without stopping frequently to catch his breath, and he is not vigorously using his accessory muscles of respiration. On reviewing his other lab tests, you note his hemoglobin (Hb) = 170, white blood cells (WBC) = 7,000, and an ECG unchanged from his previous cardiogram. The chest *x-ray* (CXR) shows hyperinflation with basal bullae but gives no evidence of cardiac failure or pulmonary infection. The patient admits to having stopped his bronchodilators in the last week. After clinical and subjective improvement with salbutamol (Ventolin®) and ipratropium bromide (Atrovent®), the patient is discharged home with a prescription for his inhalers and a follow-up visit with his family practitioner.

### Case V

Four weeks later, you are completing your emergency rotation when the patient in Case IV returns. You are alarmed at his ill appearance. His wife accompanies him and relates that he "caught a cold" a week ago and has been getting progressively worse. He has been unable to eat or sleep for the last day because of his shortness of breath. When you examine him, you find that his breathing is labored at 28 breaths$\cdot min^{-1}$ with a prolonged expiratory phase and a surprisingly quiet chest. He is diaphoretic, clammy, and has difficulty catching his breath to talk. His vital signs reveal a HR of 130 beats·min$^{-1}$, BP = 180/100, with a pulsus paradoxus of 35 mm Hg with maximal use of his accessory muscles. The emergency physician orders salbutamol with ipratropium bromide by nebulization. An intravenous is established, ABGs are drawn, monitoring is initiated (ECG, oximetry, and BP), and a portable CXR is ordered. Your classmate thinks you better intubate his trachea now. Do you agree?

As the ABGs and CXR return, the patient is observed to have become increasingly drowsy, while little clinical improvement has occurred. The ABGs on facemask oxygen at 8 L·min$^{-1}$ reveal pH = 7.10, PaO$_2$ = 66 mm Hg, PaCO$_2$ = 120 mm Hg, and a HCO$_3$ = 36 mEq·L$^{-1}$. The patient is unable to tolerate continuous positive airway pressure (CPAP) support. After topical aerosol lidocaine anesthesia to the hypopharynx and glottis, the emergency physician performs direct laryngoscopy and orally intubates the patient's trachea. Hyperventilation at 20 breaths·min$^{-1}$ is initiated in order to "blow off" the carbon dioxide. The nurse reports that the patient's systolic pressure is now 65 mm Hg, and his cardiac monitor is showing sinus tachycardia at 120 beats·min$^{-1}$ with multiple VPBs. Your classmate reviews the CXR and states that he believes the patient has a pneumothorax on the left side. How are you going to manage the patient?

Before rushing to insert a needle thoracotomy and chest tube for a possible tension pneumothorax, you review the patient's status. The emergency physician asks you to take over ventilation while he reviews the chest radiograph. Although the patient has become unresponsive to verbal stimulation, his trachea is in the midline and distant air entry is heard in both lung fields. The respiratory therapist advises a decrease in respiratory rate to 8 breaths·min$^{-1}$, and you observe that the airway pressures required to ventilate the patient have decreased. A repeat CXR is ordered to verify the ETT position. A fluid bolus of Ringer's lactate 1,000 mL increases the patient's blood pressure to 100 mm Hg systolic. The VPB's remain but are now unifocal and less frequent. A mechanical ventilator is set up to provide ventilation with an inspired O$_2$ concentration of 50%, a tidal volume of 750 mL, and an intermittent mandatory ventilatory (IMV) rate of 8 breaths·min$^{-1}$ with 5 cm of positive end expiratory pressure (PEEP).

Arrangements are made to transfer the patient to the ICU. Review of the initial CXR shows the previous basilar bullae but no evidence of a pneumothorax. The second CXR shows the ETT tip to be correctly positioned mid-trachea.

Your classmate was correct about the patient requiring tracheal intubation. Clinical examination and ABG analysis confirmed that the patient was indeed in acute respiratory failure. Analysis of the ABGs revealed a severe acute on chronic respiratory acidosis. Often we have no background information regarding the patient's usual PaCO$_2$ and HCO$_3$ levels. In patients with COPD who may retain carbon dioxide, we rely on the pH more than the CO$_2$ to guide our management (as in Case IV). A primary respiratory acidosis with a pH of ≤ 7.20 indicates that the patient is in respiratory failure and no longer able to compensate. His condition was likely precipitated by his recent chest infection superimposed on his former severe COPD. PaCO$_2$ levels > 95 mm Hg become increasingly sedating. The minimum alveolar concentration (MAC) value of CO$_2$ = 245 (see Chapter 13 re: MAC definition). The decreased level of consciousness may be accounted for by the low blood pressure and the high arterial carbon dioxide tension.

This case illustrates several common problems. The patient presented in an extreme condition following an illness which likely resulted in significant dehydration. Upon his arrival in the emergency department, his sympathetic output was placing maximal demands on his cardiorespiratory system. Following tracheal intubation, his blood pressure fell precipitously. Patients with cardiorespiratory decompensation who require urgent tracheal intubation will often demonstrate a fall in blood pressure following intubation. This occurs irrespective of being given sedative drugs prior to intubation. The fall in blood pressure may be due to:

- The sedative drugs given
- The removal of endogenous catecholamines by removing the work of breathing from the patient
- Decreasing venous return to the heart due to positive pressure ventilation
- Hyperventilation resulting in an inadequate time for complete exhalation. The result is a condition known as auto-PEEP, where breath stacking occurs and results in a progressive increase in intrathoracic pressure. The increased intrathoracic pressure decreases venous return, impairs ventricular filling, and results in systemic hypotension. Recognition of auto-PEEP as a problem is the first step in treatment. The endotracheal tube is disconnected from the AMBU® bag or ventilator to permit passive exhalation, and ventilation should then be reinstituted at a slower respiratory rate.
- All of the above, plus unmasking a significant underlying hypovolemia or concurrent illness (e.g., myocardial infarction).

The occurrence of multiple ventricular premature beats may reflect an irritable myocardium secondary to hypercapnia, hypotension, and hypoxemia. Another explanation for the appearance of the VPBs may be the result of an acutely induced hypokalemia. Mechanical hyperventilation may result in a precipitous drop in the $PaCO_2$ level. The sudden lowering of $PaCO_2$ will rapidly increase the patient's pH, shift K+ into the cells, and create an acute extracellular hypokalemia. The differential diagnosis of this patient's acute hypotension, dysrhythmias, and abnormal CXR included a tension pneumothorax. In this case, the emergency physician correctly interpreted the lucency on the CXR as chronic basilar bullae and avoided the potential disastrous consequences of a needle thoracostomy and chest tube insertion in this patient (i.e., risk of a bronchopleural-cutaneous fistula).

In retrospect, this patient fulfilled several criteria for tracheal intubation (Tables 7.1 and 7.2). This emergency was best met by first supporting ventilation of the patient's lungs. As this patient's condition was likely to require prolonged ventilatory support, this was most easily accomplished by endotracheal intubation.

## Potential Complications of Intubation

Either the laryngoscope or the ETT can cause direct injury to the airway. The lips, tongue, pharynx, larynx, and trachea are all susceptible to injury. Damage to the teeth may be caused by the laryngoscope or by biting on either the ETT or the rigid suction tip. Damage to the teeth, though rare, is still the most frequent problem resulting in litigation against anesthesiologists. Damaged teeth can fragment and may be aspirated by the patient.

The patient who experiences a sore throat following the operation (with tracheal intubation) may obtain some relief with throat lozenges. This discomfort rarely persists for > 24 hr. Beware of the patient who recalls a severely sore throat on previous operations. The patient may have a restricted airway, and the larynx may have been traumatized due to a difficult tracheal intubation. Inserting the ETT through the larynx can injure the vocal cords or even dislocate the arytenoid cartilages. Patients with arthropathies, such as rheumatoid arthritis, may have arthritis involving the arytenoid cartilages which creates a "functional laryngeal stenosis". When symptomatic, these patients may note hoarseness or pain on speaking. These patients are at an increased risk for vocal cord and arytenoid injury with tracheal intubation, and extra care and use of a smaller ETT should be considered.

If the ETT is too short, it may result in accidental extubation, and excessive advancement of the ETT into the trachea may result in an endobronchial intubation. Prolonged ETT placement may lead to vocal cord granulomas or tracheal stenosis. Although a cuffed ETT protects against gastric aspiration, it bypasses the body's natural humidifying and warming mechanisms and affords a potential conduit for pathogens to enter the lungs. In patients requiring prolonged tracheal intubation and ventilation, this may be associated with "ventilator acquired pneumonia".

Upon inserting the ETT, a patient is subjected to a significant sympathetic stress that may precipitate tachycardia, dysrhythmias, and myocardial ischemia. Pediatric patients have a relatively higher parasympathetic tone than adults; hence, tracheal intubation of infants and children may result in a significant bradycardia. In both adult and pediatric patients, medications are commonly given prior to tracheal intubation in an attempt to minimize these reflexes.

The most serious complication of tracheal intubation is an unrecognized esophageal intubation. The resulting gastric distension with ventilation subjects the patient to hypoxia, hypercarbia, impairment of chest excursion, and increases the chance of regurgitation and pulmonary aspiration.

## Criteria for extubation

The criteria for extubation are generally the reverse of those for intubation. The patient should not require an ETT for airway provision, protection, maintenance or tracheobronchial toilet, and should meet criteria for adequate oxygenation, ventilation, and lung mechanics. The condition that initially required intubation should be resolved prior to extubation. The patient should be able to protect the airway, i.e., the patient should be awake with an intact gag and cough reflex. The patient should be hemodynamically stable, and the RR should be > 8 breaths·min$^{-1}$ and < 35 breaths·min$^{-1}$. Respiratory muscles will fatigue with prolonged rates > 35 breaths·min$^{-1}$. Oxygenation should be adequate, which means a PaO$_2$ of at least 60 mm Hg on an inspired oxygen concentration of ≤ 50%. This should be accompanied with evidence of adequate ventilation with a PaCO$_2$ of < 50 mm Hg. Vital capacity should be greater than 15 mL·kg$^{-1}$ (approximately 1 L in a 70 kg patient) with a tidal volume of > 5 mL·kg$^{-1}$, and the negative inspiratory force (NIF) should be more negative than -25 cm H2O. The vital capacity, tidal volume, and NIF can be measured at the bedside with simple spirometry equipment.

**Further reading:**

Access the following *ePrimer* supplemental links to view additional case studies involving difficult airway management. These cases are presented to show how various clinical scenarios influence the choice of induction medications and the approach to airway management.

1. Elective case, difficult ventilation
   http://www.anesthesiaprimer.com/AP/Ch7IntubationDecisions/Case1DifficultVentilation.pdf
2. Closed head Injury
   http://www.anesthesiaprimer.com/AP/Ch7IntubationDecisions/Case2RaisedICP.pdf
3. Pregnant patient for an emergency Cesarean delivery
   http://www.anesthesiaprimer.com/AP/Ch7IntubationDecisions/Case3EmergCS.pdf
4. A patient with burns to 30% of his body
   http://www.anesthesiaprimer.com/AP/Ch7IntubationDecisions/Case4Burn.pdf
5. A patient with a neck injury.
   http://www.anesthesiaprimer.com/AP/Ch7IntubationDecisions/Case5NeckInjury.pdf

**References:**

1. Nunn Applied Respiratory Physiology, 3rd edition, p.248.
2. Takahata O, Kubota M, Mamiya K, et al. The efficacy of the BURP maneuver during a difficult laryngoscopy. Anesth Analg 1997; 84: 419 – 421.

**URL Resources:**

Emergency cricothyroidotomy http://www.youtube.com/watch?v=dvWy9NXiZZI

# CHAPTER 8

# The Laryngeal Mask Airway Device (LMAD)

Patrick Sullivan MD, Takpal Birdi MD, Leo M. Jeyaraj MD

## Learning Objectives

1. To become conversant with the differences between a LMAD and an ETT.
2. To become informed about the contraindications to the use of a LMAD.
3. To gain an appreciation of the role of the LMAD in airway management.
4. To gain an appreciation of the role of these devices in the management of a difficult airway.

## Key Points

| | |
|---|---|
| 1 | Laryngeal mask airway devices (LMADs), such as the LMA™, have revolutionized airway management. |
| 2 | LMADs do not protect the airway in patients at risk of gastric aspiration during anesthesia. |
| 3 | Insertion of a LMAD may be lifesaving in the patient whose lungs cannot be ventilated or whose trachea cannot be intubated. |

Prior to the 1990s, anesthesiologists provided airway management to patients under general anesthesia either by holding a face mask (with or without the aid of an oral and/or nasal airway) or by intubating the trachea.

In the 1980s, Dr. Archie Brain revolutionized airway management with his pioneering work on a new "laryngeal mask airway". The LMA™, as it is known today, became commercially available in North America in 1991 around the same time that propofol was introduced as a new general intravenous anesthetic agent. Prior to 1991, thiopental was the most common intravenous anesthetic drug used to induce anesthesia. Propofol provided a more intense depression of the pharyngeal reflexes compared with thiopental. This profound depression of the pharyngeal reflexes that propofol provided permitted placement of a LMA™ with minimal adjuvant medications. This played a key role in the widespread acceptance of LMADs and their subsequent high profile for airway management throughout the world.

## What is the difference between a LMAD and a tracheal tube?

The LMA™ is a specialized airway device made of wide bore PVC tubing with a distal inflatable non-latex laryngeal cuff (Fig. 8.1). Without the need for special equipment, the LMA™ can be inserted into the back of the

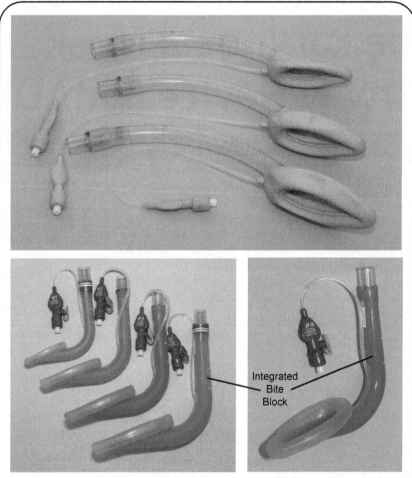

Fig. 8.1 LMA devices. LMA™ classic (top image) and AMBU aura™ LMA (bottom images). The AMBU LMA™ incorporates a bite block and has a reinforced tip to prevent backfolding of the tip on insertion.

patient's pharynx with the soft laryngeal cuff resting above the vocal cords at the junction of the larynx and esophagus. An endotracheal tube (ETT) generally requires a laryngoscope or other specialized device for proper insertion into the trachea. Unlike a LMA™, the ETT passes between the vocal cords with its tip resting in the mid-tracheal position.

A foreign body in the trachea, such as an endotracheal tube, evokes an intense irritant reflex. This results in an increase in heart rate and blood pressure and a cough reflex. The anesthesiologist routinely administers potent anesthesia medications, such as opioids and muscle relaxants, to blunt or abolish this reflex. The tracheal "foreign body" reflex

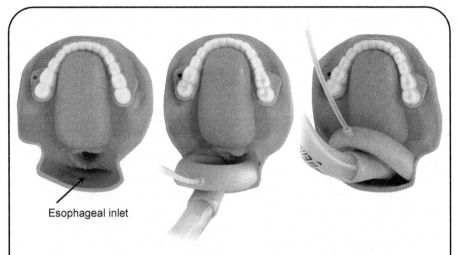

Esophageal inlet

Fig. 8.2 Laryngeal model illustrating the position of the LMA™ in relation to the tongue, larynx and esophagus. Note that the tip of the LMA™ is positioned behind the glottis in the upper esophageal inlet.

does not result from insertion of a LMAD because it does not enter the trachea. As such, a LMAD can be positioned without the use of muscle relaxants. Deep general anesthesia is required to depress the pharyngeal tone for proper positioning of the LMAD. This can be achieved with propofol alone or with one or more adjuvant medications to propofol, such as fentanyl, remifentanil[1], midazolam, or an inhalational anesthetic agent. Once the LMAD is properly positioned, anesthesia is commonly maintained using inhalational anesthetic agents, such as sevoflurane, in addition to air and oxygen. Spontaneous, supported, or controlled modes of ventilation can be used with a LMAD. When controlled ventilation is used with a LMAD, the airway pressures must be closely monitored and should be < 20 cm $H_2O$. Pressures > 20 cm $H_2O$ may result in gastric insufflation, increased gastric pressure, and an increased risk of regurgitation and aspiration.

## Does the LMAD protect the patient against gastric aspiration?

Should gastroesophageal reflux occur, a LMAD will not prevent gastric contents from entering the trachea (see Chapter 25: Unusual Anesthesia Complications: Aspiration Pneumonitis and Chapter 9: Rapid Sequence Induction).

## Which patients would be suitable candidates for general anesthesia with a LMAD?

Patients who have no identified risk factors for aspiration (see Chapter 9) and who do not require tracheal intubation and controlled ventilation are suitable candidates for the LMAD. It may be difficult to obtain an adequate seal using a face mask in patients with no teeth or those with a full beard. The LMAD is particularly useful in these patients as it provides a good seal and an unobstructed airway.

## Which patients are not suitable candidates for a LMAD?

1. Patients with risk factors for gastric aspiration.

   For example, a comatose patient in the emergency department with a full stomach would not be a good candidate for the LMAD, as the patient would be at high risk for gastric aspiration.

2. Patients with oropharyngeal pathology, retropharyngeal pathology, or foreign bodies in the hypopharynx.

   Examples include patients with oropharyngeal cancer, tonsillar abscess, epiglottitis, and trauma to the mouth.

3. Patients with a limited mouth opening (e.g., wired jaw, temporomandibular joint [TMJ] disease).

4. Patients requiring positive pressure ventilation with airway pressures of > 20 cm H20 (e.g., patients with significant restrictive or obstructive airway disease, morbid obesity, Trendelenburg position, laparoscopy).

## How do you position a LMAD?

The LMA™ is positioned after the induction of general anesthesia. The laryngeal mask should be lubricated, and the cuff valve should be checked. It is recommended that the cuff be fully deflated prior to insertion. However, our experience with the LMA Classic™ has been to use a small amount of air in the cuff (6 - 10 mL in an adult cuff) to facilitate its insertion. This approach helps to prevent the tip of the LMA™ from folding back upon insertion, which can make proper positioning of the LMA™ problematic. The patient should be placed in the supine position with the head and neck oriented in the usual "sniffing position" used for tracheal intubation.

Anesthesia is typically induced with the use of propofol. Other agents, such as thiopental, ketamine or sevoflurane, can be used to induce anesthesia. Propofol is the preferred induction agent as it is superior to thiopental for reducing laryngeal irritability and laryngospasm during LMA™ insertion.

The LMAD is placed after induction of general anesthesia. First, open the patient's mouth by creating an atlanto-occipital extension of the neck in combination with forward displacement of the jaw. Next, insert the tip of the LMA™ into the patient's mouth, and press it up against the patient's hard palate while advancing it into the pharynx with the right hand. Guide the cuff of the tube along the posterior pharyngeal wall, and then insert it as far as possible into the pharynx.

The following approach is recommended to facilitate advancing the laryngeal cuff past the tongue. Place the right index finger at the tube-cuff interface and use it to guide the cuff into the pharynx. At the same time, use the palm of the right hand to push the proximal end of the LMA™ into the pharynx. Resistance is felt when the distal tip of the cuff is positioned at the upper esophageal sphincter. An assistant may help by holding the patient's mouth open or by lifting the patient's jaw forward to open the hypopharyngeal space. The black line running longitudinally along the LMA™ tube should face the patient's upper lip. Once the LMA™ is placed in this position, inflate the cuff with air. This will cause the LMA™ to rise out of the patient's mouth a little as it settles into its correct position. The additional resources section provides a URL link of a video demonstrating the insertion of a classic LMA™.

## How do you remove the LMA™?

The LMA™ can be left in place until the patient is awake enough to remove it without assistance. Alternatively, the care provider can remove the LMA™ as the patient is emerging from anesthesia. Laryngeal cuff deflation is not necessary prior to removal. Removal of the LMA™ with the cuff inflated may actually assist in removal of upper airway secretions. Conversely, release of air may reduce the risk of cuff damage from the patient's teeth during removal, although deflation of the LMA™ cuff in the lightly anesthetized patient could result in laryngospasm due to stimulation of the vocal cords by secretions. Laryngospasm is an involuntary reflex closure of the glottis by adduction of the vocal cords. It may result in the inability to oxygenate or ventilate the patient's lungs and result in secondary hypercarbia and hypoxemia. Stridor, a high-pitched inspiratory sound produced by upper airway obstruction, may be noted during laryngospasm. Propofol can be used to deepen anesthesia, or a muscle relaxant, such as a small dose of succinylcholine, may be required to break the laryngospasm and permit positive pressure ventilation and oxygenation.

## How do you choose the correct LMA™ size?

The patient's weight is used as a rough guide for the LMA™ size. Sizes 4 and 5 are the most common LMA™ sizes used in adult anesthesia, and sizes are also available for pediatric and neonatal use. The laryngeal cuff is inflated with the minimal amount of air to provide a seal.

| LMA™ Size | Patient Weight (kg) |
|-----------|---------------------|
| 1 | Neonates < 5 |
| 1.5 | 5 – 10 |
| 2 | 10 – 20 |
| 2.5 | 20 – 30 |
| 3 | 30 – 50 |
| 4 | 50 – 70 |
| 5 | 70 – 100 |
| 6 | > 100 |

## Other Laryngeal Mask Airway Devices

The LMA™ was the original extraglottic device. Today, many different airway devices, each with their own unique features, are commercially available. In North America, modifications of the LMA Classic™ remain the most common alternatives to endotracheal intubation for patients undergoing general anesthesia.

The simplest of the extraglottic airway devices are the oropharyngeal and nasopharyngeal airways. These devices can be very useful in resolving an upper airway obstruction, and their use is a basic skill all physicians should possess.

Upper airway obstruction in an unconscious patient is most commonly caused from the tongue falling back into the hypopharynx. In the unconscious state, there is a decrease in the tone of the muscles attaching the tongue to the mandible, hyoid bone, and epiglottis. The respiratory efforts of the unconscious patient tend to pull the tongue backward and cause further airway obstruction. Furthermore, the epiglottis tends to fall downward in the unconscious patient further increasing the upper airway obstruction. Apart from tracheal intubation, there are a number of simple maneuvers that can be used to overcome an upper airway obstruction in the supine unconscious patient.

1. Clearance of foreign material from the airway.
2. Use of a chin lift maneuver.
3. Use of a jaw thrust maneuver.
4. Insertion of an oral and/or nasal airway.
5. Positioning patients on their side in the semi-prone "recovery position".

LMA devices require deep general anesthesia to be properly positioned. They are designed to maintain a patent airway in the unconscious patient. Many of these devices incorporate a distal cuff that can be used to

The deflated cuff of the classic LMA™ is advanced in a sweeping motion along the hard palate, soft palate and posterior pharyngeal wall.

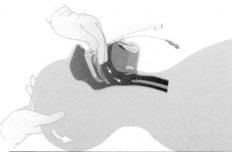

The classic LMA™ insertion technique recommends complete cuff deflation and using the tip of the index finger at the LMA™ tube / cuff interface to direct the tip of the cuff into the upper esophageal inlet.

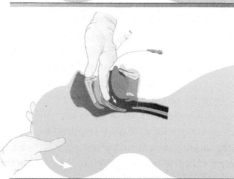

Rotation of the occiput and / or forward displacement of the mandible can be used to facilitate advancement of the LMA™ into the upper esophageal inlet.

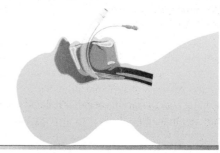

Once positioned, the LMA™ cuff is inflated to create a seal. Inflation pressures of 20 cm H₂O or less are recommended.

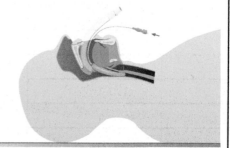

Fig. 8.3 Insertion technique for Classic LMA™.

minimize an airway leak during positive pressure ventilation.

### Modifications to the LMA Classic™

Many commercially available modifications of the LMA™ have been developed over the last two decades. The original LMA Classic™ was designed to be sterilized and reused; however, today's LMADs are available as disposable single-use airway tools or for reuse after appropriate sterilization. There are currently many new developments in LMADs offered by several different manufacturers. Some examples of these new developments include the AMBU® Aura laryngeal airway, which has a reinforced tip to reduce the incidence of "back folding" with insertion, a more common problem with the LMA Classic™. Insertion of the AMBU® Aura laryngeal airway is performed with the cuff fully deflated. This creates a very slim profile and allows ease of insertion without the aid of the operator's finger to guide the airway into the hypopharynx. Neck flexion with extension at the atlanto-occipital junction is used for insertion, similar to that used for the LMA Classic™. Gentle cephalad pressure is applied on insertion such that the tip of the AMBU® Aura airway follows the curve of the hard and soft palates into the hypopharynx. It is important to slide the airway around the patient's tongue so that it does not push the tongue backwards into the hypopharynx. Once the AMBU® Aura airway is properly seated in the hypopharynx, the laryngeal cuff is inflated, and the airway is secured with tape. Refer to the additional resources URL to view the AMBU® Aura insertion technique.

The primary advantage of the AMBU® Aura laryngeal airway over the LMA Classic™ is the incorporation of a built-in bite block. On occasion, a patient may forcibly bite on the LMA tube during light levels of anesthesia or on emergence of anesthesia. This can result

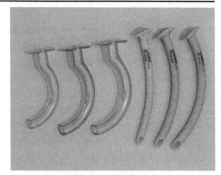

## Fig. 8.4 Oral and naso-pharyngeal airways.

in a complete airway occlusion. If the patient attempts to breathe against the occluded airway, a serious complication called negative pressure pulmonary edema can occur. The AMBU® Aura laryngeal airway has essentially eliminated this problem. See Chapter 25 for a further discussion on the pathophysiology and consequences of negative pressure pulmonary edema.

### Challenges encountered with insertion and positioning of a LMAD

A common cause of difficulty with LMAD insertion is poor timing of anesthetic drug administration. While propofol will induce a state of anesthesia in an "arm-brain" circulation time, the peak effect of propofol occurs 30 - 60 sec after the loss of eyelid reflex. Attempts to insert a LMAD immediately after loss of eyelid reflex are frequently difficult, as propofol has not yet reached its peak effect in suppressing the upper pharyngeal tone. The simple solution is to provide a brief period (30 - 60 sec) of gentle bag-mask ventilation after loss of eyelid reflex and prior to LMAD insertion.

Perhaps the next most common cause of difficult LMAD insertion is the result of an insufficient depth of anesthesia, sometimes referred to as the "APD syndrome" (Acute Propofol Deficiency Syndrome). Increasing the depth of anesthesia with propofol or other medications[1] will frequently suppress the pharyngeal tone enough to permit placement of the airway.

Failure to negotiate the laryngeal cuff around the patient's tongue may also create problems positioning the LMAD. Rather than pushing the patient's tongue inferiorly with the laryngeal airway and prohibiting proper placement, atlanto-occipital extension combined with a jaw thrust will frequently open up the hypopharyngeal space and permit the laryngeal airway to pass around the tongue.

Difficulties may also occur when the LMAD is malpositioned or an inappropriate size is used. This could cause the laryngeal cuff to push the epiglottis downward and result in a partial or complete airway obstruction. Solutions to the problem include readjusting the LMAD position, LMAD removal and reinsertion, adjusting the position of the patient's head, or changing the size of the LMAD. Stridor, partial or complete airway obstruction, and leaks with positive pressure ventilation are occasionally seen with a LMAD. If difficulties persist despite a clinically well-positioned LMAD, fiberoptic bronchoscopy can be used to provide additional detail regarding the position of the LMAD relative to the glottis. We now appreciate that the LMAD can provide a clinically acceptable airway despite being malpositioned and that difficulties with ventilation may occur despite a well-positioned LMA device. When problems persist, the best solutions may be removal of the LMA device and tracheal intubation.

The **LMA ProSeal**™ features two channels in the main airway tube. One tube is used for gas exchange while the second is directed at the upper esophageal inlet to vent the stomach or allow passage of a gastric tube into the stomach. Like the LMA Fastrach™, the LMA Proseal™ incorporates a built in bite block in its shaft. The LMA Proseal™ cuff provides a superior seal compared to the LMA Classic™, permitting positive pressure ventilation at higher pressures. The LMA Proseal™ is designed to be sterilized and reused. Unlike the LMA Classic™ and LMA Fastrach™, the LMA Proseal™ is generally not intended to be used as a conduit for tracheal intubation. The LMA Supreme™ is available as a single-use disposable LMA Proseal™.

The **King LT**® supraglottic airway is a curved silicone tube with a soft tip. The soft distal tip is designed to be inserted into the esophageal inlet. It has two cuffs that can be inflated using a single pilot balloon. While the distal cuff is positioned in the esophageal inlet, the proximal cuff is used to seal the oropharynx. The tube between the two cuffs has incorporated ventilation holes for gas exchange.

The King LT® can be used for both spontaneous and controlled ventilation. It is supplied with a special bite block that allows tube fixation with an elastic strap and prevents tube occlusion due to biting. The King LT® has become popular with paramedics for both emergency and difficult airway management. The King LTS-D™ version has a distal opening in the esophageal port to allow passage of a gastric tube into the stomach.

The **i-Gel**™ is a single-use non-cuffed supraglottic airway device that is intended for use in fasted patients. It can be used for both spontaneous and controlled ventilation and as a conduit for tracheal intubation. The i-Gel™ is manufactured in a soft gel-like plastic that molds into the hypopharyngeal space without the use of an inflatable cuff. A gastric channel allows direct suctioning or passage of a gastric tube, and an anterior epiglottic blocking ridge is intended to reduce the possibility of epiglottic down-folding on insertion.

The **Combitube**™ airway device is designed to allow blind intubation into the esophagus or trachea. It consists of two lumens

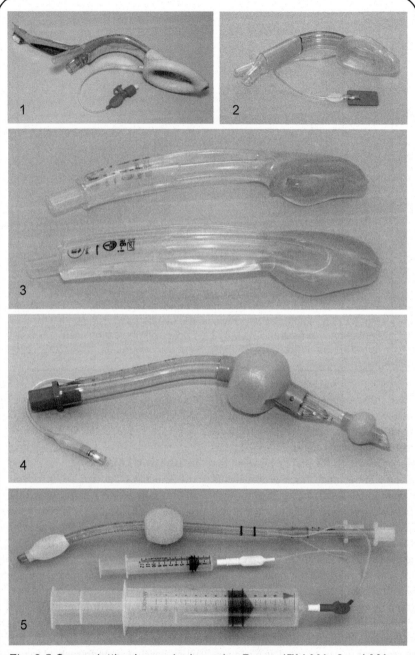

Fig. 8.5 Supraglottic airway devices. 1 = Proseal™ LMA, 2 = LMA Supreme™ (a disposable Proseal type of airway device), 3 = i-Gel™ laryngeal airway, 4 = King LT-D™Laryngeal tube, 5 = Combitube™.

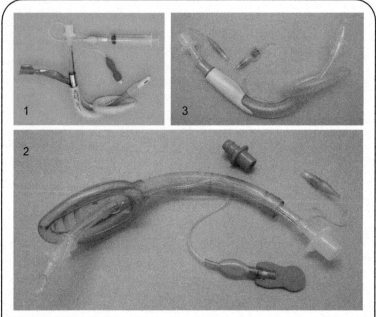

Fig. 8.6 Supraglottic airway devices that can be used as a conduit for intubation. 1 = Fastrach™ LMA, 2 = Cookgas™ intubating LMA (air-Q™), 3 = Ambu aura-i™ LMA.

with two cuffs. An open-ended distal lumen with a low-volume cuff is designed to make a seal in either the trachea or the esophagus. A second lumen is sealed at its distal end but has a series of fenestrations that lie between the distal cuff and the much larger proximal cuff. The Combitube™ should be inserted through the patient's mouth along the back of the tongue, with the tongue manually displaced, until the proximal black mark lies between the teeth. On blind insertion, the distal end will move toward and into the esophagus. Both cuffs can then be inflated, and the patient's lungs can be ventilated using the fenestrated second lumen. If the distal lumen is placed in the trachea blindly or under direct vision using a laryngoscope, it can be used as a conventional ETT. The Combitube™ is mainly intended for use in emergency airway management. Use of an esophageal detection device, a $CO_2$ detector, or capnography is necessary to help identify its placement and to distinguish the correct lumen to use for ventilation.

## Intubating LMADs

The **LMA Fastrach**™ is classified as an intubating LMA (ILMA). It was designed to address the problems encountered when attempting to intubate the trachea blindly through the LMA Classic™. Although a LMA Classic ™ can be used as a conduit for intubation, the LMA Fastrach™ incorporates features that increase the rate of successful intubation, including an insertion handle, a rigid shaft with a special anatomical curvature, and an elevating bar designed to lift the epiglottis when passing an endotracheal tube. Special silicone endotracheal tubes (sizes 7.0 ID, 7.5 ID, or 8.0 ID) are designed for use with the LMA Fastrach™. A flexible fiberoptic scope loaded

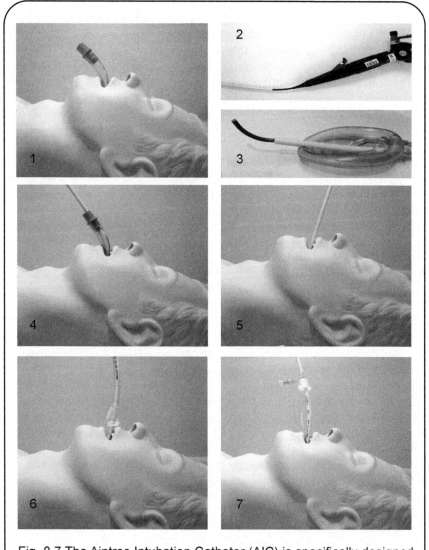

Fig. 8.7 The Aintree Intubation Catheter (AIC) is specifically designed to facilitate the exchange of a LMA device (LMAD) with an endotracheal tube. 1: The LMAD is inserted in the usual fashion.
2: The AIC is loaded onto a pediatric (3.5 mm) fiberoptic broncho-scope (FOB). 3 - 4: The FOB is advanced with the AIC through the LMAD into the trachea. 5: The AIC is held in place while the FOB and LMAD are removed. 6 - 7: An endotracheal tube (ETT) is advanced over the AIC into the trachea. The ETT is held in place while the AIC catheter is removed. Adapted from Zura A, Doyle DJ, Orlandi M. CJA 2005;52:646-649.

with an ETT can be used to direct the ETT through the LMA Fastrach™ into the trachea.

A number of LMADs are now available for use as a primary airway or to facilitate endotracheal intubation (fig. 8.6). The **Cook ILA™** is designed for use as an intubation conduit. It is shorter than the classic LMA™ allowing the ETT cuff to be passed distal to the vocal cords. It has no obstructing aperature bars and accommodates conventional ETTs. The **Ambu® Aura-i™** is a new single-use disposable LMAD that can also be used as a primary airway tool, but it is specifically designed to facilitate endotracheal intubation.

## Exchanging a LMA™ for an ETT in a patient with a difficult airway:

There are a couple of options when a LMA™ or LMAD needs to be replaced with an ETT. One option is to replace the LMAD with a LMA Fastrach™ and intubate the trachea through the LMA Fastrach™ as previously described. Alternatively, a special airway exchange catheter (Aintree) can be used to guide the ETT into the trachea (fig. 8.7). The Aintree airway exchange catheter is first loaded on a pediatric fiberoptic scope. The fiberoptic scope is then passed through the LMAD into the trachea. The Aintree catheter is then left in the trachea while the fiberoptic scope and LMAD are removed. The ETT is then advanced over the Aintree catheter into the trachea. The Aintree catheter is then removed and tracheal placement is confirmed with capnography.

## Laryngeal Mask Airway Devices in Emergency Settings

**Difficult Airway Scenario:** The American Society of Anesthesiologists Task Force on the Management of the Difficult Airway[2] recommends early insertion of an LMAD in the "can't intubate – can't ventilate" (CICV) scenario (see Chapter 7). In this setting, an extraglottic airway may be lifesaving. The extraglottic airway is used to ensure adequate oxygenation and ventilation while additional help and resources are recruited. The LMAD may be removed and exchanged for an endotracheal tube using advanced airway equipment, or alternatively, it may be used as a conduit for tracheal intubation (see Cook Aintree Catheter[3]). If use of the LMAD fails in the CICV scenario, emergency measures (e.g., cricothyroidotomy or tracheostomy) may be required to establish a surgical airway.

**Advanced Cardiac Life Support (ACLS):** The American Heart Association updates the Basic Cardiac Life Support (BCLS) and ACLS guidelines every five years. The most recent 2010 ACLS guidelines recognize the LMAD as an acceptable alternative to tracheal intubation for airway management in the cardiac arrest patient.[4] The use of a LMAD, such as an esophageal-tracheal tube (Combitube™), LMA™, and intubating laryngeal tube™ continues to be supported as an alternative to endotracheal intubation for airway management during CPR.

## References:

1. Lee MP, Fanzca JS, Chui WK et al. The use of remifentanil to facilitate the insertion of the laryngeal mask airway. Anesth Analg 2001;93:359-362.
2. Practice Guidelines for Management of the Difficult Airway: An Updated Report by the American Society of Anesthesiologists Task Force on Management of the Difficult Airway. Anesthesiology 2003; 98: 1269-77.
3. Zura A, Doyle DJ, Orlandi M. Use of the Aintree intubation catheter® in a patient with an unexpected difficult airway. Can J Anesth 2005;52:646-649.
4. Neumar RW, Otto CW, Link MS et al. Part 8: Adult Advanced Cardiovascular Life Support: 2010 American Heart Association Guidelines for Cardiopulmonary Resuscitation and Emergency Cardiovascular Care. Circulation 2010, 122:S729-S767.

# CHAPTER 9

# Rapid Sequence Induction

Christopher Mercer MD and Patrick Sullivan MD

## Learning Objectives

1. To identify risk factors for pulmonary aspiration.
2. To understand interventions that can reduce a patient's risk of pulmonary aspiration in the perioperative period.
3. To describe 5 key components of a rapid sequence induction.
4. To understand the rationale behind the "modified" rapid sequence induction.

## Key Points

| | |
|---|---|
| 1 | Rapid sequence induction (RSI) is an advanced skill. The procedure is potentially risky because it removes the patient's ability to breathe and exposes the patient to potential awareness, cardiovascular instability, hypoxemia, vomiting, and pulmonary aspiration if drug doses are not chosen correctly or difficulty with intubation occurs. |
| 2 | Incorrect application of cricoid pressure (CP) may make direct laryngoscopy more difficult. Ensure the assistant understands the correct technique for applying CP before inducing general anesthesia. Consider adjusting or removing CP if difficulty with intubation is encountered. |
| 3 | Regional or local anesthesia with monitored anesthetic care rather than general anesthesia may reduce the risk of gastric aspiration in the perioperative period. |

General anesthesia impairs the natural protective airway reflexes and exposes a patient to the risk of aspiration of stomach contents. This devastating complication is rare but potentially life-threatening and is discussed further in Chapter 25. All patients are at risk of aspiration of gastric contents under general anesthesia. To reduce the risk of aspiration, all patients undergoing elective surgery are asked to abstain from eating solid foods for a minimum of 6 hr and clear fluids for a minimum of 3 hr prior to surgery. After a suitable fasting period, most patients will have an empty stomach, which minimizes the risk of aspiration. This allows for a slow controlled induction of general anesthesia and subsequent airway management typically with a laryngeal mask airway device (LMAD) or endotracheal tube (ETT).

Recent *British Consensus Guidelines*[1] include the following recommendation for fluid therapy:

*"In patients without disorders of gastric emptying undergoing elective surgery, clear non-particulate oral fluids should not be withheld for more than two hours prior to the induction of anesthesia"* (evidence level 1a).

The current Canadian guidelines continue to recommend abstinence of clear fluids for a minimum of 3 hr prior to surgery.

A subgroup of patients remain at high risk of gastric aspiration despite an adequate fasting period. Patients requiring emergent surgery are assumed to have a full stomach and are therefore considered at highest risk of aspiration under anesthesia. The predisposing risk factors for gastric aspiration include a full stomach, depressed level of consciousness (LOC), impaired airway reflexes, abnormal anatomical features, decreased gastroesophageal (GE) sphincter competence, increased intragastric pressure, and delayed gastric emptying (Table 9.1). Patients who have any of these predisposing risk factors for gastric aspiration and who require a general anesthetic should be considered at a higher risk of aspiration during the perioperative period, and may be candidates for an RSI technique.

## Table 9.1 Predisposing Risk Factors for Aspiration

| | | |
|---|---|---|
| Decreased LOC | Drug or alcohol (ETOH) overdose<br>Anesthesia<br>Head injury | Central nervous system (CNS) pathology<br>Trauma or shock states |
| Impaired airway reflexes | Prolonged intubation<br>Local airway anesthesia<br>Decreased LOC | Myopathies<br>Cerebrovascular accident (CVA) |
| Abnormal anatomy | Zenker's diverticulum | Esophageal stricture |
| Decreased GE competence | Nasogastric (NG) tube<br>Elderly patient<br>Pregnancy | Hiatus hernia<br>Obesity |
| Increased intragastric pressure | Pregnancy<br>Obesity<br>Bowel obstruction | Large abdominal tumors<br>Ascites |
| Delayed gastric emptying | Narcotics<br>Anticholinergics<br>Fear, pain, labour, trauma | Pregnancy<br>Renal failure<br>Diabetes |

## Table 9.1 Predisposing Risk Factors for Aspiration

| Preventative measures | Preoperative fasting | NG tube prior to induction |
|---|---|---|
| | $H_2$ antagonists (↓ acidity) | CP on induction |
| | Antacids (↓ acidity) | Extubation awake on side |
| | Metoclopramide(↓ motility) | Regional or local anesthesia |
| | Antiemetics | |

This chapter is written as an introduction to the principles and technique of a RSI. It must be understood that RSI should only be performed by a clinician skilled in airway management with experience in intubation, alternative airway rescue techniques, and a thorough knowledge of the pharmacology of the drugs to be administered. Proper preparation, assistance, and backup plans are critical in ensuring a safe outcome. The procedure is potentially risky because it removes the patient's ability to breathe and exposes the patient to potential awareness, cardiovascular instability, hypoxemia, and gastric reflux or aspiration if drug doses are not chosen correctly or difficulty with intubation occurs.

## Technique for Rapid Sequence Induction

The key components of a rapid sequence induction are:
1. Preoxygenation
2. Application of CP with loss of consciousness
3. Administration of intravenous anesthetics and a muscle relaxant
4. Endotracheal intubation with a cuffed endotracheal tube (ETT)
5. Confirmation of ETT placement and release of CP

### 1. *Preoxygenation:*

Preoxygenation is performed to increase a patient's oxygen reserve prior to induction of anesthesia. This allows for a relatively longer period of apnea and airway management before desaturation occurs. The purpose of preoxygenation is to replace the nitrogen in the patient's lungs, i.e., the functional residual capacity (FRC), with oxygen. The FRC has a volume of approximately 2.5 L in an average adult and provides a reservoir of oxygen after induction of anesthesia. With a typical oxygen consumption of 250 mL·min$^{-1}$ in an average adult, the FRC provides an oxygen reservoir for the apneic period from induction of anesthesia to tracheal intubation.

Preoxygenation is achieved by breathing 100% oxygen from a tight-fitting mask for a period of 3 min or more. If time does not allow for this, four large (vital capacity) breaths of 100% oxygen will replace > 95% of the nitrogen in the patients lungs with oxygen. Room air consists of approximately 79% nitrogen and 21% oxygen. Hence, it is important to maintain a proper seal between the mask and patient during preoxygenation to avoid entraining room air (nitrogen). Preoxygenation is an important strategy to maximize the patient's oxygen reserves prior to anesthetic induction, paralysis, and intubation.

### 2. *Cricoid pressure:*

Cricoid pressure was first described by Dr. Sellick in 1961 and is often referred to as the "Sellick maneuver".[2] The maneuver involves the application of CP by an assistant at the time of anesthetic induction. The CP is not released until the airway is secured with a cuffed ETT. Cricoid pressure involves the displacement of the cricoid ring in a posterior direction towards the patient's esophagus as a way to prevent gastric contents from entering the airway during induction and tracheal intubation. It is important that the assistant receives instruction on the proper application of CP prior to induction of anesthesia. The assistant is positioned near the patient's head, placing a thumb and forefinger on the cricoid ring. With the administration of the anesthetic drugs, the clinician will instruct the assistant to apply approximately 8 – 10 lbs of pressure on the cricoid cartilage in a posterior direction. As this can be uncomfortable, more gentle pressure may be applied until the patient is rendered unconscious. Full pressure will then be maintained until the patient's airway has been secured with a cuffed ETT.

Cricoid pressure may distort the clinician's view of the larynx during intubation, especially when applied incorrectly. Manual repositioning of the assistant's hand, lightening of CP, or removal of CP may be required when visualization of the larynx is compromised. Cricoid pressure is often confused with another maneuver termed "BURP". BURP refers to a "backward, upward, and rightward pressure" on the thyroid cartilage. A BURP maneuver may be requested by a clinician as a means of improving laryngeal visualization during direct laryngoscopy and tracheal intubation.[3] A BURP maneuver is not used to prevent gastric aspiration. Fig. 9.1 illustrates the proper application of cricoid pressure.

### Clinical Pearl:

*Assistants learning the technique of applying cricoid pressure can be instructed to practice applying pressure with their thumb and first finger to the bridge of their nose until it becomes uncomfortable. The pressure at which this occurs is said to correlate roughly with 8 – 10 lbs of pressure.*

### 3. Administration of intravenous anesthetics and muscle relaxants:

Cricoid pressure is applied with the administration of an intravenous anesthetic and loss of consciousness. This is immediately followed by the administration of a neuromuscular relaxant drug (commonly succinylcholine or rocuronium) to produce profound skeletal relaxation of the oropharyngeal, laryngeal, and diaphragm muscles. Relaxation of these muscles will optimize the conditions for endotracheal intubation. While these agents are discussed in detail in other chapters of this text, a short discussion on their application in the context of RSI is warranted. Commonly used drug doses for a RSI are listed in Table 9.2. The doses of medication used should always be tailored to the clinical situation (see Chapter 7: Intubation Decisions).

i. **Intravenous anesthetic agents** are used to render the patient unconscious without delay and to induce muscle paralysis for a RSI. Factors influencing the choice of drug and dose to use include the drugs time to peak effect, duration, elimination, hemodynamic factors, and side effects. The most common induction agent is propofol. Thiopental, etomidate, and ketamine are other alternative induction agents that may be used in special circumstances.

ii. **Neuromuscular Relaxants** (NMR) are used for paralysis (muscle relaxation). Paralysis facilitates rapid tracheal intubation by relaxing the skeletal muscles and preventing laryngospasm, coughing, and vomiting. Historically, the classic neuromuscular relaxant used in a RSI technique was succinylcholine, a depolarizing NMR. The primary advantage of succinylcholine is its rapid onset and short half-life; however, it has several unique serious potential side effects that are not seen with any other

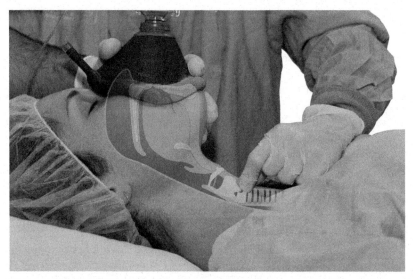

Fig. 9.1 Application of cricoid pressure. Backward pressure is applied on the cricoid cartilage to occlude the esophagus. The aim is to prevent gastric contents from entering the airway after induction of anesthesia and prior to endotracheal intubation.

relaxant. For that reason, it is especially important for the clinician to have a clear understanding of the contraindications and side effects of succinylcholine to decrease the risk of any adverse reaction to the drug. The contraindications to succinylcholine are discussed in detail in Chapter 12. Alternative nondepolarizing NMR drugs, such as rocuronium, may be used in a RSI. Their slower onset time compared with succinylcholine may be decreased by using a higher dose at the expense of a longer duration of paralysis.

iii. **Other pharmacologic agents** may be used in a RSI. An opioid, such as fentanyl, may be administered several minutes prior to a RSI to blunt the sympathetic response (frequently manifested by tachycardia and hypertension) at the time of tracheal intubation. When appropriate,

Table 9.2   Common Drug Doses Used in a Rapid Sequence Induction

| Agent | Dose | Onset | Duration (estimated) | Notes |
|-------|------|-------|----------------------|-------|
| Propofol | 1 - 2.5 mg·kg⁻¹ | ABCT* | 10 min | Hypotension |
| Etomidate | 0.2 - 0.3 mg·kg⁻¹ | ABCT* | 10 min | Less BP effect |
| Ketamine | 1 - 2 mg·kg⁻¹ | ABCT* | 10 min | Increases HR/BP |
| Succinylcholine | 1 - 2 mg·kg⁻¹ | 60 sec | 7-10 min | Increases K+ |
| Rocuronium | 0.3 - 0.6 mg·kg⁻¹ | 90 sec | 45 min | Higher dose (RSI) |
| *ABCT = arm-brain circulation time; BP = blood pressure; HR = heart rate; K+ = potassium. | | | | |

a benzodiazepine, such as midazolam, may be administered for anxiolysis and amnesia prior to induction of anesthesia. If succinylcholine is to be used in the RSI, the clinician may choose to administer a small "defasciculating" dose of a nondepolarizing NMR to minimize postoperative myalgias resulting from the fasciculations associated with succinylcholine (see Chapter 12). In special circumstances, e.g., patients with raised intracranial pressure, lidocaine in a dose of 1 - 1.5 mg kg$^{-1}$ may be administered 3 - 5 min prior to induction to attenuate the sympathetic response and raised intracranial pressure (ICP) associated with endotracheal intubation.

Prepare resuscitation drugs prior to performing a RSI. See Chapter 6 mnemonic, "A Basic Mad Poster"

### 4. *Endotracheal intubation:*

Endotracheal intubation with a cuffed ETT is the cornerstone of a RSI. Once placed, a properly positioned cuffed ETT will prevent aspiration of gastric contents. Proper preparation is required to ensure that the first attempt at tracheal intubation is the best attempt. Preparation includes placing the patient in an optimal "sniffing" position, placement of standard monitors prior to induction of anesthesia (electrocardiogram [ECG], BP, oxygen saturation [SpO2]), preoxygenation, the use of a styletted ETT, an immediately available suction unit fitted with a Yankauer suction tip, and clear backup management plans with appropriate emergency drugs and airway equipment should difficulty with intubation occur.

### 5. *Confirmation of ETT placement:*

There are only two immediately available clinical gold standards for confirmation that the ETT is in the trachea and not in the esophagus, i.e., the direct visualization of the

ETT passing between the vocal cords into the glottis and the continuous return of end-tidal carbon dioxide (ETCO2). Auscultation of the lung fields should also be performed following intubation to confirm air entry to both lung fields and to rule out an endobronchial intubation. Auscultation is also performed to detect any abnormal breath sounds, such as wheezing, after the patient's trachea has been intubated.

The rise and fall of the chest with ventilation, the absence of gastric sounds with ventilation, and misting on the ETT are frequently observed, but these are not reliable indicators to confirm correct endotracheal intubation. The ETT cuff is inflated to create a seal during positive pressure ventilation. The cuff is inflated with the minimal amount of air that will prevent an audible air leak during ventilation of the lungs (typically < 25 mmHg). Cricoid pressure should be maintained until the clinician instructs the assistant to release it after tracheal placement is confirmed.

## Modified Rapid Sequence Induction

A *"modified RSI"* is often used today. While the classic RSI technique was rapidly embraced following Sellick's description in 1961, there remains a paucity of evidence supporting its use.[2,4] Every component of the RSI technique has come under scrutiny, resulting in clinicians promoting modifications to the *"classic RSI technique"*.[5] Some clinicians may thus elect to incorporate modifications to the classic RSI.

**Cricoid pressure** has been observed in some cases to be ineffective in preventing gastric contents from entering the airway. For this reason, some clinicians may choose to eliminate CP from their RSI technique. Sellick provided a very specific description of the correct application of CP. "The head and neck are *fully extended* (as in the position for tonsillectomy). This increases the anterior convexity of the cervical spine, *stretches the esophagus, and* *prevents its lateral displacement* when pressure is applied to the cricoid". However, in some cases, the use of neck extension may be contraindicated or impractical. Without neck extension, the esophagus may lie lateral to the cricoid cartilage, and CP may not prevent gastric contents from entering the airway at induction of anesthesia.

**Bag mask ventilation (BMV)** is usually avoided after induction of anesthesia in a classic RSI. The use of BMV after induction of anesthesia may result in gastric insufflation, gastric distension, and an increased risk of regurgitation and aspiration. This is especially true when inflation pressures exceed 20 cm $H_2O$. As inflation pressures rise, the competence of the lower esophageal sphincter is overcome and gastric distension results. With progressive gastric distension, gastric pressures rise and with it the risk of regurgitation.

Despite preoxygenation, certain patients are at risk of rapid desaturation following induction of anesthesia and may require BMV to maintain a saturation level > 90%. Hence, the clinician may elect to modify the RSI and use gentle BMV with pressures < 20 cm H2O following induction of anesthesia. When electing to manually ventilate a patient in a RSI, insertion of an oral airway may improve airway patency and minimize the pressure required for effective ventilation. Even with preoxygenation, the time required to recover muscle function following 1 mg·kg⁻¹ of intravenous succinylcholine exceeds the time to desaturation (see Fig. 9.2). Significant desaturation is predicted to occur following succinylcholine if intubation is unsuccessful or there is a delay in ventilating the patients lungs.

**Nondepolarizing relaxants,** such as rocuronium, may be used in a *modified* RSI even though succinylcholine has been the relaxant of choice in a *classic* RSI. A nondepolarizing relaxant may be chosen as a means of avoiding potential side effects (e.g., arrhythmias, hyperkalemia, myalgias, and increased intracranial pressures) associated with succinylcholine. Administering a higher dose of nondepolarizing relaxant will produce paralysis in a period of time comparable with that of succinylcholine, but at the expense of a much longer duration of paralysis. This distinction must be considered as the patient will be unable to breathe unassisted should intubation be unsuccessful.

The *2010 ACLS Guidelines* state that the routine use of **cricoid pressure** during airway management of patients in cardiac arrest is **no longer recommended**. This recommendation is based on evidence of reduced effectiveness in ventilating a patient's lungs as well as increased difficulty with airway management (placement of an extraglottic airway device or performing laryngoscopy and intubation).

## Clinical Case

A 45-yr-old male is brought to the operating room for open reduction and fixation of a left femoral fracture. He is in a traction splint and is in considerable discomfort but oriented and able to provide a coherent history. He states that he was at a bar when a fight broke out, and he was hit with a baseball bat. He admits to having consumed approximately 12 beers in the preceding 3 hours, and he ate some pizza about 4 hours ago. He has no significant medical history and no known allergies; he takes no regular medications and has not had previous surgeries. He admits to smoking one pack of cigarettes per day for the last 20 years and occasionally smokes marijuana. He is moderately obese, (weight = 105 kg) and has a short thick neck with a slight limitation in his cervical extension on range of motion testing. Examination of his oropharynx reveals a Mallampati class 3 airway with full dentition and a facial beard.

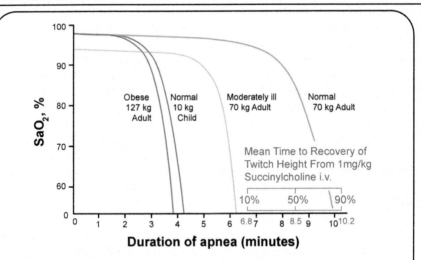

Fig. 9.2 Computerized apnea model of time to hemoglobin desaturation following preoxygenation for various patients. Note severe desaturation occurs with apnea prior to recovery from 1 mg/kg of intravenous succinylcholine. Adapted from Benumof JL et al. Anesthesiology 1999;87:979-982.

**Test your knowledge**

1. What are the airway considerations for this patient?
2. What features of the history and physical exam would alert you to an increased risk of pulmonary aspiration?
3. What can be done to decrease his risk of pulmonary aspiration?
   The following URL link provides a discussion of this clinical case.
   http://www.anesthesiaprimer.com/AP/Ch9RSI/Ch9Supplement.pdf

**References**

1. Powell-Tuck J, Gosling P, Lobo D et al. The British Consensus Guidelines on Intravenous Fluid Therapy for Adult Surgical Patients (GIFTASUP); updated 2011.
2. Sellick, BA (1961). "Cricoid pressure to control regurgitation of stomach contents during induction of anaesthesia". The Lancet Aug 19 1961; 278: 404-6. Also available at http://www.anesthesiaprimer.com/AP/Ch9RSI/Sellick.pdf
3. Takahata O, Kubota M, Mamiya K, et al. The efficacy of the BURP maneuver during a difficult laryngoscopy. Anesth Analg 1997; 84: 419 – 421.
4. Science, pseudoscience and Sellick Maltby JR, Beriault MT Ed. Can J Anesth 2002; 49: 443–447.
5. Cricoid pressure in emergency department rapid sequence tracheal intubations: a risk-benefit analysis. Ellis DY, Harris T, Zideman D. Ann Emerg Med 2007;50(6):653-665.

# CHAPTER 10

# Monitoring in Anesthesia

Patrick Sullivan MD, Ahmed Soliman MD

## Learning Objectives

1. To gain an appreciation of the standard and advanced physiologic monitors used in the perioperative period.
2. To gain an understanding of how these monitors provide information on a patient's well-being.
3. To distinguish between normal and abnormal physiologic data.
4. To gain an appreciation of the indications and limitations of physiologic monitors.

## Key Points

1. Oxygen saturation levels plummet rapidly when the $PaO_2$ decreases to < 60 mm Hg.

2. End-tidal carbon dioxide ($ETCO_2$) measurements are crucial in confirming endotracheal intubation.

3. An experienced anesthesia care provider is the most important monitor in the operating room (OR).

4. Judging the depth of anesthesia is an inexact science.

5. Recovery from muscle relaxants is judged to be adequate when the train-of-four (TOF) ratio is > 90%.

6. Surgery increases antidiuretic hormone (ADH) and renin-aldosterone levels, causing an abrupt decrease in urine output in the perioperative period.

7. Hourly urine output is a poor monitor of fluid requirements in the perioperative period.

In addition to visual and auditory observations, several automated electronic monitors are commonly used to provide information on a patient's physiological well-being in the perioperative period. These physiologic monitors provide valuable information and trends that anesthesiologists use to optimize vital organ function, tissue perfusion, and oxygenation.

A clinician must interpret the information provided by these devices in order to differentiate normal from abnormal physiology.

It is only in this context that the clinician can formulate a differential and provisional diagnosis and decide whether an intervention is required.

## What should we monitor?

Current Canadian and American *Guidelines to the Practice of Anesthesia* and patient monitoring concur that the presence, at all times, of appropriately trained and experienced anesthesia personnel is the only indispensable monitor during the conduct of general anesthesia, regional anesthesia, and monitored anesthetic care.

A preanesthetic checklist must be completed prior to commencing anesthesia. This includes a documented history and physical examination of the patient, a review of appropriate laboratory investigations, a preanesthesia evaluation, an American Society of Anesthesiology (ASA) classification, and confirmation that the *nil per os* policy has been observed if it is an elective procedure.

## Required monitoring:

Every patient receiving general anesthesia, major regional anesthesia, or monitored anesthetic care requires continuous pulse oximetry, electrocardiography (ECG) monitoring, $ETCO_2$ measurements when an endotracheal tube (ETT) or laryngeal mask airway device (LMAD) is used, and anesthetic gas monitoring when inhalational anesthetic agents are used. Blood pressure measurements (either directly with an arterial line or noninvasively) must be monitored regularly and repeatedly, generally a minimum of every 5 min.

Anesthesiologists must have exclusive ease of access to monitor the patient further at their discretion, including the ability to examine the patient visually using appropriate lighting, measure the patient's temperature, assess neuromuscular function (when neuromuscular blocking drugs are used), and

auscultate the patient with a stethoscope. Temperature monitoring is mandatory if changes in temperature are anticipated or suspected.

## I. OXYGENATION

### How can we determine whether or not the patient is well oxygenated?

Oxygenation is monitored clinically by ensuring adequate skin coloration and by pulse oximetry. The inspired oxygen concentration $(F_iO_2)$ is quantitatively monitored during all general anesthetics using an oxygen analyzer. Each analyzer is equipped with an audible low oxygen concentration alarm.

Pulse oximetry allows beat to beat analysis of the patient's oxygenation status. Oximetry is based on the differences in light absorption by hemoglobin as it binds and releases oxygen. Red and infrared light frequencies are transmitted through a translucent portion of tissue, such as the fingertip or earlobe. The signal is filtered to isolate pulsatile changes in light absorption. Microprocessors are then used to analyze the amount of light absorbed by two wavelengths of light, and this is compared with a table of measured values to determine the concentration of oxygenated and deoxygenated forms of hemoglobin. Once the concentrations of oxyhemoglobin (oxyHb) and deoxyhemoglobin (deoxyHb) have been determined, the oxygen saturation $(SpO_2)$ can be calculated. Current pulse oximeters have numeric LED displays for the heart rate and percent saturation. A pulse plethysmograph allows visual analysis of the pulse waveform, while an audible tone, which varies with the percent saturation, allows an auditory assessment of the patient's oxygenation status.

Pulse oximetry includes measurements of oxyHb, deoxyHb, methemoglobin (metHb), and carboxyhemoglobin (carboxyHb). An overestimation of the true measured $SaO_2$ may occur in the presence of significant carbon monoxide poisoning (e.g., a burn victim). Oximeters may become inaccurate or unable to determine the oxygen saturation when the tissue perfusion is poor (e.g., shock states or cold extremities), when movement occurs, when dysrhythmias are present, or when there is electrical interference (e.g., electrosurgical cautery unit).

The oxyHb dissociation curve describes a sigmoidal shape (see Fig. 10.1). A decrease in $PaO_2$ to < 60 mmHg (a $PaO_2$ of 60 mmHg corresponds to an $SpO_2$ of aproximately 90%) results in a rapid fall in the oxygen saturation. The lower limit of acceptable $SpO_2$ is 90% as this represents an arterial oxygen tension just above hypoxic values.

Under optimal lighting conditions with no excessive skin pigmentation and a normal hemoglobin level, the earliest that cyanosis can be appreciated is at an oxygen saturation of approximately 85%. This corresponds to a $PaO_2$ of 55 mmHg (see oxygen dissociation curve Fig. 10.1). At a $SaO_2$ of 70%, the $PaO_2$ will be approximately 40 mm Hg, which is considered a critically low value, and most clinicians will be able to detect the presence of cyanosis.

*Clinical Pearl:*

*The pulse oximeter's audible tone should be enabled in emergency settings in remote locations. This provides the health care team with continuous immediate feedback to the patient's heart rate and saturation level.*

## II. VENTILATION
### How can we determine whether or not the patient is breathing adequately?

For patients with an ETT or LMAD, we can monitor ventilation by observing chest excursion and reservoir bag displacement, and by listening to breath sounds over both lung fields. Ventilation is quantitatively monitored using $ETCO_2$ analysis as well as expired gas volumes (tidal volume) and respiratory rate. An audible disconnection alarm is standard for all patients whose lungs are mechanically ventilated. Arterial blood gas analysis may be used as an aid when assessing the adequacy of both oxygenation and ventilation. The anesthesiologist continually monitors the respiratory rate, tidal volume, airway pressures, $ETCO_2$ values, and $SpO_2$ levels to ensure adequate oxygenation and ventilation during general anesthesia. Desaturation, hypercarbia, and reductions in tidal volume and respiratory rate are commonly associated with inadequate ventilation and may require specific interventions. In patients breathing spontaneously without an ETT or LMAD, ventilation is monitored by observing chest excursion, respiratory rate, exhaled $CO_2$ measured at the mouth, and $SpO_2$.

## III. CIRCULATION
### How can we assess the patient's circulatory system?

The circulation can be monitored clinically by palpation of the pulse and auscultation of heart sounds. Quantitative evaluation of the circulation includes a continuous ECG signal, pulse oximetry, and regular and repeated blood pressure measurements.

A three or five-lead electrode system is commonly used for ECG monitoring in the OR. A three-lead system has electrodes positioned on the right shoulder (white "right arm" lead), left shoulder (black "left arm" lead), and chest positions (red lead). Lead II is usually monitored with a three-lead system, as the axis of this vector is similar to the P-wave axis. Identification of P-waves in lead II and its association with the QRS complex is useful in distinguishing a sinus rhythm from other rhythms. With a five-lead electrode system, the chest electrode (brown lead) is usually placed in the left anterior axillary line at the fifth interspace and is referred to as the V5 precordial lead. A five-lead electrode system adds

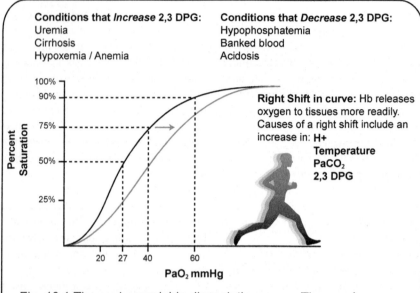

**Conditions that *Increase* 2,3 DPG:**
Uremia
Cirrhosis
Hypoxemia / Anemia

**Conditions that *Decrease* 2,3 DPG:**
Hypophosphatemia
Banked blood
Acidosis

**Right Shift in curve:** Hb releases oxygen to tissues more readily. Causes of a right shift include an increase in: **H+**
**Temperature**
**$PaCO_2$**
**2,3 DPG**

Fig. 10.1 The oxyhemoglobin dissociation curve. The running man generates heat, carbon dioxide and acid shifting the curve to the right and enhancing oxygen release to the tissues.

a right leg electrode (green lead) and positions the red lead towards the left leg. The five-lead electrode system allows monitoring of vectors I, II, III, AVR, AVL, AVF, and V5 (see Fig. 10.5) Today's anesthesia monitors are capable of analysis of the ST segment as an indicator of myocardial ischemia. Depression or elevation of the ST segment may be indicative of myocardial ischemia or infarction, respectively. More than 85% of ischemic events occurring in the left ventricle during surgery can be detected by monitoring the ST segments of leads II and V5.

The simplest way of determining the systolic blood pressure is by manually inflating a BP cuff until the pulse disappears and then slowly releasing the cuff and palpating the return of the arterial pulse. Other methods include auscultation of the Korotkoff sounds with cuff deflation. This allows both systolic

(SBP) and diastolic (DBP) blood pressure measurements. The mean arterial pressure (MAP) can be estimated from this where: MAP = DBP + 1/3(SBP - DBP).

Automated noninvasive BP measurements are routinely performed intraoperatively using a microprocessor-controlled oscillotonometer. These units have replaced routine BP measurements using auscultation or palpation techniques. They automatically inflate the BP cuff to occlude the arterial pulse at pre-set time intervals. The cuff pressure is sensed by a pressure transducer. Repeated step deflations provide oscillation measurements that are digitalized and processed as the cuff is deflated. In most circumstances, rapid accurate measurements of the blood pressure can be repeatedly obtained in less than a minute. Automated BP measurements are routinely performed every

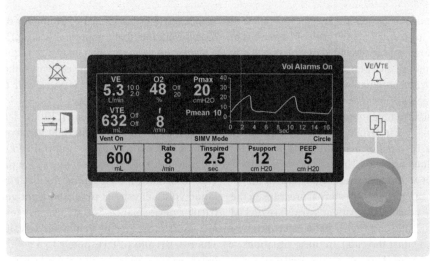

Fig. 10.2 Typical display of anesthesia ventilator settings. VE = minute ventilation, Pmax = maximum pressure, VTE = tidal volume expired, SIMV = synchronized intermittent mandatory ventilation.

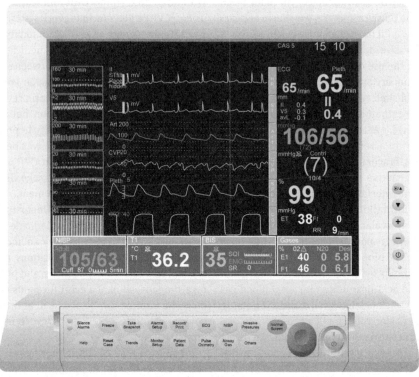

Fig. 10.3 Common cardiac and respiratory monitoring parameters.

3 - 5 min during general anesthesia. Repeated rapid measurements for prolonged periods of time are not recommended due to a small risk of a compressive peripheral nerve injury.

When automated noninvasive BP measurements are unsuccessful, simple auscultation or palpation techniques can be used with a manual cuff. In certain circumstances, an automated BP monitor may be unable to measure the blood pressure. This may occur in the setting of an irregular heart rate, patient movement, or intermittent external pressure on the cuff (e.g., when the patient's arms are tucked to their side and the surgeon intermittently leans against the cuff). In these situations, a second manual BP cuff may be used on the arm with the pulse oximeter. The pulse oximeter's waveform will disappear as the manual cuff is inflated above the arterial pressure. The SBP is obtained by slowly deflating the manual cuff until the pulse oximeter's waveform appears again or until the radial pulse is felt.

Invasive monitoring of the circulation may include the use of an arterial, central venous, or pulmonary artery catheter. An arterial line is established typically with a small (20G in adults) catheter in a peripheral artery. The radial artery at the wrist is the most common site for an arterial catheter insertion. The femoral, brachial, and dorsalis pedis arteries are alternative sites for arterial line insertion. The arterial waveform provides beat to beat information that can be used to assess the intravascular volume status of the patient. Intraoperative point-of-care testing using small samples of blood from the arterial line can be used to provide information on oxygenation and acid-base status (arterial blood gas analysis), hemoglobin level, coagulation status, as well as electrolytes and glucose.

Procedures frequently requiring direct arterial pressure monitoring include major cardiac, thoracic, vascular, and neurosurgical procedures. Patients with coexisting diseases, including significant cardiopulmonary disease, severe metabolic abnormalities, morbid obesity, and major trauma, may also require perioperative arterial line placement. A short video of an arterial insertion is provided in the additional resources section.

A central venous pressure (CVP) catheter provides an estimate of the right atrial and right ventricular pressures. Central venous pressure measurements may be used to provide information concerning the patient's blood volume, venous tone, and right ventricular performance. Serial measurements are much more useful than a single value. The HR, BP, and CVP response to a volume infusion (100 - 500 mL of fluid) can be used to evaluate right ventricular performance. Central venous pressure monitoring may be useful in patients undergoing procedures associated with large fluid shifts. Other indications for using a CVP catheter include shock states, massive trauma, significant cardiopulmonary disease, or the need for vasoactive medications. Unfortunately, the correlation between single CVP measurements and intravascular volume status is poor. A recent systematic review[1] showed a very poor correlation between CVP measurements and the ability to predict whether or not a fluid challenge was beneficial. The authors concluded that CVP measurements should not be used to make clinical decisions regarding fluid management.

The University of Ottawa Departments of Anesthesia and Emergency Medicine have developed a Web-based instructional module that discusses the anatomy, indications, preparation, technique, complications, and pitfalls regarding insertion of a central venous catheter. The module can be accessed at http://www.med.uottawa.ca/courses/cvc/e_index.html.

Unlike a CVP catheter that lies in the superior vena cava, the pulmonary artery catheter (PAC) passes through the right atrium

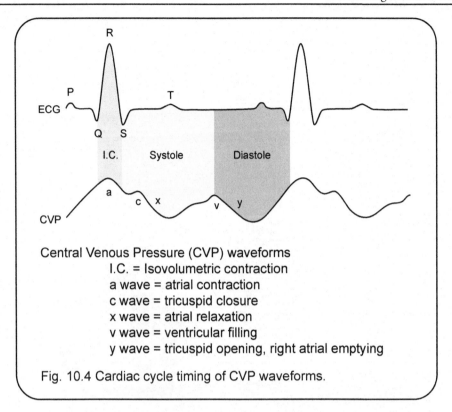

Central Venous Pressure (CVP) waveforms
I.C. = Isovolumetric contraction
a wave = atrial contraction
c wave = tricuspid closure
x wave = atrial relaxation
v wave = ventricular filling
y wave = tricuspid opening, right atrial emptying

Fig. 10.4 Cardiac cycle timing of CVP waveforms.

and right ventricle and rests in a branch of one of the pulmonary arteries (see Fig. 10.6). Inflation of a small balloon at the tip of the catheter allows occlusion of the proximal pulmonary artery and measurement of the distal pressure. This distal (back) pressure is referred to as the pulmonary artery (or capillary) wedge pressure (PCWP) or pulmonary artery occlusion pressure (PAOP) and reflects the left atrial filling pressure. Thermodilution calculations of cardiac output are performed by injecting a fixed volume of cool fluid into the right atrial port and measuring the temperature change over time from a thermistor probe at the distal tip of the PAC. A sample of blood taken from the distal tip of the PAC can be analyzed to determine the mixed venous oxygen saturation ($SvO_2$). Detailed analysis of

the patient's blood and fluid requirements as well as the adequacy of oxygen delivery can be made with the measurements obtained from a PAC. The results of manipulating the patient's hemodynamic parameters with ionotropic agents, vasopressors, vasodilators, diuretics, fluids, or blood products can then be followed.

The PAC has been used for over forty years to provide detailed information about a patient's vascular physiology. This has been used to guide interventions to optimize hemodynamics and oxygen delivery in high-risk patients undergoing major surgery. Two recent systematic reviews have validated the PAC as an effective tool to decrease perioperative morbidity and guide fluid therapy.[2,3]

Recently, minimally invasive monitors using esophageal Doppler technology and

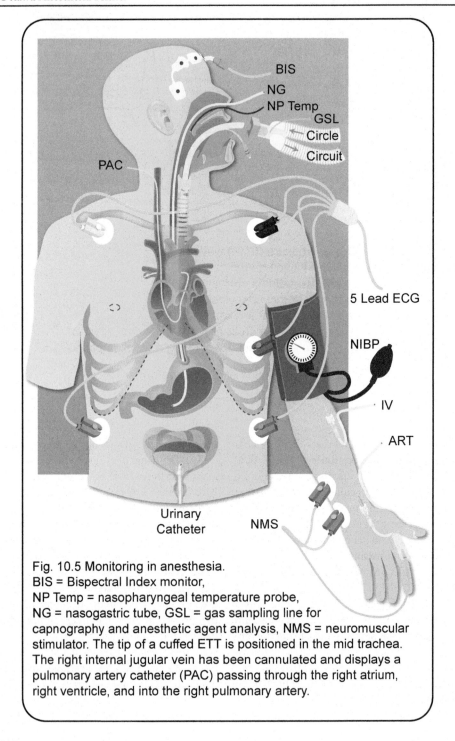

Fig. 10.5 Monitoring in anesthesia.
BIS = Bispectral Index monitor,
NP Temp = nasopharyngeal temperature probe,
NG = nasogastric tube, GSL = gas sampling line for
capnography and anesthetic agent analysis, NMS = neuromuscular
stimulator. The tip of a cuffed ETT is positioned in the mid trachea.
The right internal jugular vein has been cannulated and displays a
pulmonary artery catheter (PAC) passing through the right atrium,
right ventricle, and into the right pulmonary artery.

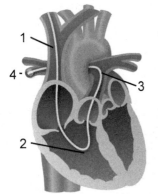
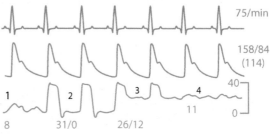

Fig. 10.6 Invasive pressure measurements. The blue waveform represents measurements obtained from a pulmonary artery catheter (PAC) as it passes through the superior vena cava (1), right ventricle (2) and pulmonary artery (3). A pulmonary capillary "wedge" pressure (PCWP) is obtained by measuring the pressure distal to the cuffed balloon at the tip of the PAC (4).

arterial pulse contour analysis have been used to guide fluid, vasopressor, and inotropic therapy to optimize hemodynamics. This technology has been shown to reduce perioperative morbidity and length of hospital stay in patients undergoing major surgery.

The PAC is one of the most invasive monitors used in the perioperative period. Despite its benefits, complications associated with the use of a PAC (e.g., central line infection, arrhythmia, pulmonary artery rupture) have limited its widespread use in the perioperative period. New completely noninvasive monitors using bioreactance technology (see Fig. 10.7) are now available. They can provide detailed cardiac performance information (equivalent to that obtained by a PAC) with continuous cardiac output monitoring capability.[4] These measurements can be obtained rapidly in the preoperative, intraoperative, or postoperative period in the awake spontaneously breathing patient or in the asleep ventilated patient. In the near future, minimally invasive and noninvasive technology will likely relegate the use of PACs to selected major cardiovascular procedures.

A comprehensive discussion of echocardiography is beyond the scope of this primer. An overview of the role of echocardiography in the perioperative period and in the acute trauma patient is provided as a URL link in the additional resources section.

## IV. ANESTHETIC DEPTH
### How do we know if we are giving too much or not enough depth of anesthetic?

Patients undergoing surgery with local or regional anesthesia are able to provide verbal feedback regarding their well-being. When we induce a state of general anesthesia, the onset of anesthesia is signalled by the lack of response to verbal commands and the loss of a "blink" reflex when the eyelash is lightly touched. Inadequate anesthesia may be signalled by facial grimacing to a painful stimulus or by movement of an arm or leg. In the case of full paralysis with muscle relaxants, inadequate anesthesia is suggested by hypertension, tachycardia, tearing, or sweating. Excessive anesthetic depth may be signalled by cardiac depression manifesting as bradycardia and hypotension. In the patient who has not

## Table 10.1 Normal Values for a Healthy Adult

| | Abbreviation | | |
|---|---|---|---|
| Systolic blood pressure | SBP | 90 - 160 | mm Hg |
| Diastolic blood pressure | DBP | 50 - 90 | mm Hg |
| Heart rate | HR | 50 – 100 | beats·min$^{-1}$ |
| Respiratory rate | RR | 8 – 20 | breaths·min$^{-1}$ |
| Oxygen saturation by pulse oximetry | SpO$_2$ | 95 – 100 | % |
| End tidal carbon dioxide tension | ETCO$_2$ | 33 – 45 | mm Hg |
| Skin appearance | | Warm, dry | |
| Color | | Pink | |
| Temperature | Temp | 36.5 – 37.5 | °C |
| Urine production | UO | > 0.5 | mL·kg$^{-1}$·min$^{-1}$ |
| Central venous pressure | CVP | 1 - 10 | mm Hg |
| Pulmonary artery pressure | PA (mean) | 10 – 20 | mm Hg |
| Pulmonary capillary wedge pressure | PCWP | 5 – 15 | mm Hg |
| Mixed venous oxygen saturation | SvO2 | 75 | % |
| Cardiac output | CO | 4.5 – 6 | L·min$^{-1}$ |

been given muscle relaxants and is breathing spontaneously, excessive anesthetic depth may result in hypoventilation with hypercapnia (increasing $PaCO_2$) and hypoxemia.

Judging the depth of anesthesia is an inexact science. Intraoperative awareness under general anesthesia is an undesired serious complication with potential long-term psychological consequences. The estimated incidence is 2 per 1,000 patients. Specific patients identified to be at risk include trauma patients, cardiac surgical patients, patients receiving total intravenous general anesthesia (TIVA), and women requiring Cesarean delivery under general anesthesia. Hence, it is important to understand the principles of assessment of anesthetic depth to avoid under or overdosing anesthetic medications.

The assessment of anesthetic depth is based on close clinical observations,

## Table 10.2 Derived Cardiopulmonary Values

| | |
|---|---|
| Body surface area (BSA) | Average = 1.9 m² (male), 1.6 m² (female) |
| Mean arterial pressure (MAP) <br> MAP = DBP + 1/3(SBP − DBP) | 80 − 120 mm Hg |
| Cardiac index (CI) = CO/BSA | 2.5 − 4.0 L·min⁻¹·m⁻² |
| Systemic vascular resistance (SVR) | 1,200 − 1,500 dynes·sec⁻¹·cm⁻⁵ |
| Pulmonary vascular resistance (PVR) <br> PVR = 80 x [(PAP [mean] − PCWP) /CO] | 100 − 300 dynes·sec⁻¹·cm⁻⁵ |
| Stroke Volume (SV) = CO/HR x 1,000 | 60 − 90 mL·beat⁻¹ |
| Alveolar oxygen tension ($P_AO_2$) <br> $P_AO_2 = ([P_B - PH_2O] \times FiO_2) - (PaCO_2/RQ)$ | 110 mm Hg ($F_iO_2 = 0.21$) (where $P_B = 760$ mm Hg, $P_{H2O} = 47$ mm Hg, RQ = 0.8) |
| Alveolar-arterial oxygen gradient (A-aO₂) <br> $A\text{-}aO_2 = P_AO_2 - PaO_2$ | A−aO₂ gradient < 10 mm Hg ($F_iO_2 = 0.21$) |
| Arterial oxygen content (CaO₂) <br> $CaO_2 = (SaO_2 \times Hb \times 1.36) + (PaO_2 \times 0.0031)$ | 21 mL·100mL⁻¹ |

CO = cardiac output; DBP = diastolic blood pressure; $F_iO_2$ = fraction of inspired oxygen; HR = heart rate; $PaCO_2$ = partial pressure of carbon dioxide; PAP = pulmonary artery pressure; $P_B$ = barometric pressure, PCWP = pulmonary capillary wedge pressure; $PH_2O$ = water vapor pressure; RQ = respiratory quotient; SBP = systolic blood pressure.

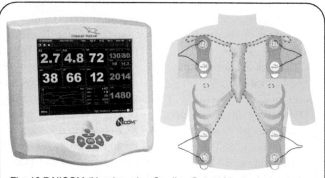

Fig. 10.7 NICOM (Non-Invasive Cardiac Output Monitoring) using bioreactance. Indices of cardiac performance and fluid responsiveness are obtained completely non-invasively and can be obtained in both the awake and anesthetized patient. Image courtesy of Cheetah Medical Inc.

physiological data (HR, RR, and BP), knowledge of the pharmacology of the anesthetic drugs, and information from special monitors (discussed below). In patients receiving general anesthesia with a volatile anesthetic gas, we are able to monitor the amount of the anesthetic gas in their breath. The anesthetic gas concentration in the patient's breath provides one more clue as to the patient's depth of anesthesia. Each anesthetic gas has a specific "minimal alveolar concentration" (MAC) value that can be related to the anesthetic depth (see Chapter 13 Inhalational Anesthesia). The MAC value can be displayed in real time on modern anesthetic monitors and provides information concerning the contribution of the volatile anesthetic gas to the depth of anesthesia. The displayed MAC value must be taken into context with other information, as it does not include the effect of other intravenous anesthetic drugs that have been administered and may underestimate the true anesthetic depth.

The bispectral Index (BIS™) monitor has been available for clinical use since 1994. It is the most common clinical monitor used to gauge the depth of anesthesia. An electrode strip attached to the patient's forehead is used to analyze the electroencephalogram (EEG) signal. A complex algorithm processes the EEG signal and provides the clinician with a single number as a measure of anesthetic depth. The value reported ranges from 0 = a silent EEG to 100 = fully awake. The manufacturer (Aspect Medical) recommends a value of 40 – 60 as an appropriate level for general anesthesia. It was hoped that this technology would provide a guide for anesthesiologists to avoid both awareness under anesthesia as well as excessive anesthetic depth. Recent studies have suggested that BIS may not reliably prevent awareness and that monitoring end tidal anesthetic gas concentrations may be equally as effective.

## V. END-TIDAL $CO_2$ MONITORING
### What is ETCO2 monitoring all about?

Capnometry is the measurement of the carbon dioxide ($CO_2$) concentration during inspiration and expiration.

A capnogram refers to the continuous display of the $CO_2$ concentration waveform sampled from the patient's airway during ventilation.

Capnography is the continuous monitoring of a patient's capnogram.

End-tidal $CO_2$ monitoring became a standard for all patients undergoing general anesthesia around 1990. Prior to this, an ETT that was incorrectly positioned in the esophagus could go unrecognized until the patient became severely hypoxic and critically ill. End-tidal $CO_2$ monitors allow for immediate detection of an esophageal intubation. It is an important safety monitor and a valuable monitor of the patient's physiologic status. Examples of some of the useful information that capnography is able to provide include:

1. Confirmation of tracheal intubation
2. Recognition of an inadvertent esophageal intubation
3. Recognition of an inadvertent extubation or disconnection
4. Assessment of the adequacy of ventilation and an indirect estimate of $PaCO_2$
5. Assistance in the diagnosis of a pulmonary embolism (e.g., air or clot)
6. Assistance in the recognition of a partial airway obstruction (e.g., kinked ETT)
7. Indirect measurement of airway reactivity (e.g., bronchospasm)
8. Assessment of the effect of cardiopulmonary resuscitation efforts.

Measurement of $ETCO_2$ involves sampling the patient's respiratory gases near the patient's airway. A value is produced using an infrared gas analysis, mass spectrometry, or a Raman scattering technique. Provided the inspired $CO_2$ value is near zero (no rebreathing

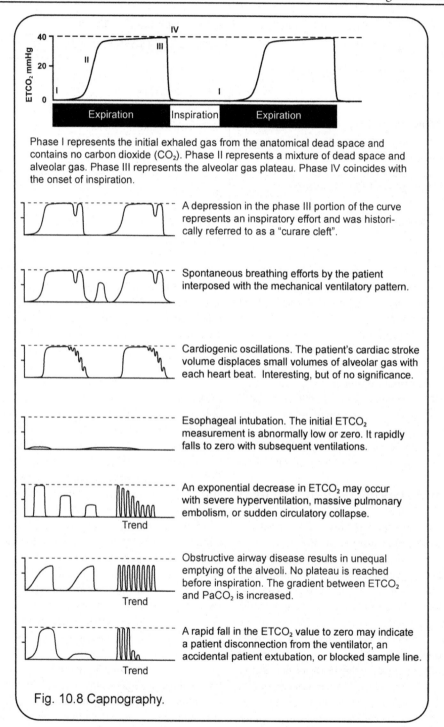

Phase I represents the initial exhaled gas from the anatomical dead space and contains no carbon dioxide ($CO_2$). Phase II represents a mixture of dead space and alveolar gas. Phase III represents the alveolar gas plateau. Phase IV coincides with the onset of inspiration.

A depression in the phase III portion of the curve represents an inspiratory effort and was historically referred to as a "curare cleft".

Spontaneous breathing efforts by the patient interposed with the mechanical ventilatory pattern.

Cardiogenic oscillations. The patient's cardiac stroke volume displaces small volumes of alveolar gas with each heart beat. Interesting, but of no significance.

Esophageal intubation. The initial $ETCO_2$ measurement is abnormally low or zero. It rapidly falls to zero with subsequent ventilations.

An exponential decrease in $ETCO_2$ may occur with severe hyperventilation, massive pulmonary embolism, or sudden circulatory collapse.

Obstructive airway disease results in unequal emptying of the alveoli. No plateau is reached before inspiration. The gradient between $ETCO_2$ and $PaCO_2$ is increased.

A rapid fall in the $ETCO_2$ value to zero may indicate a patient disconnection from the ventilator, an accidental patient extubation, or blocked sample line.

Fig. 10.8 Capnography.

## Table 10.3. Causes of Increased or Decreased ETCO2 values

| Increased ETCO$_2$ | Decreased ETCO$_2$ |
|---|---|
| **Changes in CO$_2$ Production** | |
| Hyperthermia<br>Sepsis<br>Muscular activity<br>Thyroid storm<br>Malignant hyperthermia | Hypothermia<br>Hypometabolism<br>Hypothyroidism |
| **Changes in CO$_2$ Elimination** | |
| Hypoventilation<br>Rebreathing | Hyperventilation<br>Hypoperfusion<br>Embolism |

of $CO_2$), the $ETCO_2$ value is a function of the $CO_2$ production, alveolar ventilation, and pulmonary circulation.

During general anesthesia, the $PaCO_2$ to $ETCO_2$ gradient is typically about 5 mmHg. In the absence of significant ventilation perfusion abnormalities and gas sampling errors, an $ETCO_2$ value of 35 mmHg will correspond to a $PaCO_2$ value of approximately 40 mmHg. Increases or decreases in $ETCO_2$ values may be the result of either increased $CO_2$ production or decreased $CO_2$ elimination (see Table 10.3)

## VI. MONITORING NEUROMUSCULAR FUNCTION

### How do we know whether or not a patient is paralyzed by our medications?

In order to quantify the depth of neuromuscular blockade, electromyography is commonly employed during anesthesia. This involves the application of two electrodes over an easily accessed peripheral nerve. The ulnar nerve is the most common nerve used for monitoring neuromuscular function during general anesthesia. Other nerves that may be used include the facial nerve and the common peroneal nerve. The electrodes are attached to a nerve stimulator which applies an electrical impulse to the nerve. By attaching a strain gauge to the muscle being stimulated, the muscle response to stimulation may be observed or measured. Ulnar nerve stimulation results in the contraction of the abductor pollicis muscle and a twitch in the thumb. Up to 70% of the neuromuscular receptors may be blocked by a neuromuscular blocking drug before a change in the twitch height can be observed. When 90% of the receptors are blocked, all observable twitches are eliminated.

Common methods of nerve stimulation include a single twitch stimulus, four twitch stimuli (each separated by half a second) referred to as a train-of-four (TOF) stimulus, or a continuous stimulus referred to as tetanus stimulation. The intensity of neuromuscular blockade and type of blockade (i.e., depolarizing *vs* nondepolarizing blockade) can be characterized by the response to these different types of stimuli. Clinical relaxation will occur when a single twitch or first twitch of a TOF stimulus is reduced by 75 - 95% of its original height (see Fig. 10.9).

A pure depolarizing block produces a uniform reduction in the height of a single twitch, TOF stimulus, and tetanus stimulation. If excessive amounts of succinylcholine are given (>

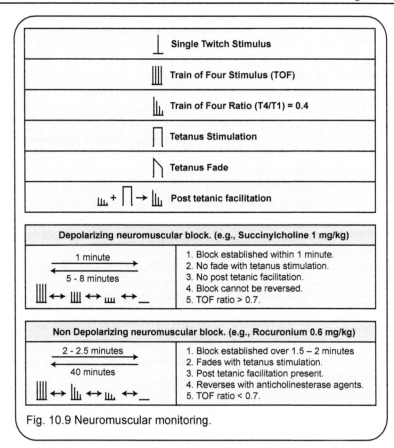

Fig. 10.9 Neuromuscular monitoring.

5-6 mg·kg⁻¹), the block may begin to resemble a nondepolarizing block and is said to be a phase II block (see succinylcholine). Tetanus stimulation of a nerve will show a continued weak contraction in the presence of a depolarizing block, but it will progressively fade with a nondepolarizing block.

In the case of a nondepolarizing blockade, there is an increasing reduction in each of the four TOF twitches. The height ratio of the fourth to first twitch (i.e., the TOF ratio) is < 0.7 in a nondepolarizing block. Also, both the single twitch and the TOF stimulus will be increased following tetanus stimulation. This is referred to as post-tetanic facilitation and occurs only with a nondepolarizing block.

The intensity of nondepolarizing neuromuscular blockade can be estimated by the height and number of twitches that are present following a TOF stimulus. When the first twitch is reduced in height by 75%, the fourth twitch disappears. With an 80% reduction in height of the first twitch, both the third and fourth twitches are lost, and with a 90% reduction in the first twitch, the remaining three twitches disappear.

When all twitches disappear, 90% of all receptors are occupied. For procedures requiring muscle relaxation, attempts are made to maintain one twitch present with a TOF stimulus. Reversal of a neuromuscular block will be easily accomplished if all four twitches of the TOF are present and will be difficult or impossible if one or no twitches are observed.

Recovery from a nondepolarizing neuromuscular blocking drug can occur spontaneously if given enough time, or it can be expedited using an anticholinesterase inhibitor (see Chapter 12 Muscle Relaxants). When the TOF ratio recovers to ≥ 90%, the patient is deemed to have recovered from the relaxant. When the TOF ratio is ≤ 70%, the patient may be at increased risk from the effects of the residual neuromuscular drug, and this may manifest itself in the recovery period with a low oxygen saturation, atelectasis, agitation, or overt muscular weakness.

## VII.    URINE OUTPUT MONITORING

Normal physiology results in a urine production from $0.5 - 1$ mL·kg$^{-1}$·hr$^{-1}$. In the perioperative setting, a cascade of endocrine responses to the stress of surgery as well as the response to anesthetic drugs results in a dramatic reduction in urine output. Aldosterone, antidiuretic hormone, renin-angiotensin II, and atrial natriuretic peptide all increase in response to surgery, resulting in the retention of salt and water. Without a fluid load, urine output is negligible under general anesthesia. As a result, health care providers frequently administer additional fluids to maintain a higher urine output due to a fear of renal failure with a low urine output. Providing hypovolemia is not present, there is no evidence supporting an association between a low urine output in the perioperative period and the development of renal failure. If a patient has a urinary catheter in place with no urine output, then an evaluation should be conducted to assess the patient's volume status and to rule out mechanical problems with the Foley catheter. There is no evidence to support the practice of using the hourly urine production as a guide to manage intravenous fluids in the perioperative period.

Is there any downside to giving additional fluids to protect against renal insufficiency? Holte et. al[6] have provided an excellent review of the consequences of giving too much fluid in the perioperative period. We now recognize that giving too little or too much fluid in the perioperative period can be associated with significant morbidity and mortality. The concept of "goal-directed fluid management" is now promoted as a logical approach to perioperative fluid management. For a further discussion on this topic please refer to the additional resources URL link for optimizing perioperative fluid therapy.

**References:**
1. Marik, P.E., Baram M, Bobbak V. Does central venous pressure predict fluid responsiveness? A systematic review of the literature and the tale of seven mares. Chest 2008; 134:172-178.
2. Gurgel ST, do Nascimento P. Maintaining tissue perfusion in high-risk surgical patients: A systematic review of randomized controlled clinical trials. Anesth Analg 2011; 112:1384-1391.
3. Hamilton MA, Cecconi M, Rhodes A. A systematic review and meta-analysis on the use of preemptive hemodynamic intervention to improve postoperative outcomes in moderate and high-risk surgical patients. Anesth Analg 2011;112:1392-1402.
4. Squara P, Denjeau D, Estagnasie P et al. Non invasive cardiac output monitoring (NICOM): a clinical validation. Int Care Med 2007; 33:1191-1194.
5. Ng A, Swanevelder J. Editorial. Perioperative echocardiography for non-cardiac surgery: what is its role in routine haemodynamic monitoring? BJA 2009;102:731-734.
6. Holte K, Sharrock N.E., Kehlet H. Pathophysiology and clinical implications of perioperative fluid excess. Brit J Anaesth 2002; 89: 622-32.
7. Modified from Gilber HC, Vendor JS. Monitoring the Anesthetized Patient. In Clinical Anesthesia 2$^{nd}$ edition, 1993. JB Lippincott Co. Philadelphia.

# CHAPTER 11

# General Intravenous Anesthetic Agents

Sarika Mann MD, M. Dylan Bould MB ChB

## Learning Objectives

1. To gain an appreciation of the advantages and disadvantages of intravenous (IV) anesthetic medications.
2. To acquire an appreciation of the pharmacokinetic and pharmacodynamic properties of intravenous anesthetic medications.
3. To gain an appreciation of the levels of sedation used for operative procedures and in critical care units.

## Key Points

| | |
|---|---|
| 1 | Intravenous anesthetic medications can be used for short or long-term sedation or to induce and maintain general anesthesia. |
| 2 | The onset of action of IV anesthetic agents is determined by the "arm-brain" circulation time. Termination of action of most IV anesthetic agents is through redistribution rather than through metabolism. |
| 3 | Propofol is the most commonly used IV anesthetic agent to induce general anesthesia. It has a rapid onset and offset and is associated with a dose-dependent decrease in blood pressure and respiration. Using a controlled infusion, propofol can be titrated to achieve light, moderate, or deep levels of sedation. |
| 4 | Ketamine has unique "dissociative" properties, which can result in unpleasant hallucinations and "emergence delirium". It has a longer duration of action compared with propofol. Ketamine has unique analgesic properties and supports cardiac and respiratory function. |
| 5 | Etomidate is useful for its rapid onset and offset, and it has minimal effect on cardiorespiratory function. It is more costly compared with propofol or ketamine and can suppress adrenal function for up to 72 hr following a single induction dose. |
| 6 | Flumazenil and naloxone can be given to antagonize the effect of a benzodiazepine and opioid, respectively. |

| 7 | Dexmedetomidine is a new (and more costly) IV sedative that can be infused for sedation, hypnosis, and analgesia with minimal respiratory depressant effects. It can be used for short-term sedation in the intensive care unit (ICU) and in the perioperative setting. Heart block and asystole have been associated with its use. |
|---|---|

Intravenous anesthetic medications can be used for short or long-term sedation or to induce and maintain general anesthesia. Induction refers to producing a state of unconsciousness, whereas maintenance refers to prolonging the anesthesia state for an indefinite period. Induction of anesthesia is commonly achieved with intravenous medications, whereas maintenance of the anesthesia state is commonly achieved with a combination of intravenous medications and inhaled anesthetic vapors (e.g., sevoflurane, desflurane, nitrous oxide; see Chapter 13). When maintenance is accomplished entirely by intravenous agents (without inhaled anesthetic gases), the technique is termed total intravenous anesthesia (TIVA).

The goals of anesthesia may include lack of awareness, amnesia, analgesia, areflexia, anxiolysis, and autonomic stability. In addition to IV anesthetic medications and inhaled anesthetic gases, additional medications, such as opioids, neuromuscular blocking agents, anxiolytics, and vasoactive medications, may be used to achieve the anesthetic goals. Opioids and anxiolytics act synergistically with IV anesthetic agents such that a reduction in the dose of these medications may be required to avoid a relative anesthetic overdose.

This chapter will present:

I. Basic pharmacological principles of intravenous anesthetic medications.

II. A discussion of commonly used intravenous induction medications, highlighting typical dose ranges, indications, pharmacokinetics, pharmacodynamics, and contraindications.

III. A discussion of the levels of sedation, ranging from light sedation to general anesthesia.

## I. Basic Pharmacological Principles

**Pharmacokinetics** refers to "what the body does to the drug" and involves absorption, uptake, distribution, metabolism, and excretion. The pharmacokinetics of most IV anesthetic medications are relatively similar (discussed below), though there are individual variations, (discussed in their relevant sections).

Intravenous administration of anesthetics results in predictable plasma concentrations. Administration of these medications will render a patient unconscious in a predictable period of time, commonly referred to as the *"arm-brain"* circulation time. The arm-brain circulation time refers to the time it takes for the drug to pass from the site of injection (typically the arm) through the right heart and pulmonary circulation to the left heart and the brain. The patient regains consciousness after several minutes, not because the drug has been metabolized, but because the drug concentration in the brain falls below a critical value as the drug is redistributed to the more slowly perfused organs.

The brain, liver, kidneys, and adrenal glands comprise the vessel-rich organs. They receive 75% of the cardiac output even though they constitute only 10% of the body mass. After an anesthetic agent reaches its peak serum level within the vessel-rich organs, it is then redistributed to other organs receiving less blood flow (e.g., muscles, fat, bone). The

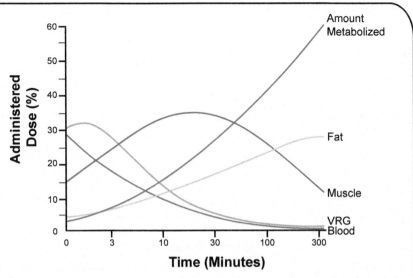

Fig. 11.1 Schematic representation typical of propofol and thio-pental intravenous drug distribution over time. Drug concentration peaks early in organs with high blood flow (i.e., vessel-rich group (VRG) of organs such as the brain and liver) with subsequent redistribution to other organs.

muscle group receives < 20% of the cardiac output, yet it comprises approximately 50% of the body mass. While peak serum concentrations of the drug are reached within seconds of injection, the fat group and vessel-poor groups may require hours before peak levels are achieved.

Metabolism occurs primarily in the liver by enzymatic reactions. The remaining drug and metabolites are excreted primarily in the urine.

Table 11.1 Organ groups relative to blood flow and body mass

| Tissue Group | Composition | Cardiac Output (%) | Body Mass (%) |
|---|---|---|---|
| Vessel-rich | Brain, heart, liver, kidney, GI tract, endocrine glands | 75 | 10 |
| Muscle | Muscle, skin | 19 | 50 |
| Fat | Fat | 6 | 20 |
| Vessel-poor | Bone, ligament, cartilage | 0 | 20 |

GI = gastrointestinal.

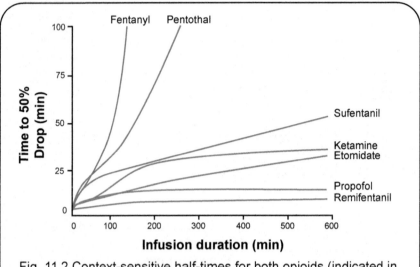

Fig. 11.2 Context-sensitive half-times for both opioids (indicated in blue) and intravenous anesthetic agents (red) as a function of their infusion duration.

The context-sensitive half-time is an important concept to understand when using intravenous sedation or a TIVA technique. This concept describes the time required for a drug's plasma concentration to decrease to a certain level following cessation of a continuous IV infusion. The context-sensitive half-time for a drug depends on its lipid solubility and mechanism of clearance. The longer the context-sensitive half-time, the longer it takes for the plasma concentration to decrease to a level compatible with awakening. Medications with short context-sensitive half-times are ideally administered with a controlled infusion. When medications are administered using a controlled infusion, dose adjustments are easily made and resolution of the medication effect is rapidly achieved when the infusion is discontinued. Combinations of IV anesthetics, medications, and opioids are often infused simultaneously. Selecting medications with similar context-sensitive half-times may be advantageous (see Fig. 11.2).

Pharmacodynamics refers to "what the drug does to the body" in the different organ systems (i.e., cardiovascular, respiratory, and central nervous systems). Pharmacodynamics describe the mechanisms of actions, drug interactions, and structure-activity relationships. These effects are discussed individually for each agent in the following sections.

**Intravenous Anesthetics**

## Table 11.2 Common Intravenous Anesthetics and Sedatives

| GABA Agonists (enhance inhibitory neurotransmission) | | NMDA Receptor Antagonist | Alpha-2 Receptor Agonist |
|---|---|---|---|
| Alkylphenol: | Propofol | Ketamine | Clonidine |
| Barbiturates: | Thiopental | | Dexmedetomidine |
| Benzodiazepines: | Midazolam | | |
| | Diazepam | | |
| | Lorazepam | | |
| Imidazole Derivative: | Etomidate | | |

NMDA = N-Methyl-D-Aspartate.

## II. Intravenous Induction Medications

### Propofol:

Propofol is currently the most commonly used IV agent for induction of anesthesia. Peak concentrations are reached rapidly following a single bolus injection, and speedy recovery ensues from redistribution. Propofol is highly protein bound and is metabolized primarily by conjugation in the liver. Although its role is not completely understood, propofol is believed to exert its primary effects through enhancement of the inhibitory neurotransmission mediated by the GABA receptor complex in the central nervous system.

### Propofol Dose:

| | |
|---|---|
| Induction: | 1 - 2.5 mg·kg$^{-1}$ iv |
| Maintenance: | 20 - 200 μg·kg$^{-1}$·min$^{-1}$ iv infusion |
| T½ re-distribution = | 2 - 8 min |
| T½ elimination = | 4 - 7 hr |

T1/2 = half-life, the period of time it takes for the amount of a substance undergoing decay to decrease by half.

A 2.5 mg·kg$^{-1}$ induction dose is used for healthy non-premedicated adults, and doses reduced to 1.0 - 2.0 mg·kg$^{-1}$ are recommended when patients are premedicated with opioids or benzodiazepines. Propofol should be used cautiously in patients with significant comorbid conditions, elderly patients, or patients with reduced cardiovascular reserve or fixed cardiac output (e.g., aortic or mitral stenosis, pericardial tamponade, hypertrophic cardiomyopathy, or shock states). Children may require higher induction doses (range 1 – 3.5 mg·kg$^{-1}$).

Maintenance of the anesthesia state can be achieved with propofol when a total intravenous anesthetic technique (TIVA) is used. Propofol is commonly combined with an opioid infusion when using a TIVA technique.

### Clinical Pearl:

*Propofol and remifentanil demonstrate potent synergism. When these drugs are used as sedatives for monitored anesthetic care, combining even small doses may result in apnea, chest rigidity, desaturation, and the inability to bag-mask ventilate the patient. Only experienced clinicians with a thorough understanding of these medications and skills in resuscitation and intubation should use these drugs for monitored anesthetic are.*

133

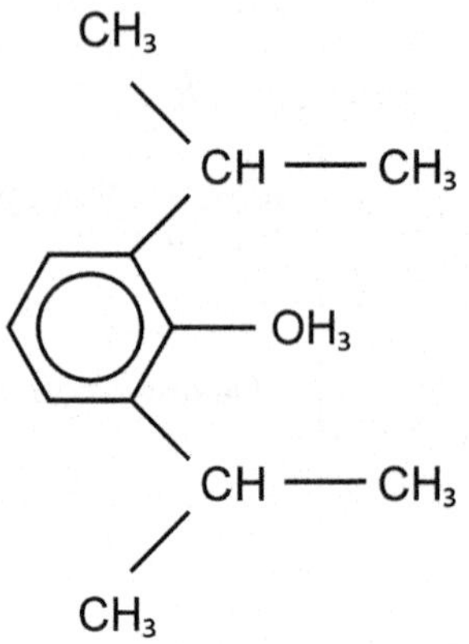

Fig. 11.3 Propofol molecule.

## Pharmacodynamics

### Cardiovascular System:

Compared with other IV anesthetic induction medications, propofol produces the greatest decrease in arterial blood pressure with reductions of up to 25 – 40% in systolic, mean, and diastolic blood pressures with standard induction doses. This decrease is attributed to a drop in systemic vascular resistance from arterial and venous vasodilation as well as a reduction in the stroke volume. The result is a reduction in preload, afterload, and cardiac output. Propofol also inhibits the baroreceptor response, limiting the normal increase in heart rate that occurs with hypotension. The cardiac depressant effect of propofol corresponds with the dose and rate of administration and may be pronounced in patients with limited cardiac reserve or reduced intravascular volume.

### Respiratory System:

Propofol depresses respiratory drive following an induction dose and produces a short period of apnea in approximately 1 in 4 patients. The drug inhibits the hypoxic ventilatory drive to breathe and reduces the normal ventilatory response to hypercapnia. Depression of the upper airway reflexes facilitates tracheal intubation and LMA™ placement even when muscle relaxants are not used. Propofol infusions bring about a decrease in tidal volume and an increase in respiratory rate with minimal change in minute ventilation.

### Central Nervous System:

Propofol decreases cerebral metabolic rate (CMR), cerebral blood flow (CBF), intracranial pressure (ICP), and intraocular pressure (IOP). It exhibits anticonvulsant properties and may be used in the treatment of seizures. Propofol-induced hypotension may result in a critical decrease in cerebral perfusion pressure (< 50mm Hg), especially in the setting of raised ICP. The cerebral perfusion pressure (CPP) can be calculated using the equation below:

CPP = MAP – ICP;

when RAP > ICP; CPP = MAP - RAP

Where: MAP = mean arterial pressure; ICP = intracranial pressure; RAP = right atrial pressure

### Complications

Pain on injection is common (up to 70% of cases) and can be distressing to the patient. Strategies to minimize the pain include the administration of propofol through a large vein, dilution of propofol, application of a tourniquet and administration of lidocaine prior to propofol, and co-administration of lidocaine with propofol (2% lidocaine 40 – 60 mg added to propofol 200 mg).

Propofol is prepared in a lipid emulsion and will support bacterial growth. Fever, chills, sepsis, and death have been linked to contaminated propofol preparations. The current U.S. Food and Drug Administration (FDA) and Center for Disease Control recommend that:

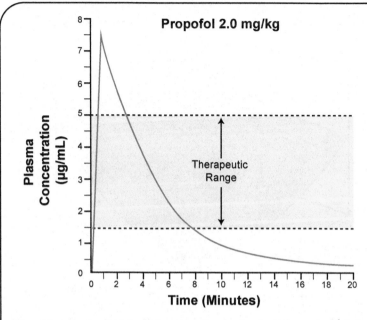

Fig. 11.4 Propofol blood levels after a single 2.0 mg·kg⁻¹ injection. The blood levels required for anesthesia during surgery are 2 - 5 µg·mL⁻¹. Awakening usually occurs at a blood level < 1.5 µg·mL⁻¹. The shape of the titration curve is similar for other IV induction agents.

- both the vial and prefilled syringe formulations must be used on only one patient;
- administration must commence immediately after the vial or syringe has been opened; and
- administration from a single vial or syringe must be completed within 6 hr of opening.

Propofol infusion syndrome (PRIS) is a complex, rare, and potentially fatal complication initially described in children receiving large infusion doses for a prolonged period. Several adult cases have now been reported. Patients typically have a neurologic injury, acute inflammatory illness, or sepsis and are receiving concomitant intravenous steroid and catecholamine support. The cardinal features are refractory bradycardia, cardiac failure, rhabdomyolysis, severe lactic acidosis, and renal failure. Other features include hyperkalemia, hyperlipidemia and hepatomegaly. Treatment is supportive following discontinuation of the infusion.

**Ketamine:**

Ketamine is an important anesthetic agent with unique properties, including analgesia, lack of respiratory depression, and cardiovascular stability. The lack of cardiac depression is believed to be the result of ketamine's sympathetic system activation. It is known as a dissociative anesthetic agent for its ability to cause a "cataleptic-type" state

135

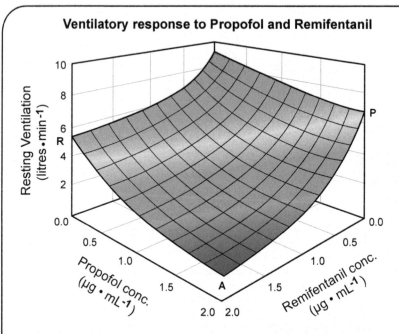

Fig. 11.5 Propofol and remifentanil synergism. Resting ventilation is depressed to a greater extent when propofol and remifentanil are co-administered as an infusion than when either agent is used alone. Significant synergism is noted at relatively low concentrations (typically used in monitored anesthetic care). Respiratory depression is greatest with the combination of remifentanil and propofol (A = apnea) when compared to propofol alone (P) or remifentanil alone (R). Adapted with permission from Dahan A, Teppema LJ. Br J Anaesth 2003;91:40-49.

where a patient may appear semi-awake but is unable to respond appropriately to sensory information. An intravenous induction dose will induce general anesthesia within an arm-brain circulation time.

Ketamine's primary effect is through inhibition of the excitatory NMDA receptor complex. Secondary effects may also occur at other receptors, including the opiate, muscarinic, cholinergic, and serotonergic receptors.

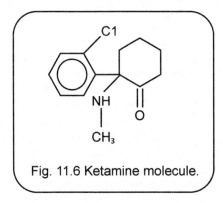

Fig. 11.6 Ketamine molecule.

**Ketamine Dose:**

| | |
|---|---|
| Induction: | 0.5 - 2 mg·kg⁻¹ *iv* or 3 - 5 mg·kg⁻¹ *im* |
| Maintenance: | 2 - 6 mg·kg⁻¹·hr⁻¹ |
| Analgesia: | 0.15 - 0.25 mg·kg⁻¹ *iv* |
| T₁/₂ distribution: | 11 - 16 min |
| T₁/₂ elimination: | 2 - 4 hr |

Ketamine may be administered by intravenous (*iv*) or intramuscular (*im*) injection, by mouth (*po*), or by rectal suspension (*pr*). It is rapidly absorbed and distributed to the vessel-rich organs following *iv* and *im* administration. Larger doses are required when administered by oral or rectal routes as the liver removes a significant amount of the drug before it reaches the systemic circulation (first-pass metabolism).

Ketamine produces a dissociative state that may result in disturbing and unpleasant hallucinations related to both the total dose and rate of administration. The resulting agitation is observed typically in the recovery phase and, as a result, has limited its use in the general population. Intramuscular or oral administration has been used in patients unwilling to tolerate intravenous access. Norketamine, the primary liver metabolite, has approximately one-third the potency of ketamine. The metabolites of ketamine are excreted in the urine.

## Pharmacodynamics

### Cardiovascular System:

Ketamine causes stimulation of the central sympathetic nervous system by inhibition of norepinephrine reuptake. This results in a transient increase in blood pressure, heart rate, cardiac output, sympathetic vascular resistance (SVR), coronary blood flow, and myocardial oxygen demand. Pulmonary vascular resistance is unchanged provided ventilation is controlled. Ketamine has a direct negative inotropic action on the heart when the normal sympathetic nervous system is blocked or exhausted (e.g., patients with a prolonged illness, sepsis, or in states of shock). In this setting, administration of ketamine may result in a decrease in cardiac output and blood pressure.

Ketamine should be used with caution in patients with coronary artery disease, uncontrolled hypertension, congestive heart failure, and arterial aneurysms. The sympathetic effects may be blunted by the co-administration of benzodiazepines, opioids, or inhaled anesthetics.

### Respiratory System:

Ketamine does not result in significant respiratory depression. Functional residual capacity, minute ventilation, tidal volume, and hypoxic pulmonary vasoconstriction are typically preserved. Ketamine maintains the respiratory response to hypercapnia and preserves the laryngeal and pharyngeal airway reflexes. Induction doses of ketamine may result in loss of airway reflexes, and they do not eliminate the risk of gastric aspiration. Transient hypoventilation or apnea may occur with the co-administration of opioids. Mild respiratory depression may occur in healthy patients following induction doses of > 2 mg·kg⁻¹ *iv*.

Ketamine is a known bronchodilator and can be a useful induction agent in patients with asthma or in an asthmatic patient requiring urgent tracheal intubation. Increased secretions occur with ketamine and can be limited with the prior administration of an anticholinergic, such as atropine or glycopyrrolate.

**Central Nervous System:**

Ketamine produces cerebral vasodilation, increasing CMR and CBF. Historically, ketamine was contraindicated in patients with increased ICP. Provided ventilation is controlled and normocapnia is maintained, ketamine may not produce an increase in ICP. Cerebral perfusion pressure is maintained with ketamine due to an increase in MAP.

Psychotomimetic effects, such as unpleasant dreams, hallucinations, or frank delirium may occur with even low doses of ketamine. This problem is particularly prone to develop in elderly patients and when large doses of ketamine are administered rapidly. The incidence of emergence delirium is decreased with the co-administration of a benzodiazepine. Other strategies to limit emergence delirium include slow administration of small doses of ketamine and having the patient recover in a quiet environment.

Ketamine has anticonvulsant properties and may be used in the treatment of seizures. Increased muscle tone with ketamine may cause myoclonic contractions and vocalizations that should not be mistaken for seizure activity.

**Endocrine System:**

Ketamine's sympathetic stimulation may result in an increase in blood glucose and plasma cortisol.

## Additional Properties

**Analgesia:**

Ketamine may be used as an adjunct for pain management in an attempt to reduce opioid use and opioid tolerance. This can be useful in patients who are either opioid intolerant or, alternatively, opioid tolerant and dependent. In this context, small doses of ketamine may improve analgesia without compromising respirations or airway patency. Analgesia can be achieved with small boluses of ketamine (2 – 5 mg) and can be maintained using a low-dose infusion of ketamine in combination with an opioid (see Chapter 17: Acute Pain).

*Clinical Pearl:*

*Heath care providers can safely use low doses of ketamine for procedures requiring sedation and analgesia.*

**Etomidate:**

Etomidate is more expensive and less commonly used as an anesthetic induction agent compared with propofol and ketamine. It produces minimal cardiovascular or respiratory depression and is void of any analgesic properties. Etomidate is associated with profound adrenocortical suppression following a single induction dose and is considered to be contraindicated in patients with sepsis. Etomidate potentiates the inhibitory effects of the GABA receptors in the central nervous system. Like propofol, etomidate commonly causes pain on injection, which can be reduced with the co-administration of lidocaine.

The duration of action is linearly correlated with the dose administered. As a general rule, $0.1$ mg·kg$^{-1}$ of etomidate will provide approximately 1.5 min of unconsciousness. Its action is terminated by redistribution to other tissues. Metabolism is due to both ester hydrolysis and hepatic conjugation forming inactive metabolites that are excreted in the urine and bile.

**Etomidate Dose:**

| | |
|---|---|
| Induction: | 0.2 - 0.6 mg·kg⁻¹ *iv* |
| T$_{1/2}$ distribution: | 2.7 min |
| T$_{1/2}$ elimination: | 2.9 - 5.3 hr |

## Pharmacodynamics

### Cardiovascular System

Etomidate has a minimal effect on the cardiovascular system, which can be advantageous when managing trauma patients or patients with significant cardiovascular disease. It also has a minimal effect on blood pressure, systemic vascular resistance, heart rate, contractility, and cardiac output. Cardiovascular depression may occur when it is administered to patients with hypovolemia.

### Respiratory System

Etomidate may produce apnea following induction, yet the depressant effects on the respiratory system are modest compared with other IV anesthetic medications.

### Central Nervous System

Etomidate decreases CMR, CBF, and ICP due to its cerebral vasoconstrictive effects. Cerebral perfusion pressure is maintained due to the lack of cardiovascular depression. Myoclonic movements can be observed in 30 - 60% of patients and may be seen as seizure-like activity on an electroencephalogram (EEG). Postoperative nausea and vomiting are more common with etomidate than with other IV induction agents.

### Endocrine System

Cortisol is a hormone released from the adrenal gland in response to stress, and it has many beneficial physiological effects. Adrenocortical suppression following etomidate can last 20 – 72 hours after a single induction dose. This is due to a dose-dependent inhibition of 11 β-hydroxylase, which is required for the conversion of cholesterol to cortisol. The suppression of cortisol is more pronounced in trauma or critically ill patients and has been associated with increased morbidity and mortality in these patients.

*Clinical Pearl:*

*Etomidate-induced adrenocortical suppression has made it a controversial intravenous induction agent in patients with sepsis. Several countries currently prohibit its use.*

### Barbiturates:

Thiopental was once the most frequently used IV anesthetic induction drug. Its use has declined with the introduction of propofol and the reduced pricing of generic brands of propofol. Indications for thiopental include rapid induction of anesthesia, treatment of increased ICP, control of convulsive states, and neuroprotection in patients with cerebral ischemia. Barbiturates act by depressing the reticular activating system and by suppressing the transmission of excitatory neurotransmission (e.g., acetylcholine) while enhancing the transmission of inhibitory neurotransmitters (e.g., GABA).

### Thiopental Dose:

| | |
|---|---|
| Thiopental: | 3 – 4 mg·kg⁻¹ *iv* |
| T$_{1/2}$ distribution = | 2 - 4 min |
| T$_{1/2}$ elimination = | 11 hr |

Since the acid dissociation constant (pKa) of thiopental (7.6) is relatively close to physiological pH (7.35 - 7.45), changes in a patient's acid-base balance can dramatically change the non-ionized or physiologically active drug proportion. In the presence of acidosis, the non-ionized fraction of the drug increases, allowing the drug to move readily through cell membranes to the effect sites. The termination of action of barbiturates is due to redistribution from the brain to other tissues and organs.

Metabolism of thiopental occurs primarily in the liver, with < 1% of the initial drug excreted unchanged in the urine.

Thiopental is an alkaline solution that precipitates when mixed with acidic formulations (e.g., neuromuscular blockers), which may cause occlusion of IV lines if administered together. Accidental arterial or subcutaneous injection causes extreme pain and may lead to tissue necrosis.

## Pharmacodynamics

### Cardiovascular

Induction doses of thiopental result in peripheral vasodilation with a decrease in preload, a compensatory increase in heart rate, and a mild reduction in blood pressure. Despite the decrease in preload, cardiac output is generally maintained due to the increased heart rate. Barbiturates cause a dose-related depression of myocardial function that may be pronounced in patients with limited cardiac reserve or hypovolemia. As with the other anesthetic agents, elderly patients require lower induction doses due to slower redistribution and the resulting higher peak plasma concentrations.

### Respiratory

Induction of anesthesia with barbiturates is associated with apnea and a moderate suppression of laryngeal and cough reflexes. There is also a dose-related depression of the ventilatory response to hypercarbia and hypoxia. The functional residual capacity is reduced by 20%, and tidal volume, respiratory rate, and minute ventilation are also reduced. Laryngospasm or bronchospasm may occur with induction of light levels of anesthesia and with airway manipulation.

### Central Nervous System

Barbiturates are cerebral vasoconstrictors that produce a decrease in both CBF and ICP. Cerebral perfusion pressure is maintained as the drop in ICP exceeds the decline in arterial blood pressure. The cerebral metabolic rate (CMR) is also reduced and is associated with a dose-dependent slowing of EEG activity. Barbiturates have anticonvulsant properties and may be used in the treatment of seizures. Barbiturates are also believed to exhibit anti-analgesic effects.

### Hepatic

Barbiturates may precipitate porphyria in susceptible individuals.

### *Clinical Pearl:*

*Thiopental and other intravenous barbiturates have recently been removed from the market and are currently unavailable for use in Canada.*

## III.    Level of Sedation

### Sedation and Monitored Anesthesia Care

Monitored anesthetic care is provided for patients undergoing procedures receiving local anesthesia, sedation, and analgesia. The primary goals are control of pain and anxiety and the provision of safe sedation. Up to 30% of all operative procedures are conducted using monitored anesthetic care delivered by anesthesiologists and other health care personnel (e.g., emergency physicians, radiologists, nurses). A spectrum from light to deep sedation is dependent on several factors, including the level of sedation desired by the patient, surgeon, and anesthesiologist, the patient's underlying medical issues, and the intensity of pain produced by the procedure. Anesthetics are titrated to allow patients to tolerate uncomfortable procedures; they provide anxiolysis and analgesia while ensuring safety. Common procedures requiring monitored anesthetic care include endoscopic procedures (e.g., colonoscopy), radiologic procedures, and surgical procedures for which local or regional anesthetic techniques are used. Various combinations of sedative-hypnotics (propofol, ketamine, or benzodiazepines) and analgesics are used with various delivery systems (e.g., intermittent boluses, infusions, or patient-controlled sedation) to provide effective sedation and monitored anesthetic care.

Delivery of monitored anesthetic care requires appropriate monitoring, a recovery unit, and trained health care personnel skilled at dealing with different levels of sedation. Combinations of medications are frequently used for monitored anesthetic care. Medication synergism and differences in patient sensitivities can make it challenging to achieve anxiolysis and patient comfort while avoiding respiratory depression and airway obstruction. Even experienced anesthesiologists will occasionally find that an unintentional deep level of sedation progresses to that of a general anesthetic (see Fig. 11.7). As such, it is important for the health care provider to have the necessary skills to recognize signs of excessive sedation and to provide the basic airway skills, hemodynamic support, and use of medications (e.g., naloxone and flumazenil). The Ramsay sedation scoring system is commonly used by health care providers as a simple way of quantifying the level of sedation during and after monitored anesthetic care (see Fig. 11.8).

### Sedation in the Intensive Care Unit

Unlike procedural sedation, sedation in a critical care unit is often maintained for longer periods of time and is required for mechanical ventilation rather than for pain. Traditional continuous sedative infusions have been associated with an increase in both the length of stay and period of duration of mechanical ventilation. Newer protocols incorporating daily interruptions in sedation have been shown to reduce length of stay. Ideally, a sedative regimen should control pain, be easily titrated, have a rapid onset and offset, and have minimal accumulation.

Benzodiazepines, midazolam, and lorazepam are safe and effective when used for short-term infusions. A propofol infusion can be easily titrated to achieve the desired level of sedation while also permitting interruptions in sedation for patient assessments and family visits.

### Benzodiazepines

Benzodiazepines are popular co-induction agents that produce amnesia and anxiolysis with minimal depressant effects on the cardiorespiratory systems. Commonly used benzodiazepines include midazolam, diazepam, and lorazepam. The range of elimination half-times for midazolam, lorazepam, and diazepam are 1 - 4 hr, 10 - 20 hr, and 21 - 37 hr, respectively.

**Midazolam Dose:**

Sedation:     $0.01 - 0.1$ mg·kg$^{-1}$ iv
Co-induction:     $0.02 - 0.04$ mg·kg$^{-1}$ iv

Flumazenil (Anexate®) is the only specific benzodiazepine antagonist available. The onset of action is within 1 - 2 min, with a peak effect reached from 6 - 10 min. It is supplied in 5 mL ampules in a $0.1$ mg·mL$^{-1}$ concentration. The recommended dose for adults is $0.2$ mg (200 µg), and this dose can be repeated until an effect is observed. Most benzodiazepines have a longer half-life than flumazenil, hence repeated doses or an infusion of up to 3 mg·hr$^{-1}$, may be required if the effect wears off.

Benzodiazepine antagonist: Flumazenil: $0.6 - 1$ mg iv (duration 20 min)

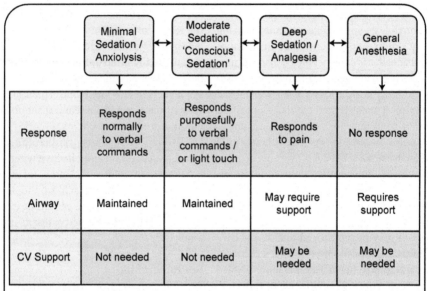

Fig. 11.7 The spectrum of sedation ranging from minimal sedation to general anesthesia can be characterized by the patient's response to verbal and physical stimuli and their requirement for airway and cardiovascular (CV) support. Definition of sedation adapted from the American Society of Anesthesiology and the Joint Commission on Acceditation of Healthcare Organizations.

Benzodiazepines inhibit the actions of glycine, facilitate the actions of the inhibitory neurotransmitter gamma aminobutyric acid (GABA), and have few systemic effects.

## Pharmacodynamics

### Cardiovascular System

Induction doses of benzodiazepines result in only a minimal reduction in blood pressure, cardiac output, and peripheral vascular resistance and result in a slight increase in heart rate.

### Respiratory System

Apnea and severe respiratory depression may occur when given intravenously or co-administered with other respiratory depressants, (particularly opioids).

### Central Nervous System

Strategies to protect the brain at risk of injury include interventions to reduce the cerebral metabolic rate (CMR), cerebral blood flow (CBF) and intracranial pressure (ICP). Benzodiazepines decrease both the CMR and CBF to a lesser extent than the reductions associated with propofol and barbiturates, and they result in little or no change to intracranial pressure. Their sedative and anticonvulsant properties are useful in treating seizure disorders, alcohol withdrawal, and seizures secondary to local anesthetic toxicity.

## Ramsay Sedation Score

1  Anxious, restless or both
2  Cooperative, oriented
3  Responds to commands
4  Brisk response to stimulus
5  Sluggish response to stimulus
6  No response to stimulus

Fig. 11.8 Ramsay Sedation Scale. From Ramsay MA et al. BMJ 1974;2:656-659.

## Clinical uses:

### Premedication:

Benzodiazepines may be used as a premedication for anxiolysis (see Chapter 4). Dose reductions should be considered in patients who are elderly, hypovolemic, or have significant comorbidities. Benzodiazepines may reduce the minimum alveolar concentration (MAC) of volatile anesthetics by up to 30%. Synergism with other induction agents, such as propofol and opioids, is common and may require dose reductions to avoid a relative anesthetic overdose.

### Dexmedetomidine

Dexmedetomidine is a highly selective intravenous alpha-2 agonist. It is useful for short-term sedation (generally < 24 hr) with assisted ventilation or for conscious sedation during short procedures without assisted ventilation. Its main usefulness is its ability to produce dose-dependent sedation and analgesia without respiratory depression.

Dexmedetomidine undergoes conjugation in the liver, and the metabolites are excreted in both the urine and bile. The elimination half-life is short (2 - 3 hr), and the context-sensitive half-time is approximately 4 hr when used as an infusion for > 8 hr.

### Dexmedetomidine Doses:

Bolus: 0.5 - 1.0 $mcg \cdot kg^{-1}$ over 10 min

Infusion: 0.2 - 0.7 $mcg \cdot kg^{-1} \cdot min^{-1}$

## Pharmacodynamics

### Cardiovascular

Dexmedetomidine has a biphasic cardiovascular effect. With an initial bolus dose of dexmedetomidine, transient hypertension and reflex bradycardia may be observed due to peripheral alpha-2 activation. The heart rate generally returns to normal after approximately 15 min and is accompanied by a decrease in blood pressure secondary to a drop in systemic vascular resistance. Severe bradycardia, heart block, and asystole have been reported with dexmedetomidine use. This effect may be reversed with the use of anticholinergics (glycopyrrolate or atropine). Patients receiving a spinal or epidural anesthetic technique with dexmedetomidine may be at an increased risk of bradydysrhythmias due to the loss of sympathetic tone produced by the regional anesthetic technique.

**Respiratory**

Dexmedetomidine results in minimal respiratory depression and may produce bronchodilation. The ventilatory response to hypercapnia is unchanged, and there are no significant changes in tidal volume or respiratory rate. Dexmedetomidine has an antisialagogue effect and has been used successfully for awake fiber-optic bronchoscopy. Its slow onset time (20 min to peak effect), increased cost, and lack of predictable effect may limit its use in this setting.

**Central Nervous System**

Sedation and anxiolysis occur with peak effect achieved within 20 min of starting an infusion. Analgesia is produced through inhibition of ascending nociceptive neurons in the dorsal horn of the spinal cord. The analgesia produced with the infusion reaches a ceiling effect that is inferior to that reached with opioids. Its opioid sparing ability may be particularly beneficial in patients with sleep apnea and those in the bariatric population

**Resources:**

Albanes J, Arnaoud S, Rey M, et al. Ketamine decreases intracranial pressure and electroencephalographic activity in traumatic brain injury patients during propofol sedation. Anesthesiology 1997; 87: 1324–1328.
Himmelsher S, Durieux ME. Ketamine for perioperative pain management. Anesthesiology 2005; 102: 211–220.
Ramaiah R, Bhananker S. Pediatric procedural sedation and analgesia outside the operating room: anticipating, avoiding and managing complications. Expert Rev Neurother 2011; 11: 755–63.
Gerter R, Brown HC, Mitchell DH, et al. Dexmedetomidine: a novel sedative-analgesic agent. Baylor University Medical Center Proceedings 2001; 14: 14-21.
**Reference Texts:**
Miller R.D., et al. Miller's Anesthesia, 7th edition, 2010.
Stoelting R.K., et al. Basics of Anesthesia, 5th edition, 2007.
Morgan G.E., et al. Lange. Clinical Anesthesiology, 4th edition, 2006.

# CHAPTER 12

# Neuromuscular Blocking Agents

Marie-Jo Plamondon MDCM, Michael Curran MD

## Learning Objectives

1. To review the physiology of neuromuscular function.
2. To gain an understanding of the pharmacology of neuromuscular blocking agents (NMBAs).
3. To review the indications and contraindications to NMBAs.

## Key Points

1. Succinylcholine is the only clinically available non-competitive depolarizing NMBA.

2. Succinylcholine can cause a number of unique and potentially serious adverse reactions that are unlike any other muscle relaxant.

3. Muscle relaxants can produce profound skeletal muscle relaxation but have no effect on consciousness.

4. Residual neuromuscular blockade is associated with an increase in postoperative respiratory complications.

5. 90% recovery of the train-of-four (TOF) stimulus is recommended to avoid postoperative respiratory complications from neuromuscular blocking agents.

6. Unlike succinylcholine, the non-depolarizing muscle relaxants can be reversed and may be used in patients with malignant hyperthermia.

Skeletal muscle contraction involves an intricate series of events. As a nerve impulse is generated, an action potential travels down the nerve to the neuromuscular junction (NMJ) (see Fig. 12.1). The action potential results in the release of acetylcholine from the nerve endings into the synaptic cleft. The acetylcholine diffuses across to the muscle's postsynaptic nicotinic receptors causing a change in the membrane's permeability to ions. The altered membrane permeability results in a sodium and potassium flux across the muscle membrane. This flux of ions decreases the muscle's transmembrane electrical potential. When the resting potential decreases from -90 mV to -45 mV, an action potential spreads over the surface of the skeletal muscle resulting in an increase in cytosolic calcium which activates

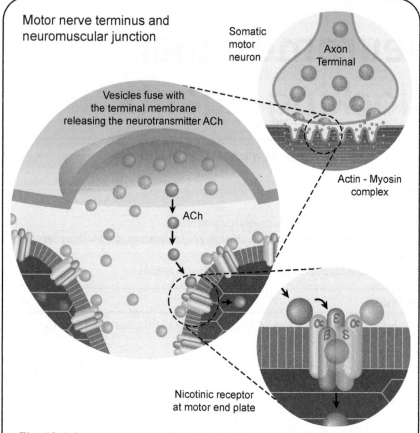

Fig. 12.1 Acetylcholine (ACh) is released from the axon terminal and either crosses the synaptic cleft to bind with post synaptic nicotinic receptors or is hydrolyzed by acetylcholinesterase. ACh binding to the nicotinic receptor results in opening of the sodium channels with muscle membrane depolarization and subsequent muscle contraction.

calcium sensitive contractile proteins resulting in a muscular contraction. Acetylcholine action is rapidly (< 15 milliseconds) terminated as it diffuses away from the muscle's end plate and is hydrolysed by acetylcholinesterase.

The neuromuscular junction (NMJ) consists of:

1. A motor nerve ending with mitochondria and acetylcholine vesicles (prejunctional).

2. A synaptic cleft of 20 - 30 nm in width containing extracellular fluid.

3. A highly folded skeletal muscle membrane (postjunctional).

4. Nicotinic cholinergic receptors located on both the presynaptic (nerve) and postsynaptic (muscle) membranes.

Muscle relaxants produce skeletal muscle paralysis by interfering with acetylcholine at the neuromuscular junction. Fortunately, involuntary muscles, such as the heart, are not affected by neuromuscular blocking drugs. Muscle relaxants have no effect on consciousness or pain threshold.

## Classification:

Muscle relaxants may be classified according to their duration of action (short, intermediate, and long) and on the basis of the type of neuromuscular block they produce. A non-competitive depolarizing muscle relaxant, such as succinylcholine, cannot be antagonized. The termination of succinylcholine's activity is dependent on hydrolysis by plasma cholinesterase (particularly by butyrylcholinesterase). All other currently used muscle relaxants are competitive non-depolarizing muscle relaxants (NDMRs). Their activity does not result in depolarization of the motor end plate or muscle fibre, and their action can be reversed by the administration of an anticholinesterase agent such as neostigmine.

## Choice of muscle relaxant

Considerations for choosing a muscle relaxant include:

1. Duration of action of relaxant and duration of required muscle relaxation.
2. Route of excretion.
3. Tendency to release histamine.
4. Cardiopulmonary side effects resulting from administration.
5. Potential adverse reactions, including bradycardia, tachycardia, bronchospasm, and hypotension.
6. The ability to reverse the neuromuscular block.
7. Cost.
8. Contraindications to any specific muscle relaxant.

9. Potential complications related to partial reversal or incomplete recovery.

Table 12.1 summarizes the duration of action of some commonly used muscle relaxants and the extent to which they depend on renal excretion.

## Non-Depolarizing Muscle Relaxants (NDMRs):

Non-depolarizing neuromuscular blocking drugs compete with acetylcholine for the cholinergic nicotinic receptor. As the concentration of muscle relaxant increases at the NMJ, the intensity of muscle paralysis increases. Anticholinesterase agents inhibit the breakdown of acetylcholine. This results in an increase in the concentration of acetylcholine at the NMJ. Anesthesiologists exploit this pharmacological action by administering acetylcholinesterase agents (e.g., neostigmine) that competitively "reverse" the effects of a non-depolarizing neuromuscular blockade.

In the 1980s, a concerted effort was made to manufacture NDMRs of short, intermediate, or long-acting duration. Examples of these drugs included mivacurium (short-acting), cisatracurium and rocuronium (intermediate-acting), and pancuronium (long-acting). Recent evidence suggests that long-acting agents contribute to postoperative respiratory complications and are now rarely used.[2,3] Intravenous infusion pumps allow precise titration of the neuromuscular block with short and intermediate duration agents.

Mivacurium is a short-acting NDMR that (like succinylcholine) undergoes hydrolysis by plasma cholinesterase. Patients who have deficiencies in the quality or quantity of plasma cholinesterase will have a prolonged duration of action with both mivacurium and succinylcholine. Mivacurium is no longer available in Canada.

Cisatracurium is classified as an intermediate-acting NDMR and is one of several

147

isomers that have been isolated from its predecessor, atracurium. Cisatracurium undergoes hydrolysis in the plasma by a non-enzymatic process referred to as Hoffman elimination and by an ester hydrolysis reaction. Significant histamine release resulting in hypotension, tachycardia, and bronchospasm that may occur after rapid administration of atracurium is not seen with cisatracurium. This lack of histamine release is the main advantage of cisatracurium over its parent compound, atracurium. The dose required to suppress 95% of the single twitch response ($ED_{95}$) of cisatracurium is 0.05 mg·kg$^{-1}$. A stable neuromuscular block can be achieved using an infusion of cisatracurium at a rate of 1 - 5 µg·kg$^{-1}$·min$^{-1}$. Cisatracurium is an ideal agent for patients with renal or hepatic insufficiency requiring muscle relaxation.

Rocuronium is an intermediate-acting NDMR that is popular for short and intermediate procedures. Rocuronium's major advantage is its ability to induce a neuromuscular block, quickly, making it suitable for a rapid induction and intubation sequence. Its administration is associated with little or no histamine release. It has an $ED_{95}$ of approximately 0.3 mg·kg$^{-1}$. The onset time (i.e., time to 90% depression of T1 twitch height) for an intubating dose of rocuronium (i.e., 2 x $ED_{95}$) is 60 - 80 sec. The onset time of rocuronium is comparable with the onset time following 1.5 mg·kg$^{-1}$ of succinylcholine (50 - 70 seconds). Hence, rocuronium matches succinylcholine's onset time and avoids its potential side effects. Nevertheless, it must be remembered that the duration of action of this dose of succinylcholine is only 8 - 12 minutes compared with 35 - 45 minutes for rocuronium. Continuous infusions in the range of 4 - 16 µg·kg$^{-1}$·min$^{-1}$ can be used to maintain a stable neuromuscular block. This should be reduced by 30 - 50% when administered in the presence of an inhaled anesthetic agent such as sevoflurane (similar to all other neuromuscular relaxants).

Rocuronium is the only NDMR that can be reversed with a selective relaxant binding agent (SRBA). Sugammadex® is a modified Y-cyclodextrin that encapsulates and effectively inactivates the rocuronium molecule.[1]

Pancuronium is a long-acting neuromuscular blocking drug. Administration of pancuronium is frequently associated with a modest (< 15%) increase in heart rate, blood pressure, and cardiac output. The increase in heart rate is due to its blockade of the cardiac muscarinic receptors as well as an inhibition of catecholamine re-uptake by sympathetic nerves. Pancuronium administration does not result in histamine release. The $ED_{95}$ of pancuronium is 0.06 mg·kg$^{-1}$. Pancuronium is much more dependent on renal excretion than the other clinically used muscle relaxants. A prolonged neuromuscular block will result when pancuronium is administered to patients with renal failure or insufficiency. Pancuronium may be used when postoperative respiratory support is planned and long duration paralysis is planned. The use of long-acting NDMRs is associated with significant postoperative respiratory complications, including atelectasis and pneumonia.[2,3]

D - Tubocurare: Curare has not been available in Canada since the early 1990s and is now of only historic interest. The muscle paralyzing properties of curare were well known to South American natives who used this drug to immobilize and kill animals with blowgun darts. In 1942, Griffith and Johnson in Montreal introduced the medical world to the paralyzing properties of curare. In the 1980s, curare was most frequently used to attenuate the muscle fasciculations and postoperative myalgia associated with the administration of succinylcholine. A small "pre-treatment" dose of curare was administered approximately 3 minutes prior to the administration of succinylcholine, resulting in its excellent "defasciculating" properties. Today, anesthesiologists may choose to attenuate the muscle fasciculations and postoperative myalgia seen with succinylcholine by administering a small (~ 1/10) "intubating dose" of a non-depolarizing muscle relaxant 3 minutes prior to succinylcholine (e.g., rocuronium 5 mg per 70 kg). "Recurarizaton" is a term that refers to the re-establishment of paralysis due to incomplete reversal or incomplete recovery from a neuromuscular block.

## Depolarizing Muscle Relaxants:

Succinylcholine is the most frequently used muscle relaxant that is administered outside the operating room by non-anesthesiology physicians. Hence, a detailed discussion of its properties is included in this chapter. Succinylcholine (Anectine®) is the only depolarizing non-competitive neuromuscular blocking agent that is clinically used. Depolarizing muscle relaxants bind and depolarize the end plate cholinergic receptors. By contrast, non-depolarizing muscle relaxants competitively block the action of acetylcholine. The initial depolarization can be observed as irregular, generalized fasciculations occurring in the skeletal muscles.

## Physical-Chemical Properties:

Succinylcholine physically resembles two acetylcholine molecules linked end to end. It has two quaternary ammonium cations that interact with the anionic sites on the muscle end plate receptors.

Ninety percent of succinylcholine undergoes hydrolysis by plasma cholinesterase before it reaches the neuromuscular junction. After binding to the end plate muscle receptors and causing skeletal muscle relaxation, it diffuses out of the NMJ. Outside the NMJ, succinylcholine is again exposed to plasma cholinesterase, and the remaining 10% is hydrolyzed. The metabolites of succinylcholine are excreted in the urine. Peak effect is reached within 60 seconds of administration, and the neuromuscular blocking effects of succinylcholine typically dissipate over the next 5 to 10 minutes.

## Phase I and Phase II Blocks:

Succinylcholine produces a prolonged acetylcholine effect. It combines with the acetylcholine receptor to depolarize the end plate, resulting in a generalized depolarization. Depolarization of presynaptic nicotinic receptors also results in asynchronous release of acetylcholine, characterized by asynchronous muscle fasciculation. The postsynaptic membrane remains depolarized and unresponsive until succinylcholine diffuses away from the end plate (due to a concentration gradient). This initial neuromuscular block is referred to as a phase I block. If large amounts of succinylcholine are given (e.g., 4 - 6 mg·kg$^{-1}$), a different neuromuscular block may occur. This block is referred to as a phase II block. Clinically, this may occur when repeated doses of succinylcholine are given or when succinylcholine infusions are used. A phase II block has features that resemble a neuromuscular block that is produced by non-depolarizing muscle relaxants. The actual mechanism of a phase II block is unknown.

### Characteristics of Phase I Blocks:
1. Similar response to a single twitch.
2. No post-tetanic facilitation.
3. Train-of-four (TOF) ratio > 0.7.
4. Muscle fasciculations prior to paralysis.
5. Decreased amplitude but sustained response to tetanic stimulus.
6. The neuromuscular block is increased when cholinesterase inhibitors are administered.

### Characteristics of Phase II Blocks:
1. Decreased response to a single twitch.
2. Post-tetanic facilitation present.
3. Train-of-four (TOF) ratio < 0.7.

4. No fasciculations with onset of paralysis.
5. Response to a tetanus stimulus fades during the stimulus.
6. The neuromuscular block can be reversed with anticholinesterase agents

The presence of a normal amount of active plasma cholinesterase is essential to terminate the effects of succinylcholine. In certain conditions, the levels of plasma cholinesterase may be low, and this is referred to as a quantitative decrease in cholinesterase levels. The consequences of a low plasma cholinesterase level are generally of little significance. In patients with severe liver disease with plasma cholinesterase levels as low as 20% of normal, the duration of a neuromuscular block resulting from the administration of succinylcholine increases threefold (e.g. 5 to 15 minutes). Liver disease, cancer, pregnancy, and certain drugs, such as cyclophosphamide, phenylzine, and monoamine oxidase inhibitors, have all been associated with low cholinesterase levels.

Abnormalities in plasma cholinesterase activity are inherited. Patients may have normal plasma levels of cholinesterase with a severely impaired enzyme activity. This is referred to as a qualitative decrease in plasma cholinesterase. Plasma cholinesterase enzyme activity is genetically determined by four alleles identified as the silent or absent allele (s), the usual allele (u), the dibucaine allele (d), and the fluoride allele (f). The normal plasma cholinesterase genotype is EuEu. Patients with abnormal cholinesterase activity are otherwise healthy and can be identified only by a specific blood test that identifies the genotype and enzyme activity. The sixteen possible genotypes are expressed as ten possible phenotypes. Six of these ten phenotypes are associated with a marked reduction in the hydrolysis of succinylcholine. Patients with the genotype EaEa have a marked reduction in the hydrolysis of succinylcholine. These patients will have a prolonged neuromuscular block that can be increased from ten minutes to several hours following a normal intubating dose of 1 - 2 mg·kg⁻¹ of succinylcholine. The EaEa genotype has a frequency of approximately 1:3200.

The treatment of postoperative paralysis secondary to deficiencies in plasma cholinesterase activity includes controlled ventilation, reassurance, and sedation. Blood samples should be taken to confirm the diagnosis and to identify the enzyme genotype. Immediate family members should be tested to determine their genotypes and susceptibility. Any patient with a significant reduction in their plasma cholinesterase activity should wear a medical alert bracelet.

## Pharmacodynamics:
### Central Nervous System (CNS):

Succinylcholine has no known effect on consciousness, pain threshold, or cerebral function. An increase in intraocular pressure (IOP) begins within 1 minute of administration of succinylcholine. A peak rise in IOP of 6 - 10 mmHg occurs at 2 - 4 minutes and subsides by 6 minutes. Factors that may increase IOP include an increase in central venous pressure; changes in pH, $PaCO_2$, and mean arterial pressure; and a direct effect from the extra ocular muscles. A normal IOP is 10 - 20 mmHg. An increase in IOP under anesthesia is undesirable in patients with an injury that disrupts the globe's integrity. These patients are at risk of vitreous extrusion and damage to the eye if the IOP increases. While succinylcholine increases IOP, crying, straining, or coughing can result in much greater increases of up to 50 mmHg. Increases in intracranial pressure (ICP) of up to 10 mmHg may occur following succinylcholine administration. The mechanism of the increase in ICP is thought to be due to the central mobilization of blood that results from succinylcholine's generalized muscle contractions.

**Respiratory (RESP):**

A progressive paralysis from the eyelids to the jaw, to the limbs, and to the abdominal, intercostal, and diaphragmatic muscles follows the administration of succinylcholine.

**Cardiovascular System (CVS):**

Succinylcholine stimulates both the nicotinic and muscarinic cholinergic autonomic receptors. As a consequence of muscarinic cholinergic stimulation, bradycardia, dysrhythmias, and sinus arrest may be observed. This vagal response is prominent among children and, after repeated doses, in adults. It may be inhibited with anticholinergics such as atropine.

**Gastrointestinal (GI):**

Succinylcholine increases the intra-gastric pressure in proportion to the intensity of the muscle fasciculations in the abdomen. It can be limited with prior use of a non-depolarizing muscle relaxant.

**Genito-Urinary (GU):**

Succinylcholine does not rely on renal excretion. Its metabolites, succinic acid, and choline, however, are excreted by the kidney. Patients with renal failure may have pre-existing hyperkalemia and may be susceptible to succinylcholine-induced hyperkalemia.

The usual serum potassium response following succinylcholine is a transient and brief increase in the extracellular K+ concentration of $\sim$ 0.5 mEq·$L^{-1}$. Generally, patients with K+ concentrations of 5.5 mEq·$L^{-1}$ should not receive succinylcholine, and all but emergency procedures should be delayed. Succinylcholine does not cross the placenta because of its low fat solubility and its ionized state.

**Musculoskeletal (MSK):**

Succinylcholine has no direct effect on the uterus or other smooth muscles. Myalgia following the administration of succinylcholine is infrequent in children, the geriatric population, and pregnant patients. The incidence of succinylcholine myalgia can be decreased with prior administration of a non-depolarizing muscle relaxant such as rocuronium (5 mg/70kg). Fasciculations result in the release of myoglobin into the serum (myoglobinemia). The excretion of myoglobin into the urine (myoglobinuria) is more common in children and can be decreased with prior treatment with non-depolarizing muscle relaxants. Succinylcholine increases the masseter muscle tone in the jaw. Some patients may respond with an abnormally high tone in masseter muscle following succinylcholine. These patients are said to have developed a masseter muscle spasm and may represent a subgroup of patients susceptible to malignant hyperthermia.

**Hyperkalemia Following Succinylcholine:**

A few cholinergic receptors are located along skeletal muscle membranes outside of the NMJ. The receptors are called extrajunctional cholinergic receptors. The number of receptors increases dramatically over a period of 24 hours whenever nerve impulse activity to the muscle is interrupted. Acute disruption of nerve activity to skeletal muscle occurs in patients who have sustained third degree burns or traumatic paralysis (paraplegia, quadriplegia). Administration of succinylcholine to these patients will result in an abnormally high flux of potassium out of the muscle cells because of the increased number of receptors. An acute rise in the serum potassium to levels as high as 13 mEq·$L^{-1}$ following succinylcholine may result in sudden cardiac arrest. Succinylcholine is absolutely contraindicated in these patients. The administration of a non-depolarizing muscle relaxant in these patients does not result in a hyperkalemic response because the receptors are simply blocked and not depolarized.

**Patients at risk of a hyperkalemic response following the administration of succinylcholine include:**

1. Patients with extensive third-degree burns. Succinylcholine should be avoided if the injury is more than 24 hours old, and it should not be given for 6 months following the healing of the burn injury.
2. Patients with nerve damage or neuromuscular diseases, such as muscular dystrophy, are susceptible to hyperkalemia and cardiac standstill with succinylcholine. The degree of hyperkalemia appears to be related to the degree and extent of muscle affected.
3. Severe intra-abdominal infections.
4. Severe closed head injury.
5. Upper motor neuron lesions.

## Specific Diseases:

Myasthenia Gravis: All muscle relaxants are best avoided, if possible, in patients with myasthenia gravis. The fluctuating fatigue and weakness in these patients is due to circulation antibodies to the nicotinic receptors at the neuromuscular junction. They are very sensitive to non-depolarizing muscle relaxants and may be sensitive or resistant to depolarizing muscle relaxants.

Myasthenic Syndrome: The Eaton-Lambert Syndrome is associated with a carcinoma of the bronchus and is due to antibodies directed against the presynaptic calcium channels resulting in fewer acetylcholine molecules being released. Unlike myasthenia gravis, muscle fatigue decreases with exercise, and the eyelids are less affected. These patients are unusually sensitive to both depolarizing and non-depolarizing muscle relaxants.

Myotonia: Patients with myotonia congenita, myotonia dystrophica, and paramyotonia congenita may develop a severe, generalized contracture if given succinylcholine. The use of a depolarizing muscle relaxant, such as succinylcholine, in these patients may result in a secondary generalized contracture of the skeletal muscles and prevent airway maintenance and ventilation.

Familial Periodic Paralysis: Succinylcholine can precipitate a generalized contracture and should be avoided in these patients.

## Dosage & Administration:

Intubating dose:

Succinylcholine has an $ED_{95}$ of approximately 0.3 mg·kg$^{-1}$. Three times the $ED_{95}$ (i.e., 0.9 mg·kg$^{-1}$ or approximately 1 mg·kg$^{-1}$) is commonly administered when rapid control of the airway is required (e.g., full stomach). The larger dose minimizes the risk of an incomplete neuromuscular blockade at 60 seconds. When a small 'pre-treatment' dose of a non-depolarizing NDMR is administered prior to succinylcholine, a larger dose of succinylcholine is recommended. When brief non-urgent neuromuscular block is required, administration of a lower dose of succinylcholine equal to 1 x $ED_{95}$ (0.3 mg·kg$^{-1}$) may be used to achieve this.

### Succinylcholine Dose:

Without rocuronium pre-treatment:
1-1.5 mg.kg$^{-1}$ iv

With rocuronium pre-treatment:
1.5-2 mg'kg$^{-1}$ iv

## Infusion:

An infusion may be used for short procedures to maintain a stable neuromuscular block. Recommended rates for infusion are 50 - 150 $\mu g \cdot kg^{-1} min^{-1}$.

## Indications:
1. Skeletal muscle relaxation during endotracheal intubation.
2. Abdominal operations of short duration.
3. Prior to electroconvulsive therapy (ECT), to prevent the possibility of seizure-induced injury (e.g., vertebral fracture).
4. Emergency treatment for laryngospasm.

## Contraindications:
### Absolute:
1. Inability to maintain an airway.
2. Lack of resuscitative equipment.
3. Known hypersensitivity or allergy.
3. Positive history of Malignant Hyperthermia.
5. Myotonia (M. Congenita, M. Dystrophica, or Paramyotonia Congenita).
6. Patients identified as being at risk of a hyperkalemic response to succinylcholine (see above).

### Relative:
1. Known history of plasma cholinesterase deficiency.
2. Myasthenia Gravis.
3. Myasthenic Syndrome.
4. Familial Periodic Paralysis.
5. Open eye injury.

## Reversal of Neuromuscular Blockade:

Muscle relaxation produced by non-depolarizing neuromuscular agents may be "reversed" by anticholinesterase agents such as neostigmine. These agents prevent the breakdown of acetylcholine in the NMJ. The increased concentration of acetylcholine at the NMJ competes with the muscle relaxant allowing the receptor once again to become responsive to the release of acetylcholine from the nerves.

The increased concentrations of acetylcholine also stimulate the muscarinic cholinergic receptors, resulting in bradycardia, salivation, and increased bowel peristalsis. Anticholinergic agents, such as atropine and glycopyrrolate, are administered prior to reversal to block these unwanted muscarinic effects. Common combinations of anticholinergic and anticholinesterase agents used to reverse a neuromuscular block are atropine 0.01 $mg \cdot kg^{-1}$ with edrophonium (Tensilon®) 0.5 - 1.0 $mg \cdot kg^{-1}$, or glycopyrrolate 0.01 $mg \cdot kg^{-1}$ with neostigmine (Prostigmin®) 0.05 - 0.07 $mg \cdot kg^{-1}$ intravenously. Edrophonium is no longer available in Canada.

## Monitoring Neuromuscular Function and Timing of Reversal:

The intensity (depth) of neuromuscular blockade may be assessed using force transduction, accelerometry, or clinical examination. The most accurate means of assessment is by measuring the muscular response to the electrical stimulation of a peripheral nerve. The most commonly used method of nerve stimulation involves train-of-four stimulus (TOF) wherein four brief electrical stimuli of 2 Hz each are applied over a period of 2 seconds. The train-of-four ratio, (T4/T1), is the ratio of the twitch response of the fourth stimulus (T4) to the first stimulus (T1). In most circumstances, adequate muscle relaxation for surgery occurs when only one of the four twitches is observed. This corresponds to a 90% blockade of the NMJ receptors. Before attempting to antagonize the neuromuscular block, clinicians must consider its intensity and anticipated duration. Reversal may be unsuccessful if only one of the four twitches is present. With inadequate reversal of muscle relaxation, patients will typically have a weak handgrip, will be unable to cough effectively, and will be unable to lift their head from their pillow for a period of 5 seconds. Treatment of inadequate reversal includes supportive ventilation, sedation, analgesia, and adequate time for the neuromuscular block to dissipate.

| Brand Name / (Trade Name) | Block | Duration (minutes) | % Dependent on renal excretion | Time to intubation (2 x ED$_{95}$ twitch suppression) | Intubating dose (mg·kg$^{-1}$) |
|---|---|---|---|---|---|
| Succinylcholine (Anectine®) | NCD | 5 – 10 | 0 | 60 seconds | 1 – 2 |
| Rocuronium (Zemuron®) | NDC | 30 – 45 | 25 | 80 seconds | 0.6 |
| Cisatracurium (Nimbex®) | NDC | 20 – 60 | 0 | 3.3 minutes | 0.1 |
| Pancuronium (Pavulon®) | NDC | 60 - 75 | 60 - 80 | 3 – 8 minutes | 0.06 – 0.1 |

Table 12.1: Properties of neuromuscular blocking agents. NCD (Non competitive depolarizing), NDC (non-depolarizing competitive).

**Test your knowledge:**
1. What is the difference between a depolarizing and a non-depolarizing muscle relaxant? Give examples of each.
2. What are the absolute contraindications for the use of succinylcholine?
3. Which patients are susceptible to hyperkalemia following succinylcholine?
4. What is the dose for intubation?
5. Which drugs can be used to antagonize a neuromuscular block?
6. What specific complications arise with inadequate recovery or reversal of neuromuscular blockade, especially with long-acting agents?

**References:**
1. Sorgenfrei IF, Norrild K, Larsen PB, et al. Reversal of rocuronium-induced neuromuscular block by the selective relaxant binding agent sugammadex. Anesthesiology 2006; 104:667-74.
2. Berg H, B, Viby-Mogensen J, Roed J, et al. Residual neuromuscular block is a risk factor for postoperative pulmonary complications. A prospective, randomized, and blinded study of postoperative pulmonary complications after atracurium, vecuronium and pancuronium. Acta Anaesth Scand 1997; 9:1095-1103.
3. Debaene B, Plaud B, Dilly MP, et al. Residual paralysis in the PACU after a single intubating dose of nondepolarizing muscle relaxant with an intermediate duration of action. Anesthesiology 2003; 98:1042-8.
4. Morgan GE, Mikhail MS, Murray MS Editors. Clinical Anesthesiology, 4th edition McGraw-Hill 2006.
5. Stoelting RK, Hillier SC. Pharmacology and Physiology in Anesthetic Practice, 4th edition. Lippincott Williams & Williams 2006.
6. Miller RD. Miller's Anesthesia 6th Edition, Churchill Livingston Elsevier 2005.
7. Murphy GS, Brull SJ. Residual neuromuscular block: lessons unlearned part 1. Definitions, incidence and adverse physiologic effects of residual neuromuscular block. Anesth Analg 2010; 111:120-128.
8. Murphy GS, Brull SJ. Residual neuromuscular block: lessons unlearned. Part 2: Methods to reduce the risk of residual weakness. Anesth Analg 2010; 111:129-140.

# CHAPTER 13

# Inhalational Anesthetics

Patrick Sullivan MD, Janet Young MD

## Learning Objectives

1. To gain an understanding of the concept of minimum alveolar concentration (MAC).
2. To become familiar with common inhalational anesthetic agents and some of their differences.

## Key Points

1. MAC refers to the minimum alveolar concentration of an inhalational anesthetic medication.

2. The MAC is used to gauge the amount of volatile anesthetic medication to provide anesthesia.

3. The MAC of an inhalational anesthetic agent is significantly reduced with the co-administration of opioid medications (see Chapter 14) and with increasing age.

4. Inhalational anesthetic agents are contraindicated in malignant hyperthermia (see Chapter 25).

5. Sevoflurane is well tolerated as an inhalational induction agent and has a better cardiovascular profile than desflurane or isoflurane.

6. Desflurane provides a rapid onset and offset of anesthesia but can be associated with sympathetic stimulation resulting in an increase in heart rate and blood pressure.

The terms inhalational anesthetic agent, volatile anesthetic, anesthetic gas, or anesthetic vapor are commonly used terms to describe anesthetic medications that are delivered to the lungs in the form of a gas. The anesthetic vapor is delivered from the anesthetic machine and anesthetic circuit to the patient's lungs where it diffuses across the alveolar capillary membrane and is dissolved in the blood. The blood then carries the anesthetic vapor to the brain and other organs in the body.

Intravenous anesthetic agents, such as propofol, are commonly used to induce a state of general anesthesia, and volatile anesthetic agents are the most commonly used drugs for maintenance of anesthesia. They are commonly used as an important component of a "balanced general anesthetic technique" where an inhalational anesthetic agent is co-administered with intravenous anesthetic medications, benzodiazepines, opioids, and muscle relaxants. In anesthesia, medications from different classes of drugs are commonly combined to minimize the side effects of any one agent and to capitalize on each agent's benefits.

Intravenous drugs are typically delivered according to a specific number of milligrams or micrograms. Inhalational agents on the other hand are administered according to a specific concentration. The concentration of a gas is expressed as a percentage of the volume of anesthetic gas to the total volume of the gas mixture. Modern anesthetic vaporizers are able to vaporize liquid inhalational anesthetic agents such that very accurate concentrations can be delivered to the patient by simply setting the vaporizer dial at the desired concentration.

The most commonly used inhalational agents today are sevoflurane, desflurane, isoflurane, and nitrous oxide ($N_2O$). The first three agents are synthetic, colorless liquids that are non-flammable and administered as a vapor from a vaporizer on the anesthesia machine.

There are several theories regarding how volatile anesthetic agents exert their effect on the central nervous system (CNS). The exact mechanism is likely multifactorial. Some of the theories include:

A volume expansion theory[1] or "Mullins critical volume hypothesis". Volatile anesthetics dissolve into lipid cell membranes in the CNS and may distort sodium channels required for synaptic transmission.

Neurotransmitter interference. Volatile anesthetics may act at the presynaptic and postsynaptic receptors inhibiting release, reuptake, or postsynaptic binding and thereby altering synaptic transmission.

Activation of gamma-aminobutyric acid (GABA) receptors and inhibition of calcium channels and or glutamate channels, resulting in inhibition of the release of neurotransmitters in the CNS.

Inhalational agents are compared with one another according to their MAC values. The MAC value of an inhalational agent is the alveolar concentration in oxygen at one atmosphere of pressure that will prevent 50% of the subjects from making a purposeful movement in response to a painful stimulus such as a surgical incision. The MAC value can be considered the effective dose in 50% of the subjects or the $ED_{50}$. Knowledge of the MAC value allows clinicians to compare the potencies of different inhalational agents. The MAC value of nitrous oxide is additive when administered with another inhalational agent, such as sevoflurane, desflurane, or isoflurane.

## Table 13.1 Common Factors Altering Anesthetic Requirements (MAC)

| Increased MAC | Decreased MAC |
|---|---|
| Hyperthermia<br>Chronic drug abuse (e.g., alcohol)<br>Acute use of amphetamines<br>Hyperthyroidism | Increasing age<br>Hypothermia<br>Severe hypotension<br>Opioids<br>Benzodiazepines<br>Acute alcohol use<br>Hypothyroidism |

Without other medications, an anesthetic depth equivalent to 1.2 -1.3 of the MAC value of a volatile anesthetic agent is required for surgical procedures. The added 20 - 30% MAC depth of anesthesia will prevent movement in 95% of patients. Table 13.1 lists factors that increase or decrease the MAC values. Advantages of volatile anesthetics are listed in Table 13.2.

## Table 13.2 Advantages of Inhaled Anesthetic Agents

| Advantages of Volatile Anesthetic Agents |
|---|
| Inexpensive<br>Easily administered<br>Rapidly titrated<br>Minimal metabolism<br>Good safety profile<br>Augment muscle relaxation<br>Able to continuously monitor levels in the body |

The rapidity with which the anesthetic state is reached depends on how quickly the anesthetic inhalational agent reaches the patient's brain to exert its partial pressure effects.

Factors determining how quickly the inhalational agent reaches the alveoli include:

1. The inspired concentration of anesthetic gas being delivered by the anesthetic machine (concentration effect).
2. The gas flow rate through the anesthetic machine.
3. The alveolar ventilation (VA); where VA = respiratory rate x tidal volume.

Increasing any of these factors will result in a faster rise in the alveolar concentration of the inhalational agent.

Factors determining how quickly the inhalational agent reaches the brain from the alveoli in order to establish anesthesia include:

1. The rate of blood flow to the brain.
2. The solubility of the inhalational agent in the brain (Fig. 13.1).
3. The difference in the arterial and venous concentrations of the inhalational agent.

Increasing any of these factors will hasten the onset of anesthesia.

Inhaled anesthetic agents are delivered from the anesthetic machine to the patient's lungs where they are rapidly absorbed into

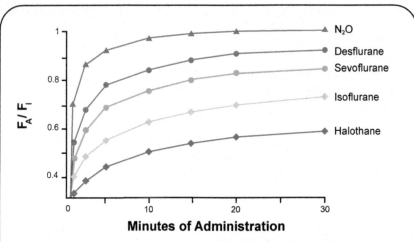

Fig. 13.1 Comparison of inhaled anesthetic solubility. Solubility determines the rate of increase in the alveolar ($F_A$) anesthetic concentration toward the inspired concentration ($F_I$). The least soluble anesthetic vapor (desflurane) shows the most rapid increase; while the most soluble anesthetic (halothane) shows the slowest increase. Adapted from Eger II, Edmond I. New Inhaled Anesthetics Anesthesiology 1994; 80:906-922.

the bloodstream. Once in the bloodstream, the anesthetic agent is delivered in a manner analogous to an intravenous medication, with the majority of medication going to the vessel-rich group of organs (see Chapter 11). The vessel-rich group of organs includes the brain, where the anesthetic gas exerts its desired effect. All modern anesthetic gases have a low molecular weight and are non-ionized, allowing them to move rapidly across neural membranes and to "wash-in" and "wash-out" rapidly from the CNS (see Fig. 13.1). The lungs are the primary site of uptake and elimination of inhaled anesthetic agents.

Patients with low cardiac output states (e.g., shock states) may experience a rapid rise in the alveolar partial pressure of an inhalational anesthetic agent. This will result in a more rapid onset of anesthesia with possible

exaggerated cardiorespiratory depressant effects.

The cascade of anesthetic partial pressure starts at the vaporizer. The gas from the vaporizer is diluted by exhaled gas to form the inspired gas. With a circle system, a fresh gas flow of 4 – 5 L·min[-1] will raise the inspired anesthetic tension (concentration) close to the vaporizer's delivered concentration (Fig. 13.2). As the body continues to take up the inhaled anesthetic gas, the alveolar anesthetic tension will remain below the inspired anesthetic tension for many hours. The brain is considered the final step in the anesthetic cascade. The brain tension will approach the alveolar tension within 8 to 10 minutes of any change. Monitoring the alveolar end-tidal concentration of the inhaled anesthetic agent provides

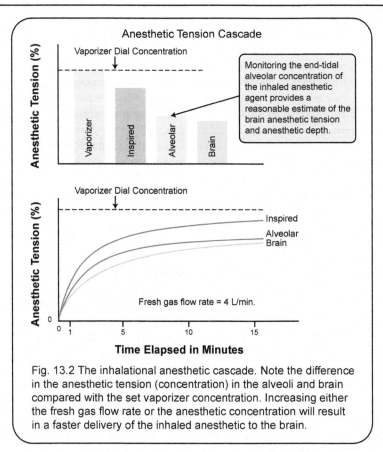

Fig. 13.2 The inhalational anesthetic cascade. Note the difference in the anesthetic tension (concentration) in the alveoli and brain compared with the set vaporizer concentration. Increasing either the fresh gas flow rate or the anesthetic concentration will result in a faster delivery of the inhaled anesthetic to the brain.

a reasonable estimate of the brain anesthetic tension.

**Isoflurane:**

Isoflurane was introduced to North America in the early 1970s and was the most common inhalational agent used for adult anesthesia in North America for many years. Isoflurane has a MAC value of 1.16%, and it has a pungent odor and a tendency to irritate the patient's airway. These irritating effects may cause patients to cough and hold their breath when isoflurane is administered too quickly; hence, it is generally not used to induce anesthesia by inhalation from a facemask. Isoflurane has favorable properties

for neurosurgical procedures as it reduces cerebral metabolic rate and causes minimal change in cerebral blood flow and intracranial pressure. Isoflurane has minimal depressant effects on the myocardium. The reduction in blood pressure produced by isoflurane is accompanied by a similar reduction in vascular resistance such that there is little change in cardiac output. In certain patients (especially young healthy patients), isoflurane may produce a significant sinus tachycardia. In a small percentage of patients with coronary artery disease, isoflurane may cause vasodilatation of the distal endocardial vessels and result in a "coronary steal". A coronary steal is produced when blood is diverted away from the collateral dependent ischemic regions of the heart to the areas of vasodilatation. The significance of this observation is still debated.

Inhalational anesthetics undergo minimal metabolism and are excreted primarily via the lungs. The effects of volatile anesthetics have traditionally been viewed as being limited to the time of exposure. Recent research suggests that these anesthetics act primarily through the γ-Aminobutyric acid type A (GABAA) receptors, and cognitive deficits can persist much longer than would be expected on the basis of their pharmacokinetics. In mice, inhalational anesthetics have been shown to impair recall of recent past memories as well as the ability to create new memories for several days following exposure to inhalational agents.[2]

**Sevoflurane**

Sevoflurane was released for use in North America in 1995. Unlike desflurane and isoflurane, sevoflurane does not have an unpleasant smell and is well tolerated for inhalational induction of anesthesia. With the use of high concentrations of sevoflurane (i.e., inspired concentrations of 5 – 8%), a patient can be taken from an awake state to a sleep state with as little as one or two vital capacity breaths. An anesthetic depth to permit laryngeal mask placement and tracheal intubation can be achieved after three to five minutes of breathing a high concentration of sevoflurane. Sevoflurane produces a dose-related reduction in blood pressure comparable with isoflurane and desflurane. This occurs due to a decrease in systemic vascular resistance without a corresponding decrease in cardiac output. Sevoflurane is a potent bronchodilator and has been used in the treatment of patients with status asthmaticus who are resistant to medical therapy and require controlled ventilation. Sevoflurane, isoflurane, and desflurane all produce uterine relaxation in a dose-dependent manner. This may be exploited to produce uterine relaxation (e.g., retained placenta), but may produce undesired relaxation in other clinical procedures (e.g., dilation and curettage [D&C]). Postoperative nausea and vomiting after sevoflurane is comparable with isoflurane and desflurane but greater than that associated with a total intravenous anesthetic (TIVA) technique using propofol.[3] Sevoflurane degrades to compound A in the presence of a carbon dioxide absorber. Compound A has been associated with nephrotoxicity in rat studies, but it has not been shown to impair renal function in adults with fresh gas flows (FGF) at or below 1 L·min$^{-1}$.

**Desflurane:**

Desflurane has the most rapid onset and offset of anesthetic effect compared with sevoflurane or isoflurane, and it offers the shortest time to emergence and orientation following anesthesia.[4] Desflurane is the most pungent of the inhalational anesthetics and is not suitable for inhalational induction due to its irritating properties. When given rapidly in high concentrations (6% or more), it may result in coughing, breath holding, laryngospasm, tachycardia, and hypertension. A marked activation of the sympathetic nervous system may occur when desflurane concentrations are increased rapidly or high concentrations are used. This is manifest as tachycardia and hypertension (and occasionally myocardial ischemia) and is associated with a surge in plasma norepinephrine, epinephrine, and anti-diuretic (ADH) levels.[5] The hemodynamic response can recur with high concentrations of desflurane or with rapid increases in concentration. Hemodynamic abnormalities typically persist for 4 – 5 minutes, while the endocrine response may persist for 15 – 25 minutes. The response is believed to be secondary to activation of upper and lower airway irritant receptors by desflurane. Desflurane anesthesia is associated with a heart rate that is approximately 10% higher than that of sevoflurane anesthesia.[6]

### Clinical Pearl:

The **"Rule of 24"** states that the risk of an adverse sympathetic surge associated with desflurane is reduced when the product of the carrier gas flow rate (fresh gas flow) multiplied by the inspired concentration of desflurane is less than 24.

**Desflurane rule of 24:** FGF (L·min⁻¹) x inspired concentration < 24

The vapor pressure of desflurane (669 mmHg at 20°C) approaches atmospheric pressure. This means that desflurane essentially boils at room temperature, making it difficult to deliver accurate concentrations of the gas. To overcome this problem, a new electrically powered vaporizer was designed to heat and pressurize desflurane to deliver a consistent and accurate concentration.

Desflurane is associated with a higher incidence of postoperative agitation and excitement in pediatric patients compared with sevoflurane anesthesia.[7] Unlike sevoflurane or isoflurane, desflurane does not produce bronchodilation. Desflurane is essentially inert with only 0.02% undergoing metabolism. Very low fresh gas flow anesthesia can be used as a desflurane cost-saving strategy as well as a means of reducing pollution secondary to waste anesthetic gases. In the presence of dry desiccated $CO_2$ absorbers, desflurane (and to a lesser extent isoflurane and sevoflurane) can degrade to form carbon monoxide (CO).[8] Carboxyhemoglobin (COHb) poisoning has been reported following $CO_2$ absorber desiccation in the presence of desflurane.[9] Newer $CO_2$ absorbers, such as Sodasorb LF®, and Amsorb Plus®, contain calcium hydroxide and are chemically unreactive, eliminating both Compound A production from sevoflurane as well as CO production from inhalational anesthetics.[10]

### Nitrous Oxide:

Nitrous oxide is an inert, inorganic, colorless, tasteless, and odorless gas. It has a rapid onset and a quick recovery of 3 - 10 minutes due to its low solubility in blood. Its low potency (MAC = 104%) limits the amount that can be administered and its usefulness when high concentrations of oxygen are required. Myocardial depression is usually minimal in healthy patients; however, significant cardiovascular depression may occur in patients with coexisting myocardial dysfunction or in patients in a shock state.

Nitrous oxide is 34 times more soluble than nitrogen. This property results in three special anesthetic phenomena. At the beginning of anesthesia, $N_2O$ leaves the alveoli much faster than nitrogen can leave the body tissues to fill the space left by $N_2O$. The result is an increase in the concentration of other gases in the alveoli (oxygen and other inhalational agents). This increase in concentration speeds the onset in inhalational anesthetic effect and is referred to as the second gas effect.

Diffusion hypoxia may result at the end of the anesthetic. As nitrous oxide is discontinued, the body stores of nitrous oxide are released and flood the alveoli, diluting the oxygen present in the alveoli. When only room air is administered at the end of the anesthetic, the dilution of oxygen may be sufficient to create a hypoxic mixture and result in hypoxemia. Other factors contributing to hypoxemia at the end of anesthesia include respiratory depression due to anesthetic agents, residual neuromuscular blockade, and pain with splinted respirations. The administration of 100% oxygen at the end of an anesthetic may avoid hypoxemia resulting from any of these causes.

## Table 13.3 Differences in Common Inhalational Anesthetic Agents

|  | **Desflurane** | **Sevoflurane** | **Isoflurane** | **Nitrous Oxide** |
|---|---|---|---|---|
| Pros | • Rapid onset<br>• Rapid emergence<br>• Rapid titration<br>• Low metabolism | • Sweet smelling, non-irritating<br>• Inhalational induction<br>• No SNS activation<br>• Potent bronchodilator<br>• No change in HR | Slower onset and offset | • Fastest onset and offset<br>• OK for MH |
| Cons | • Pungent<br>• Airway irritation<br>• SNS activation ("Rule of 24")<br>• Increased HR<br>• No bronchodilation | Compound A production | Increased HR | • Incomplete anesthesia<br>• Unfavorable in raised ICP or cerebral ischemia |
| MAC (ET %) | 6.3 | 2.0 | 1.15 | 104 |
| Metabolism | 0.02% | 5% | 0.2% | 0 |
| Contraindications | MH | MH | MH | Closed air spaces |

MAC = minimum alveolar concentration; ET = end-tidal; HR = heart rate; ICP = intracranial pressure; MH = malignant hyperthermia; SNS = sympathetic nervous system.

Finally, closed air spaces will expand in the presence of nitrous oxide due to the differences in the solubility of nitrogen and nitrous oxide. With the administration of 66% $N_2O$, a closed air space will expand twofold in volume over a period of approximately 15 minutes. For this reason, $N_2O$ is contraindicated in patients with a pneumothorax, closed loop bowel obstruction, air embolism, or any other closed air space in the body.

Nitrous oxide undergoes very little metabolism and is excreted unchanged by the lungs. As the recommended minimum concentration of oxygen delivered during general anesthesia is 30%, the maximum concentration of $N_2O$ that can be used is 70% (approximately 0.7 MAC). Hence, nitrous oxide alone is unable to provide adequate anesthesia. When nitrous

oxide is used, opioid analgesics, benzodiazepines, or another inhalational agent may be added to supplement its anesthetic effect.

A dose-related depression of cardiorespiratory function is common with each of these inhalational agents. Sevoflurane, desflurane, and isoflurane are all contraindicated in patients with malignant hyperthermia.

***Clinical Pearl:***

*How do we know if the patient is receiving enough anesthetic?*

*Our general anesthetic goal is to administer enough anesthetic to suppress the patient's awareness and pain response to surgery. Our goal is to provide adequate anesthesia (inhibit* awareness) yet, at the same time, avoid hypotension and a relative anesthetic overdose.

We can use the knowledge that the MAC values of the individual inhalational agents are additive.

Let's assume our patient is under general anesthesia and is receiving end-tidal concentrations of 63% of nitrous oxide and 1% sevoflurane, respectively. We can calculate the relative contributions of these inhalational agents to the patient's anesthetic.

63% nitrous oxide (MAC = 105%)

63/105 = 0.60 MAC

1% sevoflurane (MAC = 2%)

1 / 2 = 0.5 MAC

The combined MAC value of nitrous oxide and sevoflurane is 0.6 + 0.5 = 1.1 MAC

Providing 1.2 - 1.3 times the MAC value is needed to achieve adequate anesthesia in 95% of patients using inhalational agents alone. Opioid administration will decrease volatile MAC levels by 50 – 70% (see Chapter 14). Preoperative or intraoperative benzodiazepines will further reduce the inhalational anesthetic requirements and contribute to the depth of anesthesia. Repeated assessments for inadequate anesthesia or excessive depth of anesthesia are made during the surgery, and corresponding corrective adjustments in the anesthetic depth are made. These are based on the patient's vital signs, tearing, or obvious movement (see Chapter 10; monitoring in anesthesia).

## Resources:

1. Barash PG, Cullen BF, Stoelting RK, editors. Clinical Anesthesia 6th Ed. J.B. Lippincott Co, Philadelphia 2009.
2. Morgan, GE, Mikhail, MS, Murray, MJ. Clinical Anesthesiology 4th Ed. McGraw-Hill Co, New York 2006.
3. Miller RD, editors. Anesthesia 7th Ed. Churchill Lingstone Inc, 2010.

## References:

1. Miller KW, Paton WDM, Smith RA. The pressure reversal of general anesthesia and the critical volume hypothesis. Molecular pharmacology 1973; 9:131-143.
2. Zurek AA, Bridgwater EM, Orser BA. Inhibition of α5 γ-Aminobutyric Acid Type A Receptors Restores Recognition Memory After General Anesthesia. Anesth Analg 2012;114:845-855.
3. Gupta A, Stierer T, Zuckerman R, et al. Comparison of recovery profile after ambulatory anesthesia with propofol, isoflurane, sevoflurane and desflurane: A systematic review. Anesth Analg 2004; 98:632-41.
4. Strum EM, Szenohradszki J, Kaufman WA, et al. Emergence and recovery characteristics of desflurane versus sevoflurane in morbidly obese adult surgical patients: A prospective, randomized study. Anesth Analg 2004; 99:1848-53.
5. Weiskipf RB, Eger EI, Daniel M, et al. Cardiovascular stimulation induced by rapid increases in desflurane concentration in humans results from activation of tracheopulmonary and systemic receptors. Anesthesiology 1995; 83:1173-1178.
6. Ebert TJ, Harkin CP, Muzi M. Cardiovascular responses to sevoflurane: a review. Anesth Analg 1995; 81: S11-22.
7. Welborn LG, Hannallah RS, Norden JM, et al. Comparison of emergence and recovery characteristics of sevoflurane, desflurane, and halothane in pediatric ambulatory patients. Anesth Analg 1996; 83:917-920.
8. Coppens MJ, Versichelen LFM, Rolly G, et al. Review article. The mechanisms of carbon monoxide production by inhalational agents. Anaesthesia 2006; 61:462-468.
9. Berry PD, Sessleer DI, Larson MD. Severe carbon monoxide poisoning during desflurane anesthesia. Anesthesiology 1999; 90:613-6.
10. Kharasch ED, Powers KM, Artru AA. Comparison of Amsorb®, Sodalime, and Baralyme® degradation of volatile anesthetics and formation of carbon monoxide and compound A in swine in vivo. Anesthesiology 2002; 96:173– 82.

# CHAPTER 14

# Opioid Agonists and Antagonists

Lillia Fung MD, George Evans MD

## Learning Objectives

1. To gain an overview of the pharmacodynamics of opioid agonists and antagonists.
2. To acquire knowledge of the pharmacokinetics, indications, and suggested doses of commonly used opioids.
3. To gain an understanding of why, when, and how naloxone is used.

## Key Points

1. Opioid agonists provide analgesia, but when used alone, they are incapable of providing general anesthesia and amnesia.

2. The most feared immediate side effect of an opioid agonist is respiratory depression. Respiratory depression is commonly heralded by excessive sedation.

3. Fentanyl, sufentanil, and remifentanil are opioid medications commonly used during the induction and maintenance of anesthesia.

4. Naloxone is an effective opioid antagonist capable of reversing the effect of an opioid overdose. Most opioids have a longer duration of action compared with naloxone; hence, close monitoring, repeat dosing, or an infusion of naloxone may be required.

### Opioid Agonists and Antagonists

Opium is derived from the dried juice of the poppy plant, which contains over twenty plant alkaloids, including morphine and codeine. Opioids are exogenous substances (natural or synthetic) that bind to the opioid receptor causing analgesia and stupor without loss of touch, proprioception, or consciousness.

Opioids are a class of medications that are considered "High Alert Medications" because they increase the risk of significant patient harm when used in error. In 2007, the Institute of Safe Medication Practice (ISMP) identified the use of hydromorphone and morphine in an acute care setting as the drug treatments that most frequently cause patient harm. All opioids have the potential for misuse, abuse, and addiction. The potential for abuse is related to the release of dopamine resulting in a "brain reward" phenomenon. Opioids with a rapid onset of action (high lipid solubility) have an increased potential for abuse and addiction.

## Site of Action:

Opioid receptors are located predominately in the brain stem (amygdala, corpus striatum, periaqueductal gray matter, and medulla), spinal cord (substantia gelatinosa), and gastrointestinal tract. The binding of an opioid to an opioid receptor causes increased potassium conductance in the presynaptic membranes causing neuronal hyperpolarization. This inhibits neurotransmitter release (e.g., acetylcholine, dopamine, norepinephrine, and substance P) resulting in a depression of neurotransmission and deactivation of pain-modulating systems. The effects of stimulation of mu ($\mu_1$ and $\mu_2$), kappa ($\kappa$), and delta ($\delta$) opioid receptors are summarized in Table 14.1.

## Table 14.1 Opioid receptors; adapted from Atcheson and Lambert (1994).

| $\mu_1$ (mu1) receptor |
| --- |
| supraspinal analgesia, euphoria, bradycardia, hypothermia, urinary retention, miosis |
| $\mu_2$ (mu2) receptor |
| analgesia, respiratory depression, physical dependence, constipation |
| $\kappa$ (kappa) receptor |
| spinal analgesia, sedation, dysphoria, miosis, diuresis |
| $\delta$ (delta) receptor |
| Same as $\mu_2$ plus urinary retention |

A feature common to all opioids is a dose-related depression of respiration, sensorium, and pain perception following intravenous injection. Hepatic metabolism is the primary route of elimination, and the majority of inactive metabolites are excreted unchanged in the urine. A review of the other pharmacodynamic properties of opioids is presented below.

## Central Nervous System (CNS):

Opioids produce sedation and interfere with the sensory perception of painful stimuli. Although large doses of opioids produce unconsciousness, they are incapable of providing general anesthesia and cannot guarantee amnesia. Opioids have been shown to decrease the minimum alveolar concentration (MAC) requirement of volatile anesthetics by up to 50%.[1,2] A reaction of dysphoria rather than euphoria may occur when opioids are administered to patients who are not experiencing pain. Stimulation of the chemoreceptor trigger zone by opioids may result in nausea and emesis. Miosis resulting from opioid administration is due to activation of the parasympathetic nerves via the oculomotor nerve.

## Respiration (RESP):

Opioids produce a direct dose-dependent ventilation depressant through activation of brainstem $mu_2$ opioid receptors. This leads to a decrease in the respiratory rate and minute ventilation accompanied by a compensatory increase in the tidal volume. The result is a slow deep respiratory pattern. With increasing doses, the patient may remain conscious and will breathe when requested, but may become apneic if left alone. Respiratory depression can be reversed with naloxone. The most sensitive clinical marker of impending severe respiratory depression is excessive sedation. Opioids depress the normal compensatory increase in ventilation associated with an increase in serum partial pressure of carbon dioxide ($PaCO_2$). Patients with raised intracranial pressure (ICP) are at risk of further increases in ICP when ventilation decreases and $PaCO_2$ increases. As such, caution must be exercised when administering opioids to spontaneously breathing patients with neurological conditions.

## Cardiovascular System (CVS):

Opioids have minimal effect on cardiac function when administered at low to moderate doses. Cardiac function may be depressed when opioids are administered with either nitrous oxide ($N_2O$) or benzodiazepines. Opioids decrease systemic vascular resistance (SVR) through a decrease in sympathetic outflow or, in the case of morphine, by direct release of histamine. Morphine's tendency to release histamine produces vasodilatation with a fall in both the blood pressure and SVR. Synthetic opioids, most notably remifentanil, produce bradycardia at high doses by stimulating the vagal nucleus in the brainstem.

## Gastrointestinal/Genitourinary (GI/GU):

Opioids slow gastrointestinal mobility and may result in constipation or postoperative ileus. All opioids (particularly fentanyl and morphine) increase biliary tract tone and may precipitate biliary colic (3% incidence) in patients with cholelithiasis. This can be treated with glucagon 2 mg *iv* or naloxone 0.08 mg *iv*. By increasing the tone of the bladder sphincter, opioids may also precipitate postoperative urinary retention.

Other, less common side effects of opioids include anaphylactic reactions, bronchospasm, chest wall rigidity, and pruritis.

Morphine has been known conventionally as the "gold standard" with which all other opioids are compared. It is available in a wide variety of formulations, including oral (*po*), intravenous (*iv*), intramuscular (*im*), subcutaneous (*sc*), epidural, spinal (intrathecal), and rectal (*pr*). It can be used in the perioperative period to provide long-lasting analgesia. Recommended doses for adults range from 5 - 30 mg *po* every (*q*) 4 hours as needed (*prn*) or 2.5 - 5 mg *iv* titrated to clinical effect. Intravenous formulations should be administered slowly at a rate not exceeding 5 mg·min$^{-1}$ to avoid excessive histamine release. Intravenous patient-controlled analgesia (PCA) using morphine or hydromorphone is commonly used as part of an effective strategy to provide postoperative pain management (see Chapter 17).

Morphine is metabolized by the liver to morphine-3-glocuronide (M-3-G) and M-6-G. Most of the metabolites exist in an inactive M-3-G form. In patients with renal insufficiency, the remaining M-6-G active metabolites can accumulate to toxic levels and may require a dose reduction. A slow release oral formulation of morphine (MS Contin) is commonly used to manage chronic pain. Recommended starting doses in adults range from 10 - 30 mg *po q* 8 - 12 hr. Again, doses may need to be decreased when creatinine clearance (CrCl) is < 10 - 50 mL·min$^{-1}$.

Meperidine was the first opioid to be commercially prepared (1932). It is commonly know as pethidine (World Heath Organization nomenclature for the generic drug) or as the brand name Demerol® in North America (USA adopted name). It is indicated in the treatment of moderate to severe pain and can be administered *po*, *im*, *iv*, *sc*, or via the epidural route. Meperidine was initially considered to offer superior analgesia to patients suffering from renal colic, biliary colic, or bone pain, but it has now been shown to offer no better analgesia than morphine. It has unique properties distinct from other opioids including:

- Local anesthetic properties initially believed to be responsible for its antispasmodic activity.
- Lack of pupillary miosis, perhaps due to its structural similarities to atropine.
- Faster onset of action (i.e., more lipid-soluble) and possible higher addiction potential compared with morphine.
- A unique toxicity profile (discussed below) that is unlike other opioid agonists.

Normeperidine is an active metabolite of meperidine possessing half of meperidine's analgesic activity. Normeperidine may cause CNS excitation. In patients receiving large amounts of meperidine (> 600 mg per day) for prolonged periods of time (> 48 hr) or in patients with renal insufficiency, normeperidine levels may rise significantly and seizure activity may result.

Meperidine has similar mu receptor agonist side effects common to other opioids, commonly manifesting as respiratory depression, sedation, hallucinations, nausea, vomiting and ileus. Its unique toxic effects compared with other opioids are believed to be secondary to normeperidine accumulation with repeated doses in patients with renal insufficiency. These effects include an association with serotonin syndrome, tremor, dysphoria, delirium, and seizures. The use of meperidine has decreased significantly due to its potential toxicity compared with other opioids. Its use should be limited to < 48 hr, with a maximum daily dose of 600 mg.

Recommended adult analgesic doses are 50 – 100 mg *po*, *im*, or *sc* every 3 – 4 hr as needed (max. 600 mg per day). Meperidine is still a popular drug for procedural sedation in endoscopy and diagnostic imaging units. The recommended adult dose for procedural sedation is 50 – 100 mg *im* or *sc* ½ - 1 hr prior to the procedure. In some obstetrical units, it remains a popular drug for labour analgesia (when epidural analgesia is not an option) with a recommended dose of 50 – 100 mg *im* or *sc* every 1 – 3 hr when labour is established (max. 600 mg per day). It has also been used to inhibit postoperative shivering in a dose of 25 mg intravenously.[3]

The American Pain Society and the Institute of Safe Medication Practice recommend against the use of meperidine for pain control in patients who are elderly or in those who have reduced renal function due to the risk of seizures.

Oxycodone is available in an oral or rectal formulation and is indicated in the treatment of moderate to severe pain. Unlike morphine, oxycodone produces its analgesic effect through activation of the kappa receptors and is generally better tolerated compared with morphine. Oxycodone inhibits ascending pain pathways resulting in a change in the perception and response to pain. It is metabolized primarily by the cytochrome P450 3A4 enzyme (CYP3A4) with a minor component metabolized by the CYP2D6 enzyme. Inducers and inhibitors of CYP3A4 will reduce or potentiate the analgesic effect as well as the side effects of oxycodone. Common inhibitors of CYP3A4 include erythromycin, clarithromycin, and ginkgo. Common inducers of CYP3A4 include carbamazepine, phenytoin, and St. John's wort.

## Table 14.2 Opioid potency ratios

| Opioid | Potency Ratio |
|---|---|
| codeine | 0.1:1 |
| morphine | 1:1 |
| oxycodone / OxyContin® | 1.5 – 2:1 |
| hydromorphone / Hydromorph Contin® | 5 – 7:1 |
| methadone | 5 – 10:1 |
| buprenorphine | 75 – 100:1 |
| fentanyl | 100:1 |
| remifentanil | 250:1 |
| sufentanil | 500 – 1,000:1 |

Oxycodone is approximately 1.5 – 2 times more potent compared with morphine (Table 14.2). Recommended starting doses are 5 - 10 mg *po q* 4hr *prn*. Dose reductions in patients with renal impairment (creatinine clearance (CrCl) < 60 mL·min⁻¹) should be considered. Percocet®, a widely recognized combination pill with 325 mg of acetaminophen and 5 mg of oxycodone, is commonly prescribed for short-term pain. Percodan® contains 325 mg of acetylsalicylic acid with 5 mg of oxycodone. These medications are commonly prescribed as 1 – 2 tablets *po q* 4 – 6 hr *prn* for pain

|  | Oxycodone | Oxycontin® |
|---|---|---|
| Onset of action | 10 – 15 min | |
| Peak effect | ½ - 1 hr | |
| Duration | 3 – 6 hr | < 12 hr |
| Half-life Elimination | 2 – 3 hr | 5 hr |
| Bioavailability | 87% | 60% |
| Time to peak plasma levels | 1.4 – 1.9 hr | 4 – 5 hr |

The immediate-release formulation of oxycodone is marketed as Oxy.IR®, while the controlled-release formulation of oxycodone is called OxyContin®. The recommended starting dose for OxyContin® is 10 mg *po q*12 hr, and it must not be chewed or broken down. OxyContin® is indicated in the management of continuous moderate to severe pain for an extended period of time. It should not be used on an as needed basis in the acute postoperative setting. Abuse, misuse, and addiction are common to all opioids. While OxyContin® can provide effective analgesia in patients with chronic pain (discussed in Chapter 18), oxycodone and OxyContin® abuse, misuse, and addiction have increased dramatically in the last 20 years and have been associated with deaths, crime, and motor vehicle accidents. In many centers Oxycontin® has now been replaced by OxyNeo®. OxyNeo® tablets are produced using a unique process that hardens the tablet and makes it gel on exposure to moisture. The hardening process is intended to resist the risk of abuse by breaking, crushing, chewing or dissolving the tablet. Patients are instructed to take one tablet at a time with enough water to ensure complete swallowing immediately after placing the tablet in their mouth.

**Codeine** is a classic example of a "prodrug", i.e., an inactive form of a drug that must be metabolized in the liver by the cytochrome P450 2D6 enzyme (CYP2D6) to produce the active form, morphine. Codeine is commonly used for mild to moderate pain and has been labelled a "weak" opioid because some patients are slow metabolizers with little CYP2D6. Genetic heterogeneity is such that the CYP2D6 function may be reduced in approximately 10% of Caucasians and may be normal or enhanced in approximately 1 – 7% of Caucasians and 25% of Ethiopians. A reduction in CYP2D6 function results in a decreased conversion of codeine to morphine and a reduced analgesic effect. Alternatively, enhanced CYP2D6 function is seen in ultra-rapid metabolizers and has resulted in opioid toxicity and death in patients taking the usual recommended doses of codeine. In addition to genetic variability, a number of medications are inhibitors of CYP2D6. They prevent the conversion of codeine to its active metabolite, morphine, and thus reduce the analgesic effect.

Codeine is commonly administered as a combination pill containing acetaminophen and codeine. In Canada, acetaminophen and codeine are available as Tylenol 1, 2, 3, and 4, containing 300 mg of acetaminophen with 8, 15, 30, and 60 mg of codeine, respectively, per tablet. Each combination tablet also contains 15 mg of caffeine. The daily maximum dose of codeine combination drugs is limited by restriction of the acetaminophen total dose to less than 4 grams of acetaminophen per 24 hours (i.e., the recommended maximum dose and frequency is two tablets every 4 hr *prn*). See also Chapter 17.

*Clinical Pearl:*

*Codeine is a prodrug and its effect is unpredictable. Patients experiencing excessive sedation or respiratory depression with codeine may be "ultra-rapid" converters of codeine to morphine. These patients are at an increased risk of an overdose, and a different opioid should be considered for analgesia.*

Tramadol is a synthetic oral opioid commonly used in moderate to severe short-term pain or as an adjunct in the treatment of long-term pain. In addition to activating opioid receptors, it blocks neuronal reuptake of norepinephrine (NE) and serotonin. Norepinephrine acts on the efferent descending inhibitory pain pathway. Oral tramadol (Ultram®) is available in a 50 mg tablet. The recommended starting dose is 1 - 2 tablets *po* q 4 – 6 hr (with a maximum of 400 mg per day). The frequency should be decreased to q 12 hr in patients with renal insufficiency (CrCl < 30 mL·min$^{-1}$). Co-administration of tramadol with serotonin-norepinephrine reuptake inhibitors (SNRIs) or with selective serotonin reuptake inhibitors (SSRIs) increases the risk for developing a potentially life-threatening condition called serotonin syndrome.

Tramadol has a synergistic analgesic effect when combined with acetaminophen. In Canada, tramadol is available in combination with acetaminophen in a formulation called Tramacet®. Each tablet of Tramacet® contains 37.5 mg of tramadol with 325 mg of acetaminophen.[4] Tramacet is typically prescribed as 1 – 2 tablets *po* q 4 hr *prn* for postoperative analgesia. Tramadol preparations result in less respiratory depression and minimal effect on gastric emptying compared with other opioids. Tramadol has a half-life of 6 - 7 hr. Extended release formulations containing tramadol (Ralivia®, Zytram®, Tridural®) are now available in Canada. The costs for tramadol preparations are significantly higher than for traditional opioids and NSAIDs and may be prohibitive for some patients.

Hydromorphone (Dilaudid®) is a semi-synthetic opioid analgesic commonly used in the perioperative period. Hydromorphone is 5 - 7 times more potent than morphine, and its duration of effect is 4 - 5 hr. Starting doses are generally 1 - 2 mg *po* q 4 hr or 0.5 - 1 mg *sc* q 4 hr. Hydromorphone is metabolized to hydromorphone-3-glucuronide, which is excreted by the kidneys. This active metabolite accumulates in patients with renal failure and may cause cognitive dysfunction and myoclonus.[5] Hydromorphone is generally better tolerated in the elderly resulting in less nausea, vomiting, sedation, and pruritus compared with morphine.[6] This may be due to less accumulation of active metabolites compared with morphine. Hydromorphone is available in an intravenous form and in immediate-release and long-acting (Hydromorph Contin®) oral formulations.

Fentanyl, sufentanil, and remifentanil are common opioid agents used during induction and maintenance of anesthesia. This is due to their rapid onset and predictable duration of action.

Fentanyl is approximately 100 times more potent than morphine. Its high lipid solubility and rapid onset make it an ideal co-induction agent to blunt the hemodynamic response to direct laryngoscopy and tracheal intubation (1.5 - 5 $\mu g \cdot kg^{-1}$ *iv* bolus). Fentanyl is used extensively in operating rooms, postanesthetic units, and critical care units. It is commonly used with midazolam for procedural sedation in endoscopy and diagnostic imaging units (see Chapter 11, monitored anesthetic care). When used in high doses, fentanyl produces dose-dependent analgesia accompanied with respiratory depression, sedation, and unconsciousness. Its onset of action is rapid, peak effect at 5 min, and its duration of effect is

approximately ½ - 1 hour. Fentanyl administration should be timed such that titration is completed approximately 3 min before laryngoscopy. When used for sedation with spontaneous respiration, administration of midazolam with fentanyl greatly increases the risk of significant respiratory depression, hypoxemia, apnea, and loss of consciousness. Supplemental oxygen prior to administration as well as pulse oximetry, close observation, and titrated doses are recommended to decrease the incidence of adverse respiratory events.

Fentanyl is commonly used as part of a "balanced general anesthetic technique" where both opioids and inhalational anesthetics are used to provide anesthesia. A single bolus dose of fentanyl 3 $\mu g \cdot kg^{-1}$ *iv* decreases the MAC of inhalational agents (i.e., desflurane, isoflurane) by approximately 50%. Fentanyl requirements also decrease with age by approximately 50% from age 20 to 90. For general anesthesia, incremental doses of 0.5 – 1 $\mu g \cdot kg^{-1}$ *iv* are administered every 30 min as dictated by the clinical response and surgical procedure. Alternatively, a continuous intravenous infusion of 1 – 3 $\mu g \cdot kg^{-1} \cdot hr^{-1}$ can be used to provide stable fentanyl levels. More than 80% of fentanyl is bound to proteins (primarily albumin). The extent of binding is highly pH dependent such that there is a significant increase in unbound fentanyl in the presence of acidosis and an increase in the clinical effect as well as potential adverse effects.

Low doses of fentanyl (0.5 – 2 $\mu g \cdot kg^{-1}$) are commonly used for procedural sedation; moderate doses (2 – 20 $\mu g \cdot kg^{-1}$) are commonly used for patients requiring general anesthesia, and high doses (20 – 100 $\mu g \cdot kg^{-1}$) are less commonly used. High doses (> 750 $\mu g$) of fentanyl or equivalent doses of sufentanil and remifentanil can result in muscle rigidity and laryngeal spasm when administered rapidly on induction of anesthesia. This can result in a "stiff-chest syndrome" making ventilation difficult or impossible. The use of muscle relaxants with opioids will generally resolve the chest rigidity. Fentanyl's short duration of action is due to its redistribution from the CNS to other tissue sites in the body. It is metabolized by the liver and excreted by the kidney. Common idiosyncratic reactions with fentanyl administration include nasal pruritus and a tussive effect manifesting as a cough.

Fentanyl is also available in varying concentrations as a transdermal patch that releases a controlled hourly dose. Transdermal fentanyl is commonly used to manage patients with chronic pain (see Chapter 18) and should not be used in acute pain management or in opioid naïve patients due to the risk of an overdose. Transdermal fentanyl patches require approximately 12 hr to reach peak plasma levels and should be changed every 48 to 72 hr. Changes to the concentration of the patch should be made only after a steady-state level has been achieved (generally after 3 – 5 days). Short-acting opioids or adjuvants are added to control symptoms until steady plasma levels are achieved.

Sufentanil is the most potent opioid that is in clinical use today. It has a potency of 10 – 15 times that of fentanyl and is a highly selective mu opioid receptor agonist. Sufentanil results in a significant dose-dependent reduction in the MAC of inhalational anesthetic drugs with a maximum reduction of 70 – 90%. Respiratory depression is also dose-dependent and is especially marked in the presence of inhalational anesthetic drugs. Postoperative respiratory depression and apnea may occur with both fentanyl and sufentanil despite apparent recovery after general anesthesia. This typically occurs in the recovery room when patients are left undisturbed. It has a much smaller volume of distribution than fentanyl and is more suited to intravenous infusion techniques than fentanyl when used for long procedures

(see Fig. 11.3, context-sensitive half-life). Loss of consciousness occurs with induction doses of $1.3 – 2.8$ $\mu g \cdot kg^{-1}$. Doses of $0.3 – 1$ $\mu g \cdot kg^{-1}$ can be used to blunt the hemodynamic response to laryngoscopy and tracheal intubation but may be associated with muscle rigidity, especially in the elderly and when administered rapidly. Sufentanil is commonly used as a component of a "balanced general anesthetic technique" with either nitrous oxide or an inhalational agent. An infusion rate of $0.1$ to $0.5$ $\mu g \cdot kg^{-1} \cdot hr^{-1}$ in addition to ½ MAC of an inhalational anesthetic agent is commonly used in a "balanced general anesthetic technique".

Remifentanil is classified as an ultra-short-acting intravenous mu-opioid receptor agonist. Peak analgesic effect occurs in 1 – 3 min following administration and dissipates after approximately 10 min. Unlike other opioids, remifentanil undergoes rapid ester hydrolysis in the blood and tissues, and its recovery is due to metabolism and not redistribution. Remifentanil administration results in a dose-dependent depression of the MAC of inhalational anesthetic drugs to a maximum reduction of approximately 60%.

To avoid surgical complications, monitoring of motor-evoked responses (MERs) may be required in selected neurosurgical procedures. Remifentanil suppresses MERs to a lesser extent than midazolam, inhalational agents, and barbiturates, and it may be used as part of a total intravenous anesthetic (TIVA) technique for these procedures. In a TIVA technique, infusions of remifentanil ($0.25 – 0.5$ $\mu g \cdot kg^{-1} \cdot min^{-1}$) along with propofol ($75 – 100$ $\mu g \cdot kg^{-1} \cdot min^{-1}$) are commonly used.

The duration of respiratory depression following administration of $1.5$ $\mu g \cdot kg^{-1}$ of remifentanil is approximately 10 min. Minute ventilation typically returns to normal 5 – 15 min after discontinuing a remifentanil infusion. Adverse side effects, such as hypotension, bradycardia, muscle rigidity, and respiratory depression or arrest, may be more pronounced with remifentanil compared with other opioids because of its rapid onset of action. These side effects are dependent on dose and rate of administration. The respiratory depression and hypotension can generally be reversed with naloxone and ephedrine, respectively.

Co-administration of midazolam or propofol reduces remifentanil requirements by up to 50%. Remifentanil infusion rates of 0.01 – 0.07 $\mu g \cdot kg^{-1} \cdot min^{-1}$ can be used to provide procedural sedation and analgesia with or without premedication using 1 – 2 mg of intravenous midazolam. The combination of remifentanil with midazolam or propofol increases the risk of significant respiratory depression by up to 50% and may require airway and ventilation support.

Infusion rates of 0.1 – 0.3 $\mu g \cdot kg^{-1} \cdot min^{-1}$ of remifentanil are commonly used as part of a "balanced general anesthetic technique" along with ½ MAC of inhalational anesthetic agent. The rapid offset in action means that there will be no residual analgesic activity within 5 – 10 min after discontinuing an infusion. In procedures where postoperative pain is anticipated, other measures (local anesthesia, NSAIDs, long-acting opioid administration) should be instituted to avoid sudden pain after discontinuing a remifentanil infusion. Remifentanil administration may be associated with an "opioid-induced hyperalgesia" where patients who have received an opioid paradoxically experience more pain than expected. Opioid-induced hyperalgesia may be minimized with the co-administration of small doses of ketamine (e.g., 10 mg intravenous ketamine).[7]

Methadone is a long-acting opioid agonist with N-methyl-D-aspartate (NMDA) receptor antagonist properties. It is commonly used as an oral opioid for chronic pain and in the prevention of opioid withdrawal in rehabilitating narcotic addicts. Its use is challenged by a variable equianalgesic dose that ranges from 1 - 10 times that of oral morphine[8] as well as a variable half-life that ranges from 15 - 190 hr (average 24 hr).[9] A link to a methadone conversion tool is provided at the end of this chapter. Titration of methadone is further complicated by a variable clinical duration that may be as short as 6 - 8 hr for first time users. With time, tissues accumulate enough methadone such that once or twice daily dosing maintains stable methadone levels. Methadone is metabolized by hepatic CYP3A4. Drug interactions with inducers (e.g., dexamethasone, omeprazole, erythromycin) and inhibitors of CYP3A4 (e.g., grapefruit, midazolam, tricyclic antidepressants [TCAs]) in patients taking methadone may reduce or increase the desired effect and potential complications. Currently, only federally and provincially licensed physicians can prescribe methadone.

Buprenorphine is a semi-synthetic opioid agonist antagonist that is available in Canada in a sublingual and transdermal formulation. It is approved for moderate to severe chronic pain and opioid addiction and has a potency of 75 – 100 times that of morphine.[10] It has a ceiling effect for respiratory depression but no ceiling effect for analgesia, hence, unlike fentanyl, transdermal formulations can be used safely in opioid naïve patients.[11] The starting dose for the patch is 5 $\mu g \cdot hr^{-1}$ every 7 days and can be titrated to effect after 1 - 2 weeks. Buprenorphine has a uniquely high affinity to the mu opioid receptors, a half-life of over 2 hr, and a clinical effect lasting 6 - 8 hr. Consequently, buprenorphine is very resistant to reversal with opioid antagonists and may require large, repeated doses of naloxone. In the perioperative setting, buprenorphine may lead to a reduced analgesic effect with traditional opioid agonists.[12] The management of patients on buprenorphine in the perioperative period remains controversial.[12-14] Guidelines for the perioperative management of patients on buprenorphine who require surgury are provided at the end of this chapter.

## Opioid Antagonists:

Naloxone (Narcan®) is a pure opioid antagonist that competes with opioids at the mu, delta, kappa, and sigma receptors. Naloxone is supplied in ampoules of 0.02 mg·mL$^{-1}$, 0.4 mg·mL$^{-1}$, and 1 mg·mL$^{-1}$. The 0.4 mg·mL$^{-1}$ and 1 mg·mL$^{-1}$ ampoules should be diluted with saline to provide a concentration of 0.04 - 0.05 mg·mL$^{-1}$ for ease of administration.

Naloxone reaches its peak effect within 1 - 2 min of intravenous administration and has a clinical duration of 30 to 60 min. Perioperative surgical patients with evidence of excessive sedation or respiratory depression secondary to opioids may be given small incremental aliquots of naloxone of 0.08 – 0.1 mg $iv$ every 1 – 2 min to clinical effect. If high doses of naloxone are given, sudden reversal of the analgesic effects of opioids may result. The subsequent abrupt return of pain can result in hypertension, tachycardia, pulmonary edema, ventricular dysrhythmias, and even cardiac arrest. Continuous infusions of 3 to 10 µg·kg$^{-1}$·hr$^{-1}$ of naloxone may be required if sedation or respiratory depression recur.

## Test your knowledge:

1. What are the undesirable effects of opioids?
2. Name an opioid antagonist. What dose of this drug would be appropriate to reverse opioid-induced respiratory depression? What, if any, potential problems arise from administering too much of this antagonist?
3. What is buprenorphine and what are some concerns for the perioperative management of patients who are receiving this medication?
4. Describe the context in which remifentanil can be used.

## Suggested resources for opiod

http://itunes.apple.com/us/app/opioid-converter/id358992558?mt=8

http://itunes.apple.com/ca/app/opioids-dosage-conversion/id382383903?mt=8

## Additional Resources

## Methadone conversion tool

http://www.med.umich.edu/1info/FHP/practiceguides/pain/dosing.pdf

## Perioperative Management of buprenorphine

http://www.anesthesiaprimer.com/AP/Ch14Opioids/BuprenorphinePolicy.pdf

## Resources:

Barash PG, Cullen BF, Stoelting RK, Editors. Clinical Anesthesia 6$^{th}$ Edition, JB Lippincott, Philadelphia, 2009.

## References:

1. Atcheson R, Lambert DG. Update on opioid receptors. Br J Anaesth 1994 Aug;73:2,132-4.
2. Lang E, Kapila A, Shulugman D et al. Reduction of isoflurane minimal alveolar concentration by remifentanyl. Anesthesiology 1996;85:721-728.
3. Kranke P, Eberhart LH, Roewer N. Pharmacological Treatment of Postoperative Shivering: A Quantitative Systematic Review of Randomized Controlled Trials. Anesth Analg 2002;94:453–60.
4. Health Products and Food Branch. Summary basis of decision (SBD) Tramacet. September 17, 2008. Janssen Ortho Inc. Submission Control No. 095167.
5. Babul N, Darke AC, Hagen N: Hydromorphone metabolite accumulation in renal failure. J
6. Pain Symptom Manage 10:184, 1995.
7. Sarhill N, Walsh D, Nelson KA. Hydromorphone: pharmacology and clinical applications in cancer patients. Support Care Cancer 2001;9:84-96.
8. Joly V, Richebe P, Guignard B, et al. Remifentanil-induced postoperative hyperalgesia and its prevention with small-dose ketamine. Anesthesiology 2005 Jul;103(1):147-55.

9. Mercandante S, Caraceni A. Conversion ratios for opioid switching in the treatment of cancer pain: a systematic review. Palliat Med. 2011;25:504-15.

10.Jovey RD (ed.). Managing Pain. The Canadian Healthcare Professional's Reference. © 2002 Purdue Pharma, Toronto, Canada.

11.Sittl R. Transdermal buprenorphine in cancer pain and palliative care. Palliat Med 2006;20 (Suppl 1):s25–30.

12. Dahan A, Yassen A, Romberg R, et al. Buprenorphine induces ceiling in respiratory depression but not in analgesia. Br J Anaesth 2006;96:627–32.

13.Vadivelu N, Anwar M. Buprenorphine in Postoperative Pain Management. Anesthesiology Clin 2010;28:601-609.

14.Alford DP, Compton P, Samet JH: Acute pain management for patients receiving maintenance methadone or buprenorphine therapy. Ann Intern Med 2006; 144:127–134.

15. Roberts D, Meyer-Witting M. High-dose buprenorphine: perioperative precautions and management strategies. Anaesth Intensive Care 2005;33(1):17–25.

# CHAPTER 15

# Local Anesthetics

Teresa Furtak MD, Holly Evans MD

## Learning Objectives

1. To gain an understanding of the mechanism of action of local anesthetics.
2. To gain an appreciation of the chemical structure of local anesthetic agents and their ester and amide classification.
3. To become familiar with commonly used local anesthetic agents.
4. To gain an appreciation of the clinical signs of local anesthetic toxicity.
5. To understand strategies to reduce the risk and manage symptoms of local anesthetic toxicity.

## Key Points

1. A 1% solution contains 10 mg·mL⁻¹.

2. A 1:1,000 solution contains 1 mg·mL⁻¹.

3. A 1:200,000 (epinephrine) solution contains 5 µg·mL⁻¹.

4. Epinephrine (typically 1:200,000 concentration) combined with a local anesthetic decreases the systemic absorption and prolongs the duration of action of the local anesthetic.

5. Knowledge of the maximum safe dose of a local anesthetic, the ability to calculate the dose, and adherence to recommended doses are important strategies to decrease local anesthetic toxicity.

6. Although local anesthetic toxicity is rare, it can result in cardiovascular, respiratory, and central nervous system (CNS) depression and may be life-threatening.

Local anesthetic medications affect sensory, motor, and autonomic nerves by reversibly blocking impulses conducted through nerve fibers. They can be administered by a wide variety of techniques to provide intraoperative anesthesia and postoperative analgesia. This chapter focuses on commonly used local anesthetics and their pharmacologic properties. Strategies to recognize, prevent, and manage symptoms of local anesthetic toxicity are also presented.

## Mechanism of Action

Local anesthetics reversibly bind and block sodium channels in the nerve cell membrane. This reduces sodium ion movement across the membrane preventing the generation and propagation of action potentials along the nerve axon.

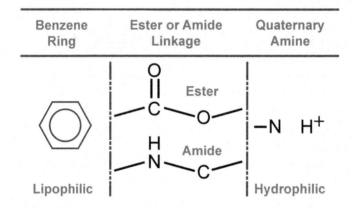

| Benzene Ring | Ester or Amide Linkage | Quaternary Amine |
|---|---|---|

Fig. 15.1 The general chemical structure of amide and ester local anesthetics consists of three basic building blocks: a benzene ring, an ester or amide linkage, and a quaternary amine.

## Basic Structure and Classification

Local anesthetic molecules consist of a lipid soluble benzene ring coupled to a water-soluble amine group by either an amide or ester link (Fig. 15.1). The lipophilic aromatic ring is responsible for the anesthetic effect. Local anesthetics are classified as either an ester or an amide on the basis of their linkage. Ester local anesthetics are metabolized by plasma cholinesterases, while amide local anesthetics are metabolized in the liver. Cocaine, prilocaine, and tetracaine are examples of ester local anesthetics. Common amide local anesthetics include lidocaine, bupivacaine, and ropivacaine. All local anesthetics exist as racemic mixtures of levo (S) and dextro (R) stereoisomers. The exceptions to this are lidocaine, ropivacaine, and levo-bupivacaine. The dextro stereoisomer may be associated with greater potency but may also have greater systemic toxicity.

## Biophysical Features

Local anesthetics are weak bases that exist in a neutral lipid soluble form or in a charged water-soluble form. Local anesthetics enter the nerve cell membrane primarily in the lipid soluble form. Once inside the cell, the charged cation form acts on the intracellular side of the sodium channel to block nerve impulses (Fig. 15.2). In an acidic environment, local anesthetics exist mainly in the charged form and diffuse poorly across cell membranes.

## Pharmacodynamics

Several factors affect how fast local anesthetics act (onset), the extent to which they block impulse generation (potency), and how long they last (duration). A faster onset of action occurs when the majority of the local anesthetic exists in an uncharged base form. In the uncharged base form, the local anesthetic readily diffuses across the plasma membrane and into the nerve cell. The pKa is the pH at which half of the local anesthetic exists in the base form and half in the cation form. The pKa can be used to estimate the proportion of the base form at physiologic pH (7.4). Local anesthetics with a pKa close to or lower than

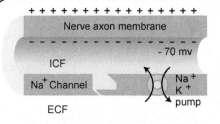

In the resting state, the sodium ($Na^+$) channel is closed, and the resting membrane potential is - 70 to - 80 millivolts. The potassium ($K^+$) concentration in the cell is approximately 10 fold greater than the extracellular concentration.

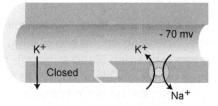

Opening of the sodium channel results in an influx of $Na^+$, a rise in the membrane potential, and depolarization of the cell. Following depolarization, the sodium channel closes.

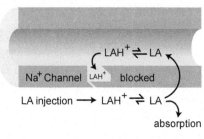

Potassium exits the cell down a concentration and electrical gradient. A $Na^+$ - $K^+$ pump helps to restore the membrane potential as the cell is repolarized.

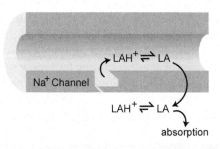

Local anesthetics (LA) exist in an acid (pH < 5) form ($LAH^+$). When injected, tissue buffering results in a rise in the pH and a portion of the drug dissociates to the free base (LA). The free base is able to diffuse across the nerve membrane. Inside the cell, the ionized form of the LA ($LAH^+$) blocks the $Na^+$ channel, preventing depolarization of the nerve membrane.

The action of the LA is terminated by diffusion out of the nerve cell due to a drop in the extracellular (ECF) LA concentration. The LA in the ECF is taken up by the capillaries and removed by the circulation.

Fig. 15.2 Local anesthetics act by blocking the sodium channel and thus preventing neural depolarization. Adapted from Principles and Practice of Regional Anaesthesia 2nd Edition 1993. Editors Wildsmith JAW, Armitage EN.

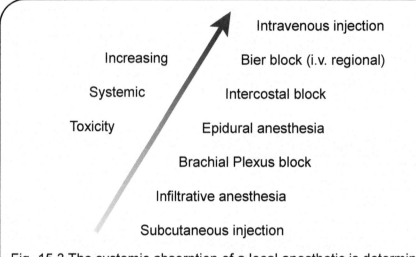

Fig. 15.3 The systemic absorption of a local anesthetic is determined primarily by blood flow which varies depending on the site of injection. Rapid absorption occurs in areas with a rich blood supply (e.g., intercostal space). Conversely, areas with a low blood supply (e.g., subcutaneous tissue) have a low potential for systemic toxicity.

physiological pH have a greater proportion of uncharged base and a more rapid onset.

Lipid solubility determines potency. A highly lipid soluble local anesthetic will penetrate the nerve plasma membrane easily to exert its effect. The duration of action of a local anesthetic is dependent on the degree of plasma protein binding. A local anesthetic that is highly protein bound will have a longer duration of action. Generally, increasing lipid solubility correlates with increasing protein binding, potency, duration, and toxicity.

## Pharmacokinetics

The systemic absorption of a local anesthetic is determined primarily by blood flow at the site of injection (Fig. 15.3). Blood flow and the rate of systemic absorption of the local anesthetic vary depending on the site of injection. High rates of absorption occur when injections are near areas with a rich blood supply (e.g., epidural space) *vs* areas with a low blood supply (e.g., subcutaneous tissue). Systemic absorption of local anesthetics can also be reduced by the addition of a vasoconstrictor. Epinephrine in a concentration of 1:200,000 (5 $\mu g \cdot mL^{-1}$) is commonly administered with local anesthetics. The presence of epinephrine reduces systemic absorption of the local anesthetic by up to 30% and increases the duration of local anesthetic effect. Many local anesthetics have intrinsic vasodilator properties. Ropivacaine, however, causes vasoconstriction reducing systemic absorption.

Following systemic absorption, local anesthetics are first distributed to highly perfused organs, such as the brain, lungs, liver, kidneys, and heart. Later, redistribution occurs to less well-perfused organs, such as muscle and fat tissue (see Chapter 11).

Ester local anesthetics are rapidly hydrolyzed by plasma cholinesterases. Some ester local anesthetics are metabolized to p-aminobenzoic acid (PABA), which may cause an allergic reaction in susceptible individuals. In contrast, amide local anesthetics are metabolized by dealkylation and conjugation in the liver. Amide metabolism is slower than ester hydrolysis. Metabolites of ester and amide local anesthetics are primarily eliminated by excretion in the urine.

## Table 15.1 Differences in ester and amide local anesthetics

| Properties | Ester Local Anesthetics | Amide Local Anesthetics |
|---|---|---|
| Metabolism | Rapid by plasma cholinesterase | Slow, hepatic |
| Toxicity | Less likely | More likely |
| Allergic reaction | Possible (PABA) | Very rare |
| Onset of action | Fast | Moderate to fast |
| pKa | Higher than pH (8.5 – 8.9) | Close to pH (7.6 – 8.1) |
| PABA = p-aminobenzoic acid; pKa = acid dissociation constant. | | |

### Clinical Application

Local anesthetics may be administered by a variety of techniques. Examples include topical administration, subcutaneous infiltration, field block infiltration, and intravenous administration (i.e., Bier block; see Chapter 16). Regional blocks with local anesthetics and neuraxial administration of local anesthetics for epidural and spinal anesthesia are discussed in Chapter 16. Local anesthetic blocks can be used to provide intraoperative anesthesia as well as postoperative analgesia.

Topical formulations of cocaine, tetracaine, and lidocaine can be used to provide anesthesia to the eye, nose, mouth, tracheobronchial tree, genitourinary tract, and skin. Lidocaine can be nebulized to provide surface anesthesia to the upper and lower respiratory tract in order to facilitate fiberoptic bronchoscopy. A eutectic mixture of local anesthetic (EMLA®) cream can be used to numb the skin for minor procedures (e.g., venipucture, arterial cannulation, lumbar puncture, and bone marrow aspiration).

Intravenous lidocaine can be used in the management of cardiac arrhythmias. It may also be used to blunt hemodynamic and airway responses and attenuate increases in intraocular pressure (IOP) and intracranial pressure (ICP) in response to tracheal intubation. This effect is believed to result from a depression of airway reflexes and calcium flux in airway smooth muscle. A lidocaine infusion can also be used to reduce postoperative pain and treat neuropathic pain.

Differential nerve blockade refers to the phenomenon where nerve conduction is inhibited in one type of nerve fiber but unchanged in another. Different types of nerves have varying sensitivities to the effects of local anesthetics. Preganglionic B fibers are the most sensitive nerves, followed by small C fibers and small to medium sized A-delta fibers (pain and temperature sensation). The large A-alpha and A-beta fibers (touch, proprioception, and motor function) are most resistant to block by local anesthetics. Typically, sensation is lost to temperature first, followed by sharp pain and then light touch.

Differential nerve block is frequently achieved with spinal and epidural anesthesia. The sympathetic block with neuraxial anesthesia often extends several segments higher than the cutaneous dermatomal block. The loss of pain and temperature sensation also often extends more cephalad than the loss of sensation to light touch. Differential blockade is exploited in obstetrical anesthesia where dilute concentrations of local anesthetic are administered into the epidural space to block the sensation of pain from uterine contractions without impairing motor function and the ability to push.

The pH of a local anesthetic solution can be raised with the addition of sodium bicarbonate. The addition of bicarbonate will increase the proportion of uncharged base molecules and facilitate diffusion into the nerve cell. In contrast, diffusion of the local anesthetic into the nerve cell will be impaired with the addition of a solution with a pH < 7.4 (e.g., commercially prepared epinephrine-containing solutions) or when a local anesthetic is injected into an acidotic environment (e.g., abscess). The addition of a small amount of bicarbonate to a local anesthetic solution has been advocated to speed the onset of action of the local anesthetic. With bicarbonate, the neutral form of the local anesthetic will increase approximately 10%, and onset of action may be decreased by 5 min. However, the addition of bicarbonate is limited by precipitation if the pH is raised to > 8 and may decrease the duration of local anesthetic effect.

## Local Anesthetic Formulations

Local anesthetic solutions exist in various concentrations (e.g., 0.5%, 1%, 2%, and 4%). In order to calculate the maximum amount of drug that can be administered, it is essential to know how to convert the percent concentration to $mg \cdot mL^{-1}$. By definition, a 1% solution has 1 g of local anesthetic per 100 mL of solution (or 1,000 mg per 100 mL = 10 $mg \cdot mL^{-1}$).

## Table 15.2 Maximum recommended local anesthetic doses.

| Drug | Onset | Maximum Dose $mg \cdot kg^{-1}$ (with Epinephrine) | Duration (with Epinephrine) |
|---|---|---|---|
| Lidocaine | Rapid | 4.5 $mg \cdot kg^{-1}$ (7 $mg \cdot kg^{-1}$) | 120 min (240 min) |
| Mepivacaine | Rapid | 5 $mg \cdot kg^{-1}$ (7 $mg \cdot kg^{-1}$) | 180 min (360 min) |
| Bupivacaine | Slow | 2.5 $mg \cdot kg^{-1}$ (3 $mg \cdot kg^{-1}$) | 4 hr (8 hr) |
| Ropivacaine | Medium | 2 - 3 $mg \cdot kg^{-1}$ | 3 hr (6 hr) |
| Chloroprocaine | Rapid | 10 $mg \cdot kg^{-1}$ (15 $mg \cdot kg^{-1}$) | 30 min (90 min) |

*Clinical Pearl:*

*A simple way to determine the number of $mg \cdot mL^{-1}$ of a solution is to multiply the percent concentration of the solution by 10.*

The concentration of epinephrine in a local anesthetic solution is expressed as a dilution (e.g., 1:1,000, 1:100,000, 1:200,000). A 1:1,000 solution means that there is 1 g of epinephrine per 1,000 mL of solution (or 1,000 mg per 1,000 mL = 1 $mg \cdot mL^{-1}$).

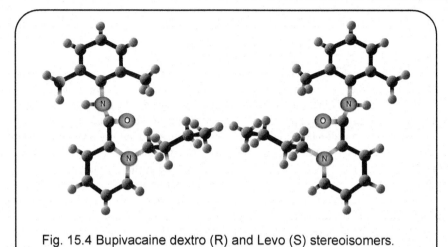

Fig. 15.4 Bupivacaine dextro (R) and Levo (S) stereoisomers.

### Lidocaine:

Lidocaine, an amide local anesthetic, is one of the most commonly used local anesthetic agents. It has a rapid onset and intermediate duration of action.

### Bupivacaine:

Bupivacaine is more potent and has a longer duration of action than lidocaine, but it is more toxic than lidocaine. Bupivacaine exists as an equal mixture of levo (S) and dextro (R) stereoisomers (fig. 15.4). The two isomers have different pharmacokinetic, pharmacodynamic, and toxicity profiles. Levobupivacaine is less cardiotoxic compared with bupivacaine. Levobupivacaine is commonly used in other countries but is not currently available in Canada.

### *Clinical Pearl:*

*A 0.25% solution of bupivacaine contains 2.5 mg·mL⁻¹ of solution. The maximum recommended dose of bupivacaine without epinephrine is 2.5 mg·kg⁻¹. As long as the number of mL injected of this solution is less than the patient's weight in kg, the maximum permissible dose will not be exceeded.*

### Ropivacaine:

Ropivacaine is similar to bupivacaine in its onset and duration of action. In contrast to many other local anesthetics, ropivacaine exists solely in the S isomer form. This results in a lower cardiotoxicity profile compared with bupivacaine.

### Cocaine:

Cocaine, a benzoic acid ester, exerts its action by blocking sodium channels and the presynaptic uptake of norepinephrine and dopamine. It has both local anesthetic and vasoconstrictor properties and can be used to provide topical anesthesia for ear, nose, and throat procedures. It is also commonly abused as a street drug and has a high potential for addiction due to its "dopamine brain reward" and euphoric effects. Intravenous and inhaled cocaine produces a more rapid effect than transmucosal application. Cocaine is a highly toxic medication due to stimulation of the sympathetic nervous system. Its use can produce hypertension, tachycardia, coronary vasospasm, myocardial ischemia, and infarction. Ventricular dysrhythmias, hyperthermia, delirium, intracranial hemorrhage, and seizures have also been associated with its use. Cocaine, like other ester local anesthetics, is metabolized by plasma cholinesterases. Cocaine has an elimination half-life of 60 - 90 min and is considered cleared in 5 - 7 hr (five half-lives). Metabolites are excreted in the urine.

**Prilocaine:**

Prilocaine is most commonly used as a topical local anesthetic. It is marketed as an equal mixture of 2.5% lidocaine with 2.5% of prilocaine in the form of EMLA® cream. EMLA® cream is applied topically in a dose of 1 to 2 g per 10 cm² of skin area and covered with an occlusive dressing. The onset of action is 30 - 60 min for superficial anesthesia and up to 2 hr for deep anesthesia.

**Local Anesthetic Toxicity**

Symptoms of toxicity occur when the blood level of a local anesthetic exceeds a certain threshold. The main determinants of the blood level are the amount of drug injected and the uptake by vessels near the site of injection. Toxicity is more likely to occur when a large dose is rapidly injected into or close to blood vessels.

Local anesthetics, such as lidocaine, produce predictable dose-dependent toxic symptoms. Central nervous system depression (confusion, sedation) and later excitation (e.g., seizures) generally precede respiratory and cardiac depression (Fig. 15.5).This sequence is less reliably observed with other local anesthetics, such as bupivacaine.

Early central nervous system symptoms may include perioral numbness, paresthesia, dizziness, tinnitus, blurred vision, and a metallic taste. As the local anesthetic plasma concentration increases, excitatory signs, such as restlessness and agitation, may occur. Further increases in plasma concentrations

can produce depressive signs, such as slurred speech, confusion, drowsiness and loss of consciousness. Finally, muscle twitching can occur as a precursor to a generalized tonic-clonic seizure. When rapid increases occur (e.g., inadvertent intravenous injection), toxicity may manifest as a sudden loss of consciousness or a seizure without any warning symptoms.

At toxic doses, local anesthetics produce cardiovascular depression, hypotension, apnea, ventricular fibrillation, and asystole. The mechanism of cardiac toxicity involves a direct effect on cardiac muscle cells, cardiac pacemaker cells, peripheral vasculature, and limbic structures of the brain important in central regulation. Relaxation of arteriolar vascular smooth muscle and direct myocardial depression can lead to hypotension. Sodium channel block of conduction fibers may result in a prolonged PR interval, prolonged QRS complex, or dysrhythmias, such as heart block or ventricular fibrillation.

A number of important strategies can be used to minimize the risk of local anesthetic toxicity. The maximum permissible dose ($mg \cdot kg^{-1}$) for the local anesthetic must first be identified (Table 15.2). The total dose to be delivered should be calculated and should be less than the maximum permissible dose. A vasoconstrictor, such as epinephrine (e.g., 1:200,000), can be added to the local anesthetic solution to minimize systemic absorption. Injection of the local anesthetic should be done slowly with frequent intermittent aspiration to minimize the risk of an inadvertent intravascular injection. Co-administration of a benzodiazepine (e.g., midazolam 1 - 3 mg *iv*) may be used to increase the local anesthetic seizure threshold.

Administration of local anesthetic must be stopped if symptoms of toxicity are identified. Local anesthetic toxicity increases in the presence of hypercarbia (increased $PaCO_2$), acidosis, and hypoxia. When seizures occur,

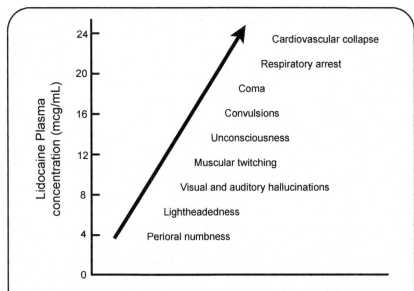

Fig. 15.5 Lidocaine systemic toxicity and plasma concentrations. Adapted from Neural Blockade. Cousins MJ, Bridenbaugh PO. 2nd Edition 1980. JB Lippincott.

basic resuscitative measures should be instituted. Apply oxygen, ensure airway patency, and hyperventilate the patient. Protect the patient against physical injury. Seizures are usually of short duration as the plasma local anesthetic levels decrease rapidly. Small doses of midazolam 1 – 3 mg *iv* or propofol 50 mg *iv* may be used for seizure control. A muscle relaxant may be required to facilitate tracheal intubation and prevent excessive increases in $PaCO_2$ secondary to muscular contractions with seizures.

In the case of life-threatening arrhythmias, Advanced Cardiac Life Support (ACLS) protocols are implemented. Lidocaine is excluded from the ACLS protocol in the treatment of ventricular arrhythmias. Lipid emulsion therapy with 20% Intralipid® is recommended. Intravenous injection of the lipid emulsion creates a lipid phase depot within the vasculature. This is believed to extract the lipid-soluble local anesthetic molecules from cardiac tissues. An initial bolus dose of 1.5 mL·kg⁻¹ of 20% Intralipid is administered intravenously over 1 min. A second bolus dose may be repeated after 3 - 5 min. A continuous intravenous infusion of 0.25 mL·kg⁻¹·min⁻¹ of 20% Intralipid® is maintained until the patient becomes hemodynamically stable or a dose of 8 mL·kg⁻¹ is reached. Arrhythmias from local anesthetic toxicity may be refractory to treatment and may require prolonged resuscitative efforts.

## Local Anesthetic Allergy

It is important to obtain a clear history of the nature of the allergic symptoms. Palpitations following local anesthetic administration may be related to an inadvertent intravenous injection of a solution containing epinephrine. Although rare, an allergy to an ester local anesthetic is more common than an allergy to an amide local anesthetic. When a reaction occurs, additives, such as para-amino-benzoic acid (PABA) and metabisulfite are commonly implicated. Cross-sensitivity may occur between the different ester local anesthetics as well as between ester local anesthetics and other PABA-containing products, e.g., sunscreen.

## Conclusion

Local anesthetics have diverse clinical applications and are used by a variety of medical specialties, including anesthesia. The safe use of local anesthetics requires a familiarity with their mechanism of action, onset time, duration of action, and metabolism. Clinicians must understand and apply strategies to prevent local anesthetic toxicity.

### Test your knowledge:

1. You are asked to suture a large scalp laceration in a 60-kg woman who has presented to the emergency department. Your supervising physician recommends you infiltrate the wound with lidocaine. What is the maximum permissible dose of lidocaine? What concentration of lidocaine would you use to provide local anesthesia? What volume of this solution can be given safely? Answer.

  http://www.anesthesiaprimer.com/AP/Ch15Local/A1.png

2. How can you minimize the risk of developing local anesthetic toxicity? Answer.

  http://www.anesthesiaprimer.com/AP/Ch15Local/A2.png

3. A young man arrives in the Emergency Department with malignant hypertension and coronary ischemia due to acute cocaine toxicity. How do you treat him? Answer.

  http://www.anesthesiaprimer.com/AP/Ch15Local/A3.png

4. You are called emergently to see a 40-yr-old woman who has a rash, facial swelling, stridor, and wheezing following dental extractions performed under local anesthesia. She has a history of allergy to PABA-containing sunscreen. Assuming this is an allergy to an ester local anesthetic, how would you manage this case? Answer.

5. http://www.anesthesiaprimer.com/AP/Ch15Local/A4.png

  Access the following link to view this chapter's clinical case presentation.

  http://www.anesthesiaprimer.com/AP/Ch15Local/ClinicalCase.png

### Additional Resources
### 2012 ASA Local Anesthetic toxicity Checklist

  http://www.anesthesiaprimer.com/AP/Ch15Local/ASRALAChecklist.pdf

### References:
Barash PG, Cullen BF, Stoelting RK et al. Editors Clinical Anesthesia 6th Edition, Lippincott Williams & Wilkins, Philadelphia, PA, 2009.
de Jong, RH. Local Anesthetics. Mosby-Year Book, St. Louis, MO, 1994.

# CHAPTER 16

# Regional Anesthesia

Daniel Dubois MD, Anne Lui MD, Desiree Persaud MD

## Learning Objectives

1. To gain an appreciation of the role and benefits of regional anesthesia.
2. To gain an appreciation of the spectrum of regional anesthesia.
3. To review the anatomy and physiology of neuraxial anesthesia.
4. To review the contraindications to regional anesthesia.

## Key Points

1. Epidural anesthesia can be used to provide prolonged postoperative analgesia.

2. Hypotension and bradycardia associated with neuraxial anesthesia are common and require prompt recognition and treatment.

3. Spinal and epidural hematomas are serious complications of neuraxial anesthesia.

4. Patients receiving medications affecting the coagulation system are at an increased risk of developing a spinal or epidural hematoma following neuraxial anesthesia.

5. Peripheral nerve blocks can be used to provide prolonged site-specific postoperative analgesia.

## Introduction

Regional anesthesia is the rendering of a specific area of the body insensate to the stimulus of surgery or injury. It can be used to provide intraoperative anesthesia, postoperative analgesia, or analgesia for labor and delivery. Regional anesthesia can also be used in the diagnosis and treatment of patients with chronic pain syndromes.

Cocaine was the first local anesthetic to be used for spinal anesthesia. In 1899, a German surgeon, Augustus Bier, injected cocaine into the spinal fluid of six patients having operations on their lower extremities.

Advancements in sterile technique, needle design, spinal anesthetic medications, and our understanding of the physiology of spinal anesthesia have improved both the safety and acceptance of this anesthetic technique. Spinal anesthesia is currently the regional anesthesia technique most commonly used in North America, and it is used widely in third world countries as a simple, inexpensive, and safe anesthetic modality.

The "physiological stress" response that occurs during and immediately after surgery is decreased by the administration of local anesthetic medications. Common adverse physiological reactions resulting from the neuroendocrine "stress response" to surgery include an increase in heart rate and blood pressure, activation of the coagulation cascade, atelectasis, and ileus. Left unmodified, these adverse perioperative responses can result in an increase in both morbidity and mortality.

## Table 16.1 Benefits of Regional Anesthesia

| Benefits of Regional Anesthesia |
| --- |
| • Increased patient satisfaction<br>• Reduced perioperative opioid requirements<br>• Decreased postoperative nausea and vomiting<br>• Reduced perioperative stress indicators (reduced catecholamines)<br>• Ability to monitor central nervous system (CNS) function in awake patients (carotid surgery, transurethral resection of the prostate [TURP])<br>• Maintenance of a protected airway and spontaneous ventilation<br>• Reduced incidence of postoperative thromboembolic events (deep vein thrombosis [DVT], pulmonary embolism [PE])<br>• Reduced perioperative blood loss (hip and knee arthroplasty, prostate surgery)<br>• Improved postoperative analgesia<br>• Cost effective |

**The Spectrum of Regional Anesthesia**

The spectrum of regional anesthesia includes topical anesthesia, infiltration anesthesia, peripheral nerve blockade, and central nerve blockade.

**Preparation for Regional procedure**

To deliver quality care and ensure patient safety, all patients having surgery require a preoperative evaluation (Chapter 3) and perioperative monitoring (Chapter 10) irrespective of the anesthetic technique used. Standard resuscitation resources (medications, equipment) and immediate access to oxygen and suction must be available prior to providing anesthesia care. Advantages and limitations of various anesthetic options are discussed with the patient prior to their surgery, including potential risks of the anesthetic technique as well as what the patient can expect to experience during and after the procedure. Developing a rapport with the patient helps to gain the patient's cooperation and facilitates performing the technical aspects of a regional block. The patient's understanding and acceptance of the technique is paramount for the success of regional anesthesia.

**Topical Anesthesia**

Various preparations of local anesthesia are available for topical use. They act by penetrating the mucous membrane, cornea, or skin surface to block sodium channel conduction and anesthesia. Cocaine 4% is often used for anesthesia of the nasal mucosa as it causes local vasoconstriction, shrinking the mucosa and facilitating local hemostasis. Lidocaine 2% jelly is commonly used for ophthalmic anesthesia and for urethral anesthesia and catheter insertion.

Common topical anesthetic creams include EMLA® and Ametop®. EMLA® is a eutectic mixture of 2.5% lidocaine and 2.5% prilocaine. Ametop® is an ester local

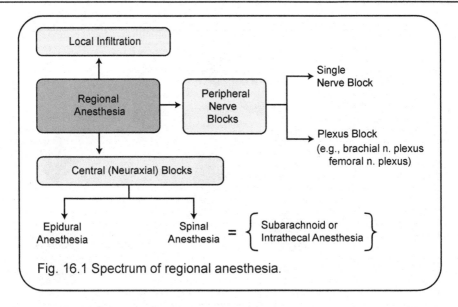

Fig. 16.1 Spectrum of regional anesthesia.

anesthetic containing tetracaine. EMLA® and Ametop® can be used for intravenous catheter insertion, blood sampling, and minor skin surgery (e.g., laser treatment, wart removal).

### Infiltration Anesthesia

Many procedures can be performed with local anesthetic infiltration. The local anesthetic medication is injected subcutaneously or into the tissues surrounding the area to be blocked. Local anesthetic solutions containing epinephrine (e.g., a 1:200,000 concentration) will prolong the duration of the block and decrease systemic absorption. When large areas are involved, a dilute solution will permit a larger volume of anesthetic medication to be used for infiltration without exceeding the maximal recommended dose of the local anesthetic (see Chapter 15).

*Clinical Pearl:*

*The maximum recommended dose of bupivacaine is 2.5 mg·kg$^{-1}$ (3 mg·kg$^{-1}$ with epinephrine). A 0.25% solution of bupivacaine contains 2.5 mg· mL$^{-1}$; hence, the maximum recommended volume (in mL) of this solution is equal to the patient's lean body weight in kilograms.*

### Intravenous Regional Anesthesia (Bier block)

Intravenous regional anesthesia (IVRA) is a simple and reliable technique used for procedures performed on the distal arm or leg and lasting less than one hour. Electrocardiogram, blood pressure, and pulse oximetry monitors are applied prior to performing the block. An intravenous catheter is secured in the nonoperative extremity to administer sedative medications and for emergency use, and a second small intravenous catheter is placed on the distal operative limb close to the surgical site. A tourniquet is applied to the limb and tested for its ability to abolish the extremity's pulse by maintaining a pressure of 100 mmHg above the systolic pressure. The operative limb is elevated, wrapped with an elastic (Esmarch) wrap to exsanguinate the limb, and the tourniquet is inflated. The Esmarch wrap is then removed, loss of arterial pulse confirmed,

189

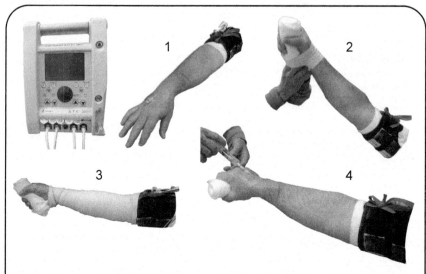

Fig. 16.2 Intravenous regional anesthesia (commonly referred to as a "Bier block"). Standard monitors are applied; an intravenous is established in the non-operative limb. 1. A double cuffed tourniquet is applied and tested on the operative limb. A small bore IV is inserted in the distal extremity. 2 - 3. The arm is elevated and wrapped tightly with an esmarch wrap to exanguinate the limb. 4. The tourniquet is inflated, the wrap removed and plain lidocaine is injected in the distal intravenous to provide operative anesthesia.

and a solution of 0.25 – 0.5% lidocaine plain (without preservative) is slowly injected into the operative limb's intravenous catheter. A volume of up to 40 mL (arm) or 70 mL (leg) is injected up to a maximum of 3 mg·kg$^{-1}$ of lidocaine. The local anesthetic diffuses from the venous vascular bed into the tissues to provide operative anesthesia within five minutes. Unintentional tourniquet release must be avoided to prevent local anesthetic toxicity. A minimum tourniquet time of 20 min is needed to allow adequate tissue uptake of the local anesthetic and avoid systemic toxic symptoms when the tourniquet is deflated.

## Peripheral Nerve and Plexus Blocks

Peripheral nerve blocks are accomplished by injecting local anesthetic medications adjacent to the peripheral nerves. Blocks may be used as the primary anesthetic technique providing painless surgery and postoperative analgesia. A thorough knowledge of the anatomy of the peripheral nervous system is essential to perform peripheral nerve blocks safely. The success of a block is greatly increased by positioning the needle as close to the nerve as possible before injecting the local anesthetic. When the tip of the needle is positioned next to a peripheral nerve, the patient may report a paresthesia, which can be used to guide administration of the local anesthetic.

Nerve stimulation for regional anesthesia has allowed the localization of a peripheral nerve without the need to elicit a paresthesia. An insulated blunt regional block needle and a peripheral nerve stimulator that generates a current to produce a motor response are commonly used to position the needle tip safely next to a peripheral nerve. Correct placement of the insulated needle is confirmed by observing muscle contractions within the motor distribution of the desired nerve with stimulation at a low current (0.3 - 0.5 mA) and a low pulse width (0.1msec).

More recently, ultrasound has been used to visualize the nerves and adjacent structures directly. Ultrasound offers a noninvasive, practical method to identify and target peripheral nerves, and it may improve the success and safety of regional blocks. The use of dynamic ultrasound is increasingly used to provide real-time visualization of local anesthetic administration and catheter placement adjacent to a major nerve plexus (e.g., brachial plexus, popliteal nerve, femoral nerve).

The most serious complications of peripheral nerve blocks arise from systemic local anesthetic toxicity and direct injury to nerves or adjacent structures. The prevention of systemic local anesthetic toxicity is discussed in Chapter 15. Key strategies to minimize the chance of an inadvertent intravascular injection are strict adherence to administration of less than the maximum recommended dose of local anesthetic, incremental administration, and frequent aspiration.

Recommended strategies to minimize nerve injuries include:
1. Aseptic technique
2. Minimal sedation
3. Use of specialized (short bevel) regional block needles
4. Avoidance of local anesthetic preservatives
5. Avoidance of high pressure injections
6. Cessation of injection if pain is encountered

## Neuraxial Anesthesia (Spinal & Epidural)

Neuraxial anesthesia refers to the administration of anesthetic medications into the epidural or intrathecal (subarachnoid) space. Contraindications to neuraxial anesthesia are listed in Table 16.2.

## Table 16.2 Contraindications to Neuraxial Anesthesia

| Absolute Contraindications | Relative Contraindications |
|---|---|
| • Patient refusal<br>• Coagulopathy<br>• Anticoagulation therapy (see American Society of Regional Anesthesia [ASRA] guidelines)<br>• Increased intracranial pressure (ICP)<br>• Allergy to local anesthetics<br>• Lack of resuscitative equipment and medications<br>• Lack of familiarity with the procedure | • Uncooperative patient<br>• Neurological deficit or demyelinating disease<br>• Significant hypovolemia<br>• Sepsis or local infection<br>• Fixed cardiac output states (aortic stenosis [AS], mitral stenosis [MS], idiopathic hypertrophic subaortic stenosis [IHSS])<br>• Previous spinal instrumentation<br>• Spinal deformities |

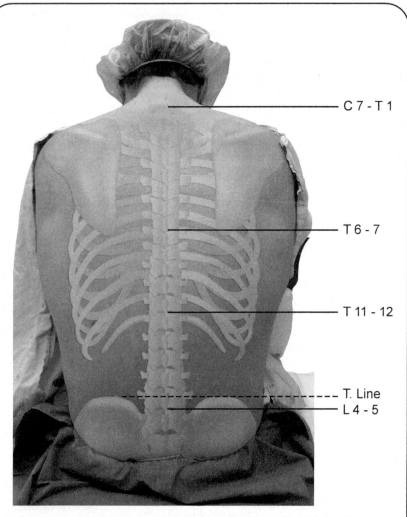

Fig. 16.3 Surface anatomy of the spine. Tuffier's line (T. Line) can be created by drawing a line across the superior aspect of the iliac crests. It passes through the L 4 vertebra and is commonly used to identify the L 3 - 4 and L 4 - 5 interspaces.

## Anatomy

The spinal cord consists of 31 pairs of spinal nerves (8 cervical, 12 thoracic, 5 lumbar, 5 sacral, and 1 coccygeal). Spinal surface landmarks are identified by palpating the spinous processes at the desired level of blockade. The three most easily identified spinous landmarks are the 7th cervical, 7th thoracic and the 4th lumbar vertebra (C7, T7, and L4 respectively).

When it is flexed, the spine of C7 is the most prominent spinous process in the neck. The 7th thoracic spinous process is generally at the level of the inferior tip of the scapula. A line drawn across the superior aspects of the iliac crests (Tuffier's line) usually intersects the body of the 4th lumbar vertebra (above the L4/L5 interspace). Tracing the 12th rib back to its spinal attachment can be used to identify the 12th thoracic vertebra. From these reference points, other levels can be identified by palpating and counting the spinous processes above and below the reference levels.

The termination of the spinal cord (conus medullaris) occurs between the 1st and 2nd lumbar vertebrae (L1-L2 level). Spinal anesthesia is performed below this level to avoid direct spinal cord injury from the spinal needle. The epidural space extends from the foramen magnum to the sacral hiatus. Epidural anesthesia may be performed at the cervical, thoracic, and lumbar levels. Flexion of the spine distracts the spinous processes, which increases the distance between them and facilitates access to the epidural and spinal space. Prior to performing neuraxial anesthesia, patients may be asked to curl up and round their back "like an angry cat" to open the spaces between the spinous processes.

## Neuraxial Physiology and Pharmacology

Refer to Chapter 15 for a discussion on the mechanism of action of local anesthetic medications. The action of a local anesthetic on spinal and epidural nerves is dependent on the size of the nerve fiber, the presence or absence of myelin, and the concentration of the local anesthetic. A concentration gradient occurs with the site of injection having the highest concentration of anesthetic and progressively decreases as the distance from the site of injection increases. Small unmyelinated fibers are blocked much more easily than

larger myelinated fibers. Sequential neural blockade proceeds from the small sympathetic nerves (fastest onset) to the large myelinated motor nerves (slow onset). This can result in a differential nerve blockade manifesting as a loss of sensation to temperature, light touch, and pain at different levels (Fig. 16.5).

### Clinical Pearl:

*Epidural analgesia may provide analgesia to pain (small neural fiber blockade) with preservation of light touch and motor function (larger neural fibers). Loss of temperature sensation is a more sensitive indicator than light touch when evaluating epidural analgesia.*

Local anesthetics injected into the subarachnoid (spinal fluid) space act directly on the unmyelinated "bare" spinal nerves, blocking sodium channels and nerve conduction. This results in a rapid and intense nerve blockade with a relatively small dose of local anesthetic.

The level and duration of the block is related to drug dose and spread of the local anesthetic. The two most influential factors affecting the height of block are the baricity of the local anesthetic and the patient's position immediately after injection. Baricity is the density of a liquid compared with that of the cerebrospinal fluid (CSF). Local anesthetic solutions that are denser, equally dense, and less dense than CSF are termed hyperbaric, isobaric, and hypobaric, respectively. Hyperbaric local anesthetic solutions tend to flow in the direction of gravity, settling in the most dependent areas of the spinal fluid. Hypobaric solutions tend to flow to the nondependent area of the CSF. Anesthesiologists control the spread of a spinal block by taking advantage of differences in local anesthetic baricity and patient positioning.

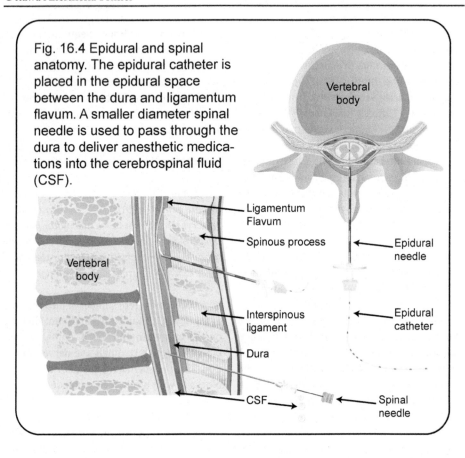

Fig. 16.4 Epidural and spinal anatomy. The epidural catheter is placed in the epidural space between the dura and ligamentum flavum. A smaller diameter spinal needle is used to pass through the dura to deliver anesthetic medications into the cerebrospinal fluid (CSF).

In the epidural space, the nerve roots are protected in a myelin sheath as they exit the spinal cord. Local anesthetics in the epidural space must diffuse through this myelin sheath to exert their anesthetic effect. As a result, epidural anesthesia typically has a slower onset and requires larger doses (5 – 10 times more) of anesthetic compared with spinal anesthesia to achieve the same sensory block.

Opioids are commonly co-administered with local anesthetics during spinal and epidural anesthesia. Extremely small doses of neuraxial opioids (e.g., 0.2 mg and 2 mg of spinal and epidural morphine, respectively) can provide profound and prolonged postoperative analgesia. Neuraxial opioids improve postoperative analgesia and labor analgesia and are discussed further in Chapters 17 - 19. The three most common spinal and epidural opioids used are fentanyl, morphine, and hydromorphone. Their clinical differences are presented in Table 15.3.

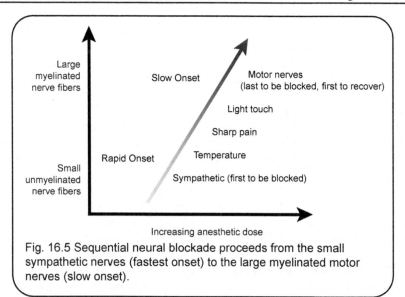

Fig. 16.5 Sequential neural blockade proceeds from the small sympathetic nerves (fastest onset) to the large myelinated motor nerves (slow onset).

## Table 16.3 Clinical Differences in Neuraxial Opioids

|  | Fentanyl | Hydromorphone | Morphine PF |
|---|---|---|---|
| Onset | 5 – 10 min | 10 – 15 min | ½ – 1 hr |
| Duration | 2 – 5 hr | 6 – 15 hr | 12 – 24 hr |
| Action | Level of injection | Intermediate spread | Rostral spread |
| Spinal dose | 10 – 25 µg | 50 – 100 µg | 0.1 – 0.3 mg |
| Epidural dose | 50 – 100 µg | 0.2 – 0.6 mg | 1 – 3 mg |

PF = preservative free. Rostral spread may lead to delayed respiratory depression.

### Cardiovascular Effects of Neuraxial Anesthesia

Hypotension with neuraxial anesthesia is a result of both vasodilation (arteries) and venodilation (veins). Venodilation decreases venous return and preload, and vasodilation reduces peripheral resistance. The incidence of significant hypotension with spinal anesthesia is estimated to be 30 – 40% and increases with general anesthesia, age > 50 years, and hypovolemia. Fluid administration and vasopressor support (e.g., ephedrine 5 – 10 mg *iv* or phenylephrine 100 µg *iv*) are commonly used to treat hypotension when the blood pressure decreases to > 25% below baseline or the systemic pressure decreases to < 90 mmHg.

Significant bradycardia is reported in 10 – 15% of patients receiving neuraxial anesthesia. It is more common with high thoracic blocks and occurs as a result of a vagally mediated decrease in heart rate secondary to reduced venous return (Bezold-Jarisch reflex) and

195

blockade of the sympathetic cardioaccelerator fibers originating from the T1 – T4 spinal segments. Risk factors for significant bradycardia with spinal anesthesia include American Society of Anesthesiology (ASA) physical class I, age < 50 years, first degree heart block, and concurrent use of beta blockers. Bradycardia is frequently treated with an anti-cholinergic agent, such as atropine or glycopyrrolate, if the patient's heart rate decreases to < 50 beats·min$^{-1}$. Severe bradycardia and asystole have been reported to occur with spinal anesthesia, and these conditions require immediate aggressive vasopressor and fluid therapy.

## Other Non-Cardiovascular Effects of Neuraxial Anesthesia

Neuraxial anesthesia is generally well tolerated in patients with significant respiratory disease. The primary muscle of respiration is the diaphragm, which is innervated by the phrenic nerve and originates from cervical roots 3, 4, and 5. Neuraxial anesthesia generally leaves diaphragmatic function intact. A small decrease (approximately 20%) in vital capacity occurs with the loss of abdominal muscle contraction during forced expiration. As the level of anesthesia progresses cephalad, there is a loss of sensation in the chest wall and patients may complain of a sensation of difficulty with breathing. Oxygenation is generally well preserved; however, in patients with severe lung disease, the loss of intercostal muscle use and abdominal muscle tone may result in respiratory insufficiency.

Neural blockade of the abdominal sympathetic tone results in a small contracted gut with active peristalsis due to a relative increase in vagal tone and may result in a faster return of normal gastrointestinal function after surgery. Neural blockade above the T8 level blocks innervation to the adrenal medulla and blunts the catecholamine "stress" response to surgical trauma. The loss of sympathetic tone may also result in difficulty with voiding and postoperative urinary retention. Peripheral vasodilation as a result of the decreased sympathetic tone may result in increased heat loss from the body and result in a lowering of body temperature.

## Neuraxial Technique

Neuraxial regional anesthetic procedures are performed using a strict aseptic technique with a hat, mask, and sterile gloves. After positioning the patient, clean the patient's skin with an antiseptic solution (typically chlorhexidine or povidone) and apply sterile drapes. Local anesthesia is injected into the skin and subcutaneous tissues over the area where the spinal or epidural needle is to be inserted.

A midline or, less commonly, paramedian approach is used to perform neuraxial anesthesia. Using a midline approach, the needle is entered between the spinous processes and directed towards the spinal canal. The needle is directed cephalad approximately 10 – 15 degrees and advanced through the skin followed by subcutaneous tissue, supraspinous ligament, interspinous ligament, and ligamentum flavum. Epidural anesthesia may be performed at any interspace in the cervical, thoracic, or lumbar spine. For epidural anesthesia, the epidural space is identified immediately after advancing the needle through the ligamentum flavum using a loss of resistance to air or saline technique. The epidural space is filled with discreet pockets of fat and veins. The veins are located primarily in the anterior and lateral epidural space and are essentially absent where the needle enters in the posterior epidural space. An epidural catheter is frequently passed through the needle into the epidural space. The catheter is then left in the epidural space and the needle is removed. Once the correct space is identified, local anesthetics, with or without opioids, are injected. Administration of local anesthesia through an epidural catheter permits slow titration of the local anesthetic into the epidural space. Intermittent aspiration is performed to ensure that the epidural catheter has not inadvertently entered a blood vessel or the spinal fluid. Slow intermittent administration of epidural local anesthetics is performed to avoid dispensing a large bolus into the spinal fluid or epidural vein. Catheter techniques may be used to maintain analgesia for labor pain or during and after major surgery. Continuous epidural infusions can be used to provide prolonged postoperative analgesia facilitating mobilization and physiotherapy. Patients receiving postoperative epidural analgesia with an epidural catheter are assessed on a regular basis by the anesthesiologist and acute pain service. In the postoperative period, patients are gradually weaned off postoperative epidural infusions over a period of several days. Prior to removal of the epidural catheter, oral analgesic medications are given to ensure adequate pain control.

For spinal anesthesia, an interspace below L2 is identified for insertion of the spinal needle. Spinal anesthesia is performed using a much thinner needle than the epidural needle, and the spinal needle is advanced past the epidural space through the dura and into the intrathecal space containing the CSF. The dose of local anesthesia for spinal anesthesia is generally about 20% of that used for epidural anesthesia, and because of the smaller dose of local anesthetic, there is essentially no risk of local anesthetic systemic toxicity with spinal anesthesia.

The use of ultrasound for neuraxial anesthesia is increasingly used to improve the success of spinal and epidural blocks. The University of Toronto has developed a free web-based interactive 3-D model to facilitate teaching clinicians the skills to use ultrasound for neuraxial anesthesia[A]. Their website can be accessed at http://pie.med.utoronto.ca/vspine.

## Complications

Misconceptions of the risks of epidural and spinal anesthesia are common amongst the public and the medical profession. The risk of a life-threatening or serious debilitating complication occurring due to epidural or spinal anesthesia is probably less than the risk of serious injury occurring when we drive in a car.

In experienced hands, the discomfort associated with the performance of most epidural or spinal blocks is comparable to that of an intravenous catheter insertion. The incidence of low back pain in patients who delivered vaginally, whether or not they had regional anesthesia, is not significantly different. In fact, patients with chronic back pain problems benefit from epidural injections of local anesthetics and steroids.

A    Niazi AU, Tait G, Carvalho J, Chan VW. On-line 3-D model to improve early ultrasound scanning of the spine. Abstract 1327726 presented at the Canadian Anesthesia Meeting June 2012.

## Table 16.4 Complications Related to Neuraxial Anesthesia

| Common | Rare |
| --- | --- |
| Backache (mild and self-limited) Hypotension Failure Postdural puncture headache (0.4 – 2%) Urinary retention | Infection (arachnoiditis, meningitis, abscess) Epidural hematoma Neurologic injury Total spinal anesthesia Systemic toxicity |

## Postdural Puncture Headache

One of the most common and debilitating complications of neuraxial anesthesia is a postdural puncture headache (PDPH). The incidence ranges anywhere from 0.4-2% with small bore non cutting needles. It is classically described as a severe, dull headache in the frontal-occipital region, which is exacerbated by an upright position and relieved when supine. It may be associated with other symptoms, such as nausea and vomiting, as well as visual and auditory disturbances. Measures to decrease the incidence of PDPH include using smaller bore pencil point needles, directing the needle bevel parallel to the ligament fibers, and limiting neuraxial anesthesia to older patients. For instance, young patients whose dura are accidentally punctured with a large bore (17G) epidural needle have about a 50% chance of developing a headache, while elderly patients do not seem to be prone to this complication.

The two main needle designs are the cutting needles (Quincke) and the pencil point tip needles (Whitacre). Cutting needles allow easy insertion through non-osseous tissues but have the downside of increased incidence of PDPH. Large-bore Quincke needles are typically reserved for patients > 60 years old, where the risk of a PDPH is much lower. The higher risk of PDPH is suggested because cutting needles transect dural fibers leaving a hole for CSF to flow out. Conversely, pencil point needles bluntly separate dural fibers and are thought to allow faster re-approximation after needle removal.

The natural history of the headache is that it will resolve spontaneously with time. Within the first week, 75% will resolve, and 88% will have resolved by six weeks. Bed rest, hydration, caffeine, and analgesics are the mainstay of conservative treatment. Patients who fail early conservative management may be offered an "epidural blood patch". The success rate of this procedure varies from 50-75% (see chapter 19)and results in quick resolution of the headache.

## Transient Neurologic Symptoms (TNS)

Transient neurologic symptoms, also referred to as transient radicular irritation (TRI), have been reported following lidocaine spinal anesthesia. The reported incidence with lidocaine is approximately 15% but ranges from 4 – 36% in various studies. Risk factors for TNS include lidocaine spinal anesthetic, lithotomy position, and ambulatory surgery, but not the concentration of the lidocaine used. Patient's typically report an ache or pain in their buttocks, lower back, or posterior thighs on postoperative day one. The symptoms can be considerably distressing, may be accompanied by abnormalities in sensation, and may persist for up to two weeks. Analgesics and nonsteroidal anti-inflammatory drugs (NSAIDs) have been used to treat the symptoms. The incidence of TNS following other

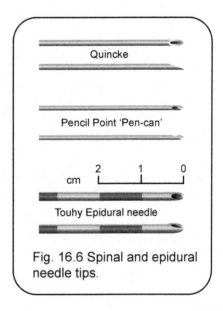

Fig. 16.6 Spinal and epidural needle tips.

spinal anesthetic agents, such as bupivacaine and ropivacaine, is < 1%.[1]

Although neurological injury is the most serious of complications, actual damage to a nerve root or the spinal cord is very rare. An awake patient will experience severe pain if the spinal cord or a nerve root is touched, at which point the clinician should withdraw and reposition the needle to avoid injury. Potential causes of permanent neurological injury include: direct nerve trauma, infection introduced into the spinal canal, a neurotoxic drug injected in error, or an epidural hematoma that develops and compresses the nerve roots.

## Table 16.5

| Risk Factors* for the Development of a Spinal or Epidural Hematoma | |
|---|---|
| platelet count | < 80,000 |
| international normalized ratio (INR) | > 1.5 |
| intravenous heparin | < 4 hours |
| clopidogrel | < 7 days |
| ticlopidine | < 14 days |
| Coumadin® | < 5 days or INR > 1.4 |
| low molecular weight heparin (LMWH) (prophylactic dosing) | < 12 hours |
| LMWH (therapeutic dosing) | < 24 hours |

*NSAIDS are not a risk factor provided no other anticoagulants are used.

An epidural hematoma is a rare and potentially avoidable complication. Early detection is critical because a delay of > 8 hr for decompression may lead to irreversible neurological deficits. Patients present most commonly with lower extremity weakness and later develop signs of cauda equine syndrome. Coagulation defects are the principal risk factors for the development of hematoma. The American Society of Regional Anesthesia (ASRA) published the third consensus statement in 2010 to assist anesthesiologists considering regional anesthesia in patients who have been taking medications affecting the coagulation system.[2]

### Regional Anesthetic Blocks

A variety of regional anesthetic blocks can be used as the sole anesthetic technique, in conjunction with intravenous sedation or with general anesthesia to provide prolonged postoperative analgesia. Common regional anesthetic blocks are listed in table 16.6. The mnemonic 'navel' can be used as an aid to recall the orientation of the neurovascular bundle in the groin when performing a femoral nerve block or catheterizing the femoral vein or artery.

Table 16.6 Common Regional Anesthesia Blocks

| Regional Blocks | Anatomy | Indications | Precautions | Side Effects |
|---|---|---|---|---|
| **Basic** | | | | |
| Topical Block | 3 mm penetration | Intravenous catheter insertion, minor surgery | Methemoglobinemia with prilocaine (EMLA®) | Vasoconstriction with EMLA®. Vasodilation with Ametop® |
| Bier Block (intravenous regional anesthesia) | Distal vein in hand or foot | Hand and foot surgery | Avoid epinephrine and cardiotoxic bupivacaine local anesthetics | Tourniquet pain may be reduced with a double tourniquet |
| Ankle block | Five nerves innervate the ankle: the saphenous, sural, posterior tibial, superficial, and deep peroneal nerves. | Foot | Avoid epinephrine | Altered proprioception |
| **Intermediate** | | | | |
| Axillary Block | Nerves around the axillary artery | Hand and forearm surgery | Musculocutaneous nerve must be blocked separately | Insensate and weak upper arm; support with a sling |
| Transversus Abdominus Plane (TAP) Block | Fascial plane between the internal oblique and transversus abdominus muscles, midaxillary line | Abdominal wall surgery. Useful alternative when epidural anesthesia is contraindicated | Bowel, liver perforation | Watch total dose of local anesthetic |
| Femoral Block | Insertion point is 2.5 cm lateral to the femoral artery at the inguinal ligament. Recall 'VAN' anatomy mnemonic. | Thigh and knee surgery | Hematoma: avoid pointing needle in medial direction towards the femoral artery | Quadriceps weakness, risk of fall; use crutches, zimmer splint |

Table 16.6 Common Regional Anesthesia Blocks (continued)

### Intermediate Blocks

| Block | Location/Insertion | Indication | Note | Complication/Comment |
|---|---|---|---|---|
| Popliteal Fossa Block | Apex of the popliteal fossa, also lateral and intertendinous approaches. | Surgery below the knee. | Saphenous nerve can be blocked for medial innervation of leg. | Drop foot, risk of fall; use crutches. |

### Advanced

| Block | Location/Insertion | Indication | Note | Complication/Comment |
|---|---|---|---|---|
| Interscalene Block | Insertion at the level of the cricoid cartilage between the anterior and middle scalene muscles. Blocks cervical roots. | Shoulder surgery | Consistently blocks the phrenic nerve and may cause respiratory distress in patients with chronic obstructive pulmonary disease (COPD). | Pneumothorax, Horner's syndrome, phrenic nerve palsy, weak upper extremity; support with sling. |
| Supraclavicular Block | Subclavian artery between the clavicle and the 1st rib. Blocks the cervical trunks. | Surgery below the shoulder. | Same as interscalene. | Higher incidence of pneumothorax compared with interscalene block. |
| Infraclavicular Block (coracoid) | Insertion point 2 cm caudad and 2 cm medial to the coracoid process. | Surgery below the shoulder. | Vascular puncture. | Lower incidence of pneumothorax; support extremity. |
| Paravertebral Block | Insertion 2.5 cm lateral to the spinous processes and 1 cm deeper than the transverse process. | Breast surgery, rib fracture analgesia, thoracotomy. | Pneumothorax, discomfort with multiple injections. | Unintentional epidural or spinal injection. |
| Sciatic Block | Anterior, posterior, and parafemoral approaches. | Above knee amputation. | May miss posterior cutaneous nerve of the thigh. | Weak lower extremity; support required for ambulation. |

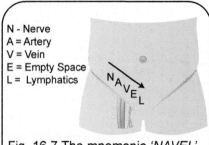

N - Nerve
A = Artery
V = Vein
E = Empty Space
L = Lymphatics

**Fig. 16.7 The mnemonic 'NAVEL' can be used as an aid to recall the orientation of the neurovascular bundle in the groin.**

## Summary

When choosing a regional technique, clinicians must consider relevant anatomy, patient positioning, choice of local anesthetic, physiologic changes, technical procedure, as well as proper patient education and consent. A careful risk-to-benefit assessment of regional anesthesia compared with alternative perioperative anesthesia and analgesia techniques should be considered. Appropriate follow-up after performing a regional block can facilitate a better understanding of the relative effectiveness of the block and allow early recognition of complications.

The lack of large randomized studies to show significant improvements in mortality or morbidity of regional anesthesia over general anesthesia has led to a continuing debate regarding the best type of anesthetic. Perhaps how well the anesthetic is administered is more important than the choice of anesthesia.

Regional anesthesia requires expertise and should be performed only under the guidance of a trained anesthesiologist. It is an important part of multimodal analgesia. The ultimate goal is to decrease perioperative opiate requirements and assist in the patient's early rehabilitation.

**Test your knowledge:**
1. Describe, in detail, how you would prepare a patient for regional anesthesia?
2. Describe the differences between a spinal and epidural anesthetic?
3. List the risk factors for a postdural puncture headache and describe how the condition is managed.
4. List 5 complications of regional nerve blocks.

**References:**
1. Cochrane Anaesthesia Group. Transient neurologic symptoms (TNS) following spinal anaesthesia with lidocaine versus other local anaesthetics. Published Online 15 April 2009.
   http://onlinelibrary.wiley.com/doi/10.1002/14651858.CD003006.pub3/pdf
2. Horlocker TT, Wedel DJ, Rowlingson JC et al. Regional anesthesia in the patient receiving antithrombotic or thrombolytic therapy. American Society of Regional Anesthesia and Pain Medicine Evidence-Based Guidelines (Third Edition). Reg Anesth Pain Med 2010;35: 64-101.

**Resources:**
3. Hadzic, A. Textbook of Regional Anesthesia and Acute Pain Management. McGraw-Hill 2007.
4. Cousins, MJ, Bridenbaugh, PO. Neural Blockade in Clinical Anesthesia and Management of Pain. Third edition 1997. Philadelphia, PA: Lipincott-Raven.
5. Morgan, GE. et al. Clinical Anesthesiology Fourth edition 2006. U.S.A : Mcgraw-Hill.
6. Barash, PG. et al. Clinical Anesthesia Sixth edition 2009. Philadelphia, PA: Lippincott Williams & Wilkins.

**Recommended URL Resources:**
www.nysora.com
www.usra.ca

# CHAPTER 17

# Acute Pain Management

John Penning MD, Doris Leung MD

## Learning Objectives

1. To gain an understanding of the anesthesiologist's role in hospital-based acute pain management.
2. To acquire a basic understanding of the pathophysiology of acute pain.
3. To gain an understanding of the concepts of multimodal analgesia and the ladder approach to acute pain management.
4. To be conversant with the role of more advanced acute pain modalities, such as patient controlled intravenous opioids, neuraxial opioids, and epidural infusions.

## Key Points

1. The quality and effectiveness of acute pain control in trauma and surgery is directly related to patient outcomes. Poor pain control not only leads to unnecessary suffering but also adds to the financial burden of the health care system.

2. Multimodal analgesia refers to the use of different classes of drugs to optimize analgesia while minimizing individual drug side-effects.

3. Foundational analgesics include acetaminophen and non-steroidal anti-inflammatory drugs (NSAIDs). They form the first step in the analgesic ladder for acute pain. They should be the first drugs to be introduced and the last to be discontinued when treating acute pain.

4. COX-2 inhibitors (e.g., celecoxib) have no effect on platelet function and cause less gastric upset and ulceration when compared with non-selective NSAIDs.

5. Tramadol or tapentadol are currently the most logical "step two" analgesics for treating acute pain in many patients. They provide analgesia with less respiratory depression and constipation than standard opioid medications.

6.   Codeine is a prodrug of morphine. Genetic polymorphisms of the CYP450/2D6 system result in a vast range of morphine blood levels in different patients.

7.   Pronociceptive modulation is an important concept that can result in the phenomena of hyperalgesia, opioid tolerance, and opioid-induced hyperalgesia. In certain patients, it plays an important role in exacerbating acute pain. New classes of drugs, such as N-Methyl-D-aspartate (NMDA) antagonists (e.g., ketamine) and gabapentinoids (e.g., pregabalin, gabapentin) can be used to reverse the pronociceptive hyperalgesia and improve pain control.

## Introduction

There have been tremendous improvements in our understanding and management of acute pain for hospitalized patients in the last 30 years. New and effective treatment modalities include intravenous opioid patient-controlled analgesia (PCA), neuraxial opioids, and continuous epidural and regional plexus catheter infusions. In the late 1980s, acute pain services were developed under the direction of departments of anesthesiology at leading health care centers worldwide. We now understand that control of acute pain improves patient satisfaction, shortens hospital stay, and improves patient outcomes. Poorly controlled pain is casually related to perioperative morbidity and mortality. Investing in acute pain management is a cost-effective strategy for hospitals, and it benefits the patient and society as a whole.

In the last few decades, tertiary health care centers worldwide have enlisted the assistance of acute pain services (APS) to manage pain after major surgery and trauma. This initiative has been spurred by various national health guidelines and anesthesiology association guidelines that recognize how quality pain control after surgery and trauma plays a key role in achieving rapid patient convalescence, earlier discharge, and a potential reduction in the incidence of post-surgical chronic pain.

## Acute Pain Neuronal Pathways and Mechanisms

**Nociception** refers to the detection, transduction, and transmission of noxious stimuli that are perceived in the brain as pain. A chain of three neurons links the periphery to the brain. The first neuron, i.e., the primary afferent nociceptive neuron, courses from the periphery to the spinal nerve root and into the spinal cord. It synapses in the spinal cord with a second-order afferent nociceptive neuron located in the substantia gelatinosa of the dorsal horn. Axonal projections from this second-order neuron cross to the other side of the spinal cord forming the spinothalamic tract, which then projects up to the thalamus. The second-order neuron synapses in the thalamus with a third-order neuron that transmits to the sensory cortex where the stimulus is interpreted by the patient as pain. This simple unidimensional model provides the basis for our understanding of how patients perceive acute pain. There is tremendous variability among patients in terms of how nociception is actually perceived as pain. Pain experienced by a patient is never static or "hard-wired" but is dynamic and constantly changing over time.

Additional dimensions of complexity are required to explain the variability in a patient's perception of pain. The second dimension involves inhibitory pathways that modulate and decrease transmission across the synapses of nociceptive afferent neurons. This results in a decrease in the amount of pain perceived by the patient. These inhibitory neuronal pathways originate in the brainstem regions and descend along the spinal cord to terminate in the substantia gelatinosa, either presynaptically at the termination of the primary afferent or postsynaptically at the origin of the secondary afferent. The main inhibitory neurotransmitters involve opioid, noradrenergic, and serotonergic receptor mechanisms. These neurotransmitters have an antinociceptive effect and promote a state of analgesia. To help maintain balance and normal function, a third dimension facilitates nociceptive transmission. In this third dimension of pain, excitatory neurotransmitters are released and their actions are pronociceptive, promoting a state of hyperalgesia (increased pain). Hence, the degree of pain experienced is a balance between the pronociceptive and antinociceptive modulating systems. Although the mechanisms involved are complex, the important principle is that the system is dynamic and not static. This dynamic modulation of nociceptive signals is but one aspect of the brains neuroplasticity.

While the basic afferent nociceptive mechanisms are quite uniform, much of the variability in pain experienced by patients may be explained by the varied level of activity in the more complex dimensions of "anti" and "pro" nociceptive modulation.

To learn more about the pathophysiology of pain mechanisms, students are directed to a Web-based self-learning module at www.managingpaintogether.com/pathophysiology.

## Clinical Relevance of Acute Pain Pathophysiology

Inadequate pain control following surgery and trauma may increase suffering, morbidity, and mortality. Nociceptive activation of the neural "network" increases motor neuron and autonomic nervous system activity. The result is a predictable neuroendocrine "stress response" to surgery and trauma. The response is mediated through a number of systems, including the endocrine, metabolic, coagulation, and inflammatory systems. It results in the development of a hypercoagulable state that can lead to thromboembolic complications (deep venous thrombosis [DVT], pulmonary embolism [PE] and myocardial infarction [MI]) in the postoperative period. Further changes associated with the stress response include a decrease in immune function, an increase in metabolism, and a generalized catabolic state. These changes may impair wound healing, increase the risk of infection, and result in general malaise and fatigue. Sympathetic tone increases as a result of spinal and supraspinal nociceptive stimulation. This can result in hypertension, tachycardia, and an increase in myocardial contractility. The combination of an increase in myocardial oxygen demand in the setting of a decrease in oxygen supply (i.e., postoperative anemia and hypoxemia) may contribute to an increase in myocardial ischemia or infarction.

Other important secondary pathophysiological changes occur as a result of nociceptive activation. These include activation of motor neurons producing an increase in muscle tone, which may result in muscle spasms at the spinal level of the nociceptive stimulus. This can be seen as "muscle splinting" following surgery with spasms of the muscles of the chest wall and abdomen. Muscle splinting impairs the patient's ability to breathe deeply, cough, and clear secretions, which increases the risk of atelectasis, hypoxemia, and postoperative pneumonia. The muscle splinting is a reflex response to nociceptive stimuli at the level of the spinal cord and can be reduced with appropriate analgesic therapy.

## Assessment of the Acute Pain Patient

Approximately 5 – 10% of patients requiring acute pain management in the perioperative period have a background history of chronic (non-cancer) pain. These patients are frequently taking opioid and non-opioid medications to control their chronic pain. A pain history is a fundamental prerequisite to the successful diagnosis and management of pain.

The mnemonic "OPQRST" can be used to elicit a pain history. The letter O stands for the onset of the pain. The letter P stands for the factors that provoke the pain. Q stands for the quality of pain, which may be described as sharp, dull, throbbing, burning, aching, or shooting. R stands for the region the patient perceives the pain and whether the pain radiates or is referred to any other area of the body. S stands for the severity of the pain, which is documented by patients rating their pain on a visual analogue scale (VAS) ranging from 0 to 10 (0 = no pain; 10 = severe pain). The VAS score can be rated at rest or with dynamic movement. T stands for the treatments the patient has received and the patient's response to the treatments.

| "OPQRST" Pain History Mnemonic | |
| --- | --- |
| O | Onset |
| P | Provoking factors |
| Q | Quality |
| R | Radiation |
| S | Severity |
| T | Treatments |

A preoperative anesthesia consult should be considered for patients who have chronic pain and are scheduled for elective surgery. The Brief Pain Inventory self-assessment tool can be used to assess the nature of a patient's pain experience and the impact it has on the patient's life. Daily VAS scores of 8 – 10 are not unusual in chronic pain patients. This information is crucial in discussing realistic perioperative goals for pain management with the patient. A detailed analgesic history should include the total opioid use per day, the frequency and type of opioids used, as well as any non-opioid pain management therapies. Opioid tolerance is common in chronic pain patients and an increase in the amount of opioid provided in the postoperative period is often required. The patient's usual chronic pain medications should be continued in the perioperative period.

Realistic goals of analgesic therapy might include:

1. A VAS score at rest < 3 and < 6 with dynamic activity.
2. Pain control permitting deep breathing, coughing, mobilization, and sleep.
3. Patient satisfaction.

Repeated assessments following initiation of analgesic therapy serve to identify any adverse effects of treatment and provide an opportunity for patients to report their degree of satisfaction. Repeat assessments also provide an opportunity to fine tune treatments, ensuring the goals of therapy are achieved.

The most common reasons for inadequate pain control following surgery or trauma are suboptimal use of standard treatment options and opioid tolerance in patients with a history of chronic opioid use.

### Clinical Pearl:

*Chronic pain patients should continue to take their usual pain medications in the perioperative period.*

When escalating analgesic therapy fails to achieve adequate pain control, **re-evaluate the pain diagnosis** and entertain the possibility that escalation of the patient's pain may result from confounding surgical or medical complications. Common examples include a surgical site infection, dehiscence of bowel anastomosis, compartment syndrome, or unrelated complications (e.g., cholecystitis or pancreatitis). Surgical re-examination may assist in eliminating other confounding diagnoses.

Psychological, social, cultural, and spiritual dimensions of a patient also contribute and impact on the "total pain" experience of a patient. Allied health professionals may be able to offer new insights and expertise to optimize and manage this multidimensional aspect of a patient's pain.

## Pharmacological Management of Acute Pain

Two fundamental concepts essential to the provision of effective analgesia are *multimodal analgesia* and the *analgesic ladder approach* to acute pain management.

## Multimodal Analgesia

Time-tested historical principles of treatment include "First do no harm" and the "Cure" must not be worse than the "Disease". Simple analgesics, such as acetaminophen and NSAIDs, suffice for mild to moderate pain but lack the efficacy required to treat severe pain. They have an analgesic ceiling beyond which an increased dose only leads to increased side effects. Opioids are better at treating severe acute pain; however, their use is limited by their side effects. Patients have varying sensitivities to opioid side effects. Some patients with severe pain will experience serious dose-limiting side effects from opioids before benefiting from their analgesic action. A rational approach to the treatment of acute severe pain is the use of several modes of analgesia. The multimodal analgesic model combines drugs from different classes to optimize analgesia while minimizing the side effects of each class. In theory, the analgesic effect from each class of drug is additive or even synergistic, while their individual side effects and toxicities (which are distinct to each class) are minimized.

## The Analgesic Ladder for Acute Pain

The World Health Organization (WHO) first presented the well-known analgesic ladder for cancer pain in 1986. We base our modified analgesic ladder for acute pain on this original ladder.

The acute pain analgesic ladder has four steps. Step one, the **foundational analgesic** step on the ladder, is the introduction of acetaminophen and a nonselective nonsteroidal anti-inflammatory drug (NSAID) or cyclo-oxygenase-2 (COX-2) inhibitor. Additional steps on the ladder are built on top of this foundation of analgesia. Step two, classically referred to as the "weak opioid" step, is the introduction of several possible medications, including tramadol, tapentadol, low doses of regular opioids, and the old standby, codeine. Step three of the analgesic ladder is the introduction of increasing doses of opioids, such as hydromorphone, morphine, and oxycodone. Step four adds long-acting opioids, such as a fentanyl patch and extended-release opioids. Adjuvant medications may be added at any point on the four steps.

# I. Foundational Analgesics

## Step One of the Analgesic Ladder

Step one medications include acetaminophen and a nonselective NSAID or COX-2 inhibitor. Step one medications are referred to as the foundational analgesics. They form a foundation upon which additional medications and modes of analgesia may be added. They are the first medications to be started and the last to be discontinued. Historically, these medications were referred to as analgesic adjuvants and were used "as needed" (*prn*). We now understand the importance of using these medications on a regular basis. Compared with the use of opioids alone, they improve pain scores, especially during activity, and they improve patient satisfaction. Foundational analgesics will decrease the amount of opioids required to treat severe pain by approximately 50%. Foundational analgesics reduce opioid use and the associated side effects, such as sedation and respiratory depression. Care must be used when foundational analgesics are introduced after the patient has received significant amounts of opioids. The **late addition** of foundational analgesics (e.g., intravenous ketorolac) to relieve pain may significantly increase analgesia and place the patient at an increased risk of severe opioid-induced respiratory depression. Hence, the recommended approach is to provide a foundation of analgesia using step one medications either before or at the same time as step two analgesics are introduced.

### Acetaminophen

Acetaminophen has modest analgesic properties. It is well tolerated and is the first drug on our acute pain ladder. Its mechanism of action remains unclear but is thought to involve direct and indirect inhibition of central cyclooxygenases as well as activation of the endocannabinoid system and spinal serotonergic pathways. An intravenous formulation of acetaminophen is available in Europe and Australia. In Canada, it is currently available only in oral and rectal formulations. The bioavailability of oral acetaminophen is good at 63 - 89%, while the rectal bioavailability is more unpredictable and ranges from 24 - 98%.[1] Short-term dosing of acetaminophen is 325 - 1,000 mg every ($q$)4 hr up to a daily recommended maximum of 4 g in healthy patients. The dose should be reduced to 2.6 g daily for long-term administration. The maximum daily dose for children is 90 mg·kg$^{-1}$. The daily maximum dose needs to be observed in order to minimize the risk of potentially fatal liver toxicity. The dose of acetaminophen should be reduced in patients with active liver disease or a history of heavy alcohol use.

### Nonsteroidal anti-inflammatory drugs (NSAIDs)

The importance of NSAIDs in the management of acute pain following surgery has only recently been appreciated. Prostaglandins are ubiquitous throughout the body and play a key role in many physiological functions. NSAIDs work as antiprostaglandins. While their pharmacology is complex, their actions are somewhat more straightforward in the realm of acute pain.

Tissue trauma causes the release of lipid fragments from cell membranes. The production of products (e.g., prostaglandin E2) that stimulate and sensitize peripheral nociceptors result from a series of biochemical events referred to as the arachidonic acid cascade. NSAIDs block the synthesis of prostaglandin E2 by inhibiting cyclooxygenase. NSAIDs also inhibit prostaglandins involved with central sensitization processes and hyperalgesia at the spinal cord level.

A minority of patients will develop serious side effects from NSAIDs. The most common side effect results from a decrease in the mucous barrier of the stomach. This may present as dyspepsia or ulceration of the stomach and duodenum. While dyspepsia with acute NSAID administration is common, fortunately, serious upper gastrointestinal (GI) bleeding is rare when NSAIDs are used to treat acute pain for < 7 days. Fatal upper GI bleeding is a rare but well-known complication of chronic NSAID therapy.

The discovery of two major subtypes of the cyclooxygenase inhibitor, COX-1 and COX-2, led to the development of COX-2 selective inhibitors, often referred to as "coxibs". The GI risks are reduced but not eliminated with the

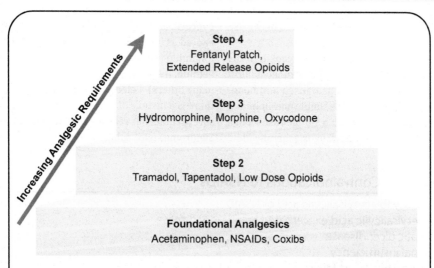

Fig. 17.1 The analgesic ladder. A foundation of non-opioid analgesics is the basis of pain management. Medications from step 2, 3 and 4 are sequentially introduced to control more intense pain. Based on the World Health Organization analgesic ladder used in the treatment of chronic pain.

use of COX-2 selective drugs. Platelet dysfunction appears to be mediated primarily through COX-1 inhibition. While nonselective NSAIDs may increase perioperative bleeding, selective COX-2 inhibitors do not affect platelet function, and from the perspective of bleeding risk, they can be used safely in the perioperative period.

NSAIDs impair renal function by inhibiting prostaglandin-induced vasodilation of the afferent glomerular arterioles. Risk factors that determine perioperative renal impairment with NSAIDs include elderly patients, hypovolemic states, exposure to intravenous contrast, and the use of angiotensin converting enzyme inhibitors (ACEIs) and angiotensin receptor blocking medications (ARBs). In hypovolemic states, the kidney maintains the glomerular filtration rate (GFR) by vasodilation of the afferent glomerular arterioles (a prostaglandin-mediated process that is inhibited by NSAIDs) and vasoconstriction of the efferent glomerular arterioles. The ACE and ARB drugs add insult to injury by blocking angiotensin-mediated vasoconstriction of the efferent glomerular arterioles.

COX-2 inhibitors and nonselective NSAIDs have received a lot of media attention concerning a possible increase in risk of thrombotic complications. These risks are extremely low but may be relevant in some patients using these medications on a long-term basis. For the vast majority of patients, the benefit of short-term NSAID use for acute pain management exceeds their risks.

Acetylsalicylic acid (e.g., Aspirin®) exacerbated respiratory disease (AERD) refers to the precipitation of bronchospasm and angioedema of the upper airway by acetylsalicylic acid. While this is a rare problem, the risk of acetylsalicylic acid cross-sensitivity with NSAIDs and COX-2 inhibitors may exist, so caution is warranted.

Is it safe to administer celecoxib in the patient with a "sulfa" allergy? Fortunately, most alleged allergies, such as nausea and headache, can be dismissed as simple non-immunological side effects. Even a simple rash from a sulfonamide antibiotic drug is generally of no concern, and celecoxib may be safely administered as it belongs to a different class of sulfonamide (similar sulfonamide class as furosemide, hydrochlorothiazide, glyberide and many others). Celecoxib is best avoided when there is a history of life-threatening allergy or severe cutaneous reaction (i.e., Steven-Johnson Syndrome) with sulfonamides.

## Table 17.1 Contraindications to NSAIDs

| |
|---|
| Allergy to acetylsalicylic acid or NSAID |
| Acetylsalicylic acid exacerbated respiratory disease |
| Peptic ulcer disease |
| Renal insufficiency |
| Congestive heart failure |
| Active inflammatory bowel disease |
| Pregnancy - may promote premature closure of ductus arteriosus |
| Bleeding disorders (COX-2 inhibitors generally OK) |
| Wound or bone healing may be impaired in at-risk patients |

## Table 17.2 Common NSAIDs and COX-2 Doses

| NSAIDs | Classification | Dosage |
|---|---|---|
| Ibuprofen | nsNSAID | 600 - 2,400 mg daily in divided doses *tid - qid* |
| Naproxen | nsNSAID | 500 - 1,000 mg daily in 2 - 3 divided doses |
| Diclofenac | nsNSAID | 75 - 150 mg daily in 2 - 3 divided doses |
| Ketorolac | nsNSAID | Only NSAID available in a parenteral formulation; 10 - 30 mg *im/iv* q6hr |
| Celecoxib | COX-2 inhibitor | 200 - 400 mg daily in 2 divided doses |

ns = nonselective.

## II. Step Two of the Acute Pain Analgesic Ladder

Step two of the acute pain analgesic ladder has traditionally been referred to as the "weak opioid" step. Codeine has been used as the classic weak opioid. Fixed doses of combination medications, such as oxycodone with acetaminophen (e.g., Percocet®) or codeine with acetaminophen (e.g., Tylenol® 3) have also been used as weak opioid choices. Several other drugs can also be considered as alternative weak opioid choices for step two of the analgesic ladder. These include tramadol, low doses of step three opioids, and tapentadol. An immediate-release formulation of tapentadol has recently been released in Canada. All step two analgesics have some limitations, making the choice of a step two drug more complex than the choice of medication for the first and third steps of the acute pain ladder.

### Tramadol and its inherent multimodal action

While tramadol might be considered a logical choice as a second step weak opioid, it is not suitable for use in all patients. Tramadol was synthesized in the late 1970s in an effort to create an opioid-type analgesic with less potential for addiction and fewer opioid side effects. Its analgesic efficacy is due in large part to its inherent multimodal antinociceptive action. It acts at opioid receptors and also inhibits norepinephrine and serotonin reuptake. Tramadol has been used extensively in Europe, Australia, and USA since the 1980s, and it may well be the most commonly prescribed centrally acting analgesic worldwide. There are intravenous tramadol formulations available in other countries, but they are currently not available for use in Canada. The oral formulation has been available for use in Canada for the last 10 years.

Tramadol's pharmacology is somewhat complex. Its three mechanisms of analgesic action are derived from distinct aspects of the molecule. The drug is a mixture of the S and R stereo isomeric forms that mediate norepinephrine and serotonin reuptake inhibition, respectively. Tramadol has poor affinity for the mu opioid receptor, rendering the parent compound devoid of clinically significant opioid activity. Tramadol's opioid efficacy is dependent on metabolism to an active metabolite. The enzyme responsible for this is cytochrome P450/2D6, the same pathway that demethylates codeine into morphine. In summary, tramadol trades in its opioid efficacy for its norepinephrine and serotonin-mediated analgesia. The result is fewer opioid side effects while preserving relatively good analgesic efficacy.

Tramadol is available in Canada in five oral preparations. Tramadol alone is marketed in Canada as Ultram® in scored 50 mg tablets. Tramacet® is a fixed combination medication containing 37.5 mg of tramadol and 325 mg of acetaminophen. Extended-release tramadol preparations are available in Canada in various strengths as Tridural®, Zytram®, and Ralivia®.

## The Pros of Tramadol

1. Reduced opioid side effects (e.g., reduced constipation, postoperativeileus, and respiratory depression). The reduced risk of respiratory depression may be especially beneficial in patients with obstructive sleep apnea (OSA).

2. Significantly reduced opioid abuse, diversion, and misuse compared with hydromorphone and oxycodone.

3. Tramadol is not a scheduled narcotic. As a result, physicians are able to phone in a prescription and are able to dispense physician samples.

4. Tramadol does not antagonize the actions of pure mu opioid agonists. Tramadol is not a mixed partial agonist/antagonist like pentazocine, butorphanol, buprenorphine, or nalbuphine.

## The Cons of Tramadol

1. Tramadol is a prodrug in terms of the opioid component of its analgesic efficacy. Like codeine, the parent compound has virtually no affinity for the mu opioid receptor and requires demethylation by the same metabolic pathway as codeine for binding to occur at the opioid receptor. Hence, patients with no CYP450/ 2D6 activity lose about 30% of the drug's analgesic efficacy (the opioid component).The norepinephrine and serotonin mechanisms are not metabolism dependent.

2. Patients may find the cost of tramadol prohibitive. The Ontario Drug Benefit program does not currently cover tramadol.

3. Tramadol has been associated with a serious and potentially life-threatening serotonin syndrome. Consider avoiding tramadol in patients currently taking other serotonin medications.

4. The maximum recommended daily dose of tramadol is 400 mg. Troublesome nausea occasionally limits the dose that can be tolerated. High doses increase the risk of serotonin syndrome and seizures.

### Tapentadol

Tapentadol immediate release (Nucynta-IR®) has recently been released in Canada. An extended release formulation (Nucynta-CR®) is also available for the treatment of chronic pain. Reports of its use are encouraging. The basic pharmacology of tapentadol is similar to tramadol but with some clinically important improvements.

Tapentadol is more efficacious as an opioid when compared with tramadol. It is a scheduled narcotic and is not a prodrug, and it has no active metabolites. It is a mu opioid receptor agonist and a norepinephrine reuptake inhibitor. Serotonin reuptake activity is trivial, removing the clinical concern of serotonin syndrome. Since a large portion of tapentadol's analgesic efficacy is mediated via its norepinephrine mechanisms, the relative opioid side-effect burden is significantly reduced relative to pure opioids.

### Low-Dose Potent Opioid Use in Step Two of the Analgesic Ladder

Another strategy for the second analgesic step is to use a lower dose of the step 3 opioids. A typical step 3 dose of hydromorphone for a healthy patient is 2 – 4 mg *po* q4hr. For this same patient, 1 – 2 mg *po* q4hr would qualify as a weak opioid level. The advantages of this strategy include simplicity and reliable efficacy. In addition, dosing can be easily increased to the step 3 analgesic level if required. The disadvantages include the risks of drug addiction, drug diversion, and potential overdose. Also, this leads to a substantial amount of potent opioids being sent to the community.

| The Pros of a Low Dose of Potent Opioid for Step Two Analgesia | |
|---|---|
| 1. | Simple and easy to escalate to higher opioid levels with the same drug if required. |
| 2. | Inexpensive. Covered by the Ontario Drug Benefit program. |

| The Cons of a Low Dose of Potent Opioid for Step Two Analgesia | |
|---|---|
| 1. | Higher opioid side effect burden relative to tramadol and tapentadol. |
| 2. | Addiction, diversion, and misuse in some patients. |
| 3. | Sending more potent opioids into the community relative to other choices. Diversion of medically prescribed hydromorphone is the most commonly abused opioid in Canada (greater than heroin!). |

### Codeine as a Second Step Analgesic Option: Codeine is a Prodrug and not a Weak Opioid

Codeine has an exceptionally low affinity for the mu opioid receptor, and its analgesic effect is dependent on its metabolic conversion to morphine. Codeine is referred to as a *prodrug* because it must be converted to morphine to exert its analgesic effect. Usually morphine is only a minor metabolite of codeine. In certain patient's, codeine conversion to morphine may be either reduced or enhanced. High serum concentrations of morphine can occur in patients who rapidly metabolize codeine, and several deaths have been linked to unexpectedly high levels of morphine after codeine use.[2] Many pediatric hospitals have removed codeine from their formulary.

The two major cytochrome P450 isoenzymes involved with codeine metabolism are the 3A4 and the 2D6 isoenzymes. Both are subject to genetic polymorphism, and both may have their activities increased by drug induction or decreased by drug inhibition. Under usual circumstances, 90% of codeine is metabolized to inactive glucuronides by the 3A4 isoenzyme process, while only 10% of codeine is converted to morphine by the 2D6 isoenzyme process. This means that an oral dose of 60 mg of codeine is converted to the equivalent of about 6 mg of parenteral morphine. However, the potential range is from as little as < 1 mg morphine to > 30 mg of a parentally equivalent dose of morphine.

Genetic polymorphisms in CYP2D6 are well characterized. About 10% of the Caucasian population have minimal 2D6 activity and therefore attain no analgesic effect from codeine. We have known this for about 20 years. On the other hand, the presence of

213

a genotype associated with ultra-rapid 2D6 activity, resulting in much higher rates of conversion to morphine, has only recently been appreciated. The prevalence of this 2D6 isoenzyme's higher than usual activity depends largely on the patient's genetic background. It occurs in 1% of patients of northern European descent, in about 10% of the Mediterranean population, and in up to 30% of east Africans. In the context of our modern global village, genetic heterogeneity in pharmacology is a significant clinical issue that warrants our attention in prescribing medications.[3]

## The Pros of Codeine as a Second Step Analgesic

1. It may be prescribed by telephone when combined with acetaminophen. The most common formulation prescribed is Tylenol 3 (codeine 30 mg, acetaminophen 300 mg, caffeine 15 mg).

2. Less diversion and risk of abuse compared with potent opioids.

## The Cons of Codeine as a Second Step Analgesic

1. Prodrug issues: Large variability in rate of conversion to morphine makes analgesic efficacy and side effects quite varied. It helps if the patient is able to relate their past experience with codeine medications.

2. Highly constipating, which is a huge issue for many elderly patients.

3. Opioid efficacy is limited by the maximum dose of acetaminophen when prescribed as a combination drug.

4. May still require a more potent opioid in the setting of severe pain.

5. Concern over acetaminophen toxicity when combination drugs are used.

**Oxycodone-acetaminophen combination**

Oxycodone is a potent oral opioid but can be used as a weak opioid option when a modest dose is combined with acetaminophen (e.g., oxycodone 5 mg with acetaminophen 325 mg). This combination drug is commercially available as Percocet®. Oxycodone 5 mg is equivalent to approximately 60 mg of codeine. Hence, two tablets of Percocet® have twice the opioid effect of two tablets of Tylenol 3.

Oxycodone is available only as an oral medication. Like codeine, oxycodone undergoes metabolism in the liver by cytochrome P450 enzymes to its active metabolite oxymorphone; however, the conversion of oxymorphone may be more reliable when compared with the conversion of codeine. Oxymorphone is ten-times as potent as its parent drug.

## Pros of Choosing Oxycodone-acetaminophen as a Second Step Analgesic

1. Greater opioid efficacy compared with codeine-acetaminophen.

## Cons of Choosing Oxycodone-acetaminophen as a Second Step Analgesic

1. Too potent for many patients, especially the elderly. If the elderly patient divides the dose in half, the acetaminophen dose received will be less than the recommended dose.

2. Diversion and misuse common. Oxycodone-acetaminophen tablets are are a popular street drug, commonly referred to as "percs".

3. Acetaminophen toxicity becomes a concern in patients taking more than the recommended dose of Percocet®.

## Step Three of the Analgesic Ladder: Strong Opioids

Opioids operate at several levels in the nervous system. Firstly, they directly dampen spinal nociceptive transmission across the synapse between primary and secondary nociceptive afferent neurons. This occurs in the dorsal horn of the spinal cord by binding to presynaptic, postsynaptic, and interneuron opioid receptors in the substantia gelatinosa. Secondly, opioids also activate noradrenergic and serotonergic inhibitory modulatory pathways that originate in the brainstem (periaqueductal grey matter) and travel down the spinal cord. They terminate pre and post synaptically on afferent nociceptive neurons in the dorsal horn of the spinal cord, releasing inhibitory neurotransmitters, such as noradrenaline, serotonin, and GABA. Thirdly, opioids modulate mood and anxiety via opioid receptors in the limbic regions of the brain. This helps alleviate the suffering component of the perceived pain. Finally, opioid receptors located in peripheral tissues, such as skin and synovial tissue inside joints, have been shown to mediate some analgesic effects in states of inflammation.

Foundational analgesics and weak opioids (step one and step two analgesics) are generally inadequate in controlling moderate to severe pain. Higher doses of opioids, such as hydromorphone, morphine, and oxycodone are commonly used to achieve analgesia in patients with severe pain.

The Institute of Safe Medication Practice (ISMP) has identified opioids as a high-risk medication, as errors in identification and dosage have been shown to have serious consequences. In this context, it may be reasonable for an institution to standardize the use of either hydromorphone or morphine as their default standard strong opioid. Hydromorphone has some advantages in that it has a more rapid onset than morphine. It is associated with less pruritus, has fewer issues with active metabolites, and hence, may be better tolerated in the elderly.

Recommended starting dosages for an opioid naïve patient suffering from moderate to severe pain are:

| | |
|---|---|
| • Hydromorphone 2 mg tablet | 1 to 2 tablets $q$4 hr |
| • Morphine 10 mg tablet | 1 to 2 tablets $q$4 hr |
| • Oxycodone 5 mg tablet | 1 to 2 tablets $q$4 hr |

The potency ratio of hydromorphone to oxycodone to morphine is 2:5:10. Elderly patients who are opioid naïve should be started at 50% of the above recommended doses.

The Ottawa Hospital Acute Pain Service opioid conversion chart offers a convenient reference for the conversion of oral and intravenous doses of hydromorphone, oxycodone, and morphine; See URL link at end of the chapter.

## Prescribing for the Analgesic Ladder

One of the disadvantages of multimodal analgesia is the complexity of drug regimens.

Ideally, drug regimens should be simple for the physicians to order and easy for nurses and patients to follow. Avoiding combination drugs helps keep things simple. In general, foundational analgesics (acetaminophen, NSAIDs, COX-2 inhibitors) should not be ordered on an as needed basis (*prn*). Below is an example of analgesic orders for an average, fit, opioid naïve patient having moderate to severe pain. This regimen should work well when combined with nursing and patient education. Dosages may need to be decreased for the elderly.

## Afferent Pathways of Nociceptive Transmission

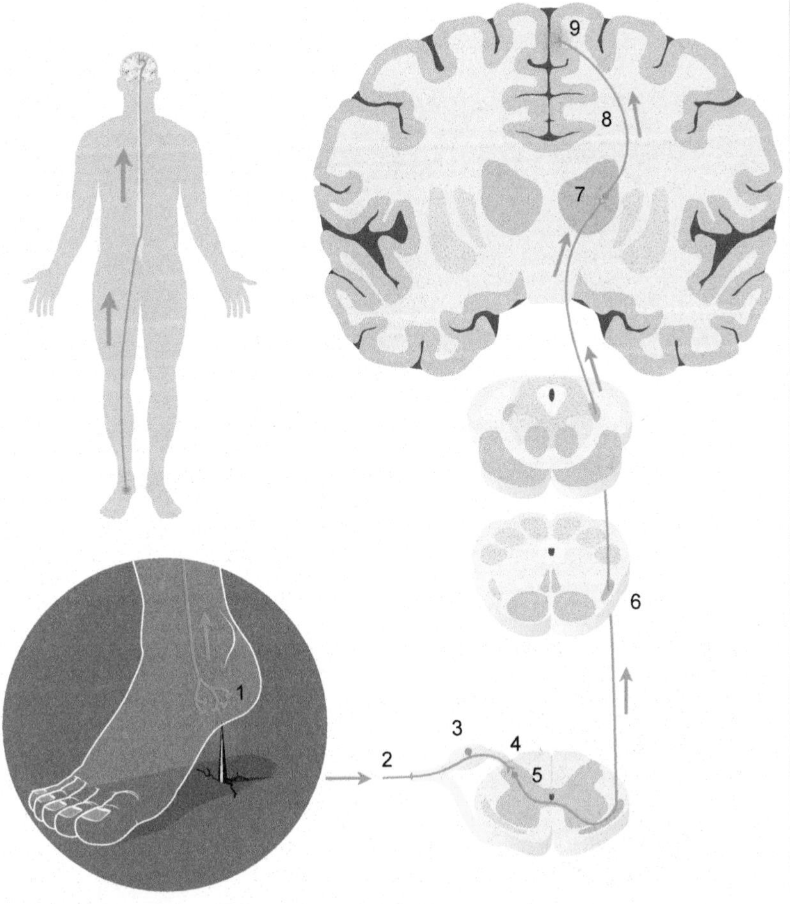

Fig. 17.2 Afferent nociceptive pathways. Adapted from Lubenow TR, Ivankovich AD, Barkin RL: Management of acute postoperative pain; in Clinical Anesthesia 5th ed., JB Lippincott, Philadelphia 2006; 1406.

1 = Peripheral nociceptor
2 = Peripheral primary afferent neurons (A delta and C fibers)
3 = Dorsal root ganglion
4 = Dorsal horn
5 = Second order neurons
6 = Spinothalamic tract
7 = Thalamus
8 = Third order neurons
9 = Sensory cortex

## Efferent Modulating Pathways

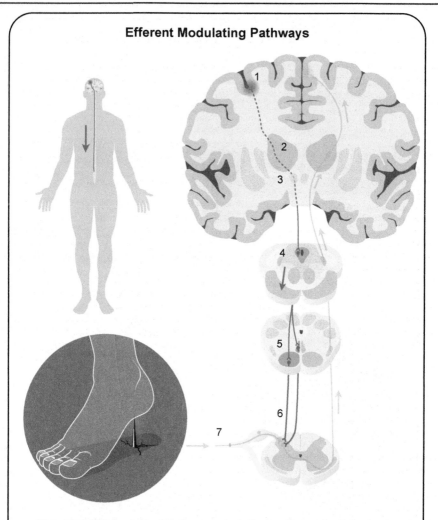

Fig. 17.3 Efferent modulating nociceptive pathways originate in the cerebral cortex and brainstem nuclei. Adapted from Lubenow TR, Ivankovich AD, Barkin RL: Management of acute postoperative pain; in Clinical Anesthesia 5th ed., JB Lippincott, Philadelphia 2006; 1409.

1 = Cerebral cortex
2 = Thalamus
3 = Hippocampus
4 = Periaqueductal grey
5 = Reticular formation
6 = Dorsolateral fasciculus
7 = Nociceptive neuron

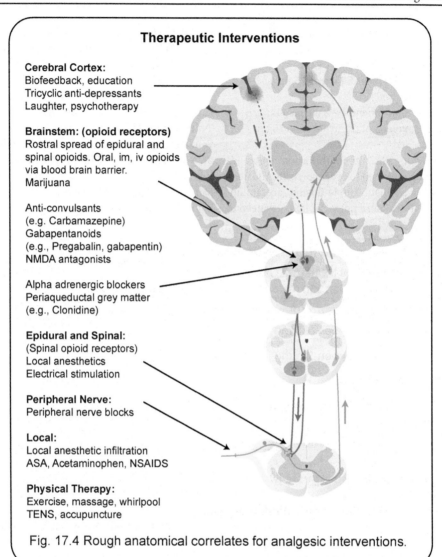

**Therapeutic Interventions**

**Cerebral Cortex:**
Biofeedback, education
Tricyclic anti-depressants
Laughter, psychotherapy

**Brainstem: (opioid receptors)**
Rostral spread of epidural and
spinal opioids. Oral, im, iv opioids
via blood brain barrier.
Marijuana

Anti-convulsants
(e.g. Carbamazepine)
Gabapentanoids
(e.g., Pregabalin, gabapentin)
NMDA antagonists

Alpha adrenergic blockers
Periaqueductal grey matter
(e.g., Clonidine)

**Epidural and Spinal:**
(Spinal opioid receptors)
Local anesthetics
Electrical stimulation

**Peripheral Nerve:**
Peripheral nerve blocks

**Local:**
Local anesthetic infiltration
ASA, Acetaminophen, NSAIDS

**Physical Therapy:**
Exercise, massage, whirlpool
TENS, accupuncture

Fig. 17.4 Rough anatomical correlates for analgesic interventions.

1. Acetaminophen 1,000 mg po q6hr
2. Naproxen 250 mg *po tid* with meals **OR** celecoxib 200 mg *po q*12hr
3. Tramadol 25 or 50 mg or 75 mg *po q*4hr as required
4. Hydromorphone 1 – 2 mg *po q*4hr *prn* to supplement tramadol once 75 mg reached

Ironically, the combination drugs are more complicated to order correctly. You need to warn against "double-dosing" acetaminophen, also, a more potent opioid may need to be ordered in case the combination drug (e.g., Tylenol® 3 or Tramacet®) is not able to provide enough analgesia.

Below is an example of an acute pain analgesic ladder using a combination drug (CD). The choices of a combination drug are Tramacet®, Tylenol® 3, and Percocet®. Foundational analgesia is provided with either an NSAID or COX-2 inhibitor. The patient is instructed to take one of the four choices from the analgesic ladder below every 4 - 6 hr depending on the pain they are experiencing.

| Combination Drug (CD) – Hydromorphone Ladder |
|---|
| 1. Foundation of NSAID or COX-2 Inhibitor. (e.g., naproxen 250 mg *po tid* or celecoxib 200 mg *po q*12 hr) |
| **One of the following four choices every 4 – 6 hours as needed** |
| 1. Acetaminophen 650 mg |
| 2. Acetaminophen 325 mg + 1 tablet CD |
| 3. 2 tablets CD |
| 4. 2 tablets CD + hydromorphone 2 mg |
| CD = combination drug<br>CD choices = Tramacet®, Tylenol® 3, or Percocet® |

## Sophisticated Analgesic Modalities

### Intravenous Patient-Controlled Analgesia

Intravenous patient-controlled analgesia (PCA) was introduced into clinical practice in the early 1990s. Before this, patients with severe pain after surgery or trauma received opioids by intermittent intramuscular or subcutaneous injection. For the most part, it was a one dose fits all approach, with patients spending little time in the therapeutic range and most of the time either in pain waiting for their next dose or experiencing side effects when drug levels exceeded the therapeutic window.

The IV PCA pump is programmed so that the patient can self-administer small IV boluses of opioid on a frequent basis. The rapid onset of analgesia allows the PCA modality to respond quickly to conditions where breakthrough pain may occur (e.g. chest physiotherapy or ambulation). Intravenous PCA has been a huge improvement in optimizing patients' postoperative analgesia. The regular administration of acetaminophen and a NSAID or COX-2 inhibitor should still be used as a foundation upon which intravenous PCA therapy is instituted.

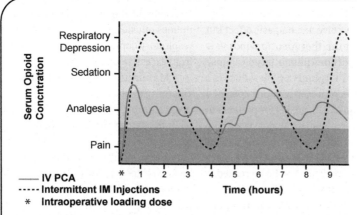

Fig. 17.5 Wide fluctuations in serum opioid concentrations are associated with intermittent intramuscular administration. This results in periods of over-sedation alternating with periods of poor pain control. By contrast, intravenous PCA opioid administration can be rapidly adjusted by the patient after surgery. This permits analgesic concentrations in the serum to be maintained for prolonged periods of time, avoiding excessive sedation.

Advantages of PCA Analgesia
1. Rapid onset of analgesia.
2. Reduced time waiting for a nurse to administer pain medication (assess patient, procure medication, and administer the drug).
3. Patient spends more time in the therapeutic range due to the elimination of the wide fluctuations in plasma opioid concentrations.
4. Adjusts to variability between patients.
5. Reduced medication errors.
6. Patients benefit psychologically when they have control over their analgesic therapy.
7. Avoids painful injections, which can be a huge issue for children.
8. Avoids risk of needle-stick injury to health care workers.
9. Improves patient-nurse relations (patients regard the nurse as a professional who is helping them optimize PCA use rather than someone who is withholding pain medications).
10. Improved analgesia permits more rapid recovery, better patient outcomes, and earlier discharge.

**The PCA pump parameters**

It is important for the patient with severe pain to receive an ample loading dose of opioid before the intravenous PCA pump is started. The administration of small IV PCA boluses will take too long to achieve the required plasma concentration. A typical loading dose of hydromorphone is 0.02 – 0.05 mg·kg$^{-1}$ administered over 10 - 20 min. Most postoperative patients receiving IV PCA will have received a significant amount of opioids during their surgery, making the loading step unnecessary.

**The Bolus dose:** This is the amount of opioid delivered when the PCA demand button

221

is pressed. The dose should be large enough for patients to perceive an analgesic effect but not so large that the therapeutic window is exceeded. For hydromorphone, a typical dose is 0.2 mg, and for morphine, a typical dose is 1 mg. Note that this represents about 20% of a typical *im* or *sc* dose. The goal is for patients to be able to maintain adequate analgesia with no more than 3 or so boluses per hr. If the patient repeatedly requires 3 or more PCA boluses per hr, the bolus dose may need to be increased.

**The Lockout Interval:** After delivering a bolus of medication, the PCA pump goes into a "lockout" mode. In the lockout mode, a "demand" is recorded when the patient presses the PCA button but no opioid is delivered. This feature ensures that enough time has passed for the drug to have an effect before a repeat bolus is available. For hydromorphone and morphine, the PCA lockout interval is usually set at about 6 min. For safety reasons, it is essential that only the patient press the PCA button. Family members and friends are strictly forbidden from pressing the PCA button. The lockout interval provides a degree of safety but does not eliminate the possibility of an opioid overdose, especially if the button is pressed when the patient is not experiencing pain. The pump records the number of demands as well as the amount of medication delivered.

**Continuous Infusion:** The PCA pump may be programmed to deliver a continuous opioid infusion. This programming mode is optional. Typical infusion rates are the equivalent of a single bolus infused over an hour. There is debate over the benefits of a continuous infusion with PCA. Proponents of this technique argue that it prevents patients from waking in the night with severe pain because they have not received pain medication for several hours. It may be particularly helpful with chronic pain patients already on long-term opioids who are not able to take their usual opioids by mouth.

However, in the opioid naïve patient, a continuous infusion may place the patient at risk of respiratory depression and other complications from excessive opioid use.

**Maximum One-Hour Limit:** This parameter provides an extra safeguard against a programming error. It also allows the physician to restrict the available dose of opioid to less than the bolus size multiplied by the maximum number of boluses permitted by lockout interval. For example, a hydromorphone bolus of 0.2 mg and a lockout of 6 min permits a total of 2 mg·hr$^{-1}$. The 1 hr limit may be set at significantly < 2 mg if desired. The pump goes into a lockout mode when the 1 hr limit is reached. Typical 1 hr limit orders are 80% of the potential hourly maximum. Patient-controlled analgesia pumps usually offer several time periods to choose from for the "dose limit". Some centers prefer to use 2 or 4-hr dose limits rather than a 1-hr dose limit. For purposes of safety and clarity, it is important that the center choose only one option.

Intravenous PCA therapy may be transitioned to oral opioids when the patient's opioid requirements are ≤ 2 boluses·hr$^{-1}$ and the patient is tolerating a regular diet.

## Neuraxial Opioids and Local Anesthetic Infusions

Neuraxial techniques include intrathecal and epidural injections. The highest concentrations of antinociceptive opioid receptors are located in the dorsal horn of the spinal cord. Administration of a small dose of opioid at the spinal level produces intense analgesia while reducing the extent of supraspinal side effects, such as sedation and respiratory depression. Opioids that are water soluble (e.g., morphine and hydromorphone) have an advantage as they reside within the aqueous cerebrospinal fluid (CSF) for up to 24 hr after a single dose injection. The intrathecal administration of 0.2 mg of morphine together with foundational analgesia (i.e., acetaminophen, NSAID, or COX-2 inhibitor) can provide excellent analgesia for up to 24 hr after major surgical procedures. A similar patient receiving IV PCA morphine might require > 40 mg of intravenous morphine in the same time period. Neuraxial morphine and hydromorphone migrate within the CSF to higher brain stem regions and produce sedation and respiratory depression. Supraspinal effects producing sedation and respiratory depression peak 6 hr after administration but can result in delayed respiratory depression for up to 24 hr. Careful monitoring is required for at least 6 hr following neuraxial morphine and hydromorphone administration. Single-shot neuraxial opioid techniques are well-suited for patients at low risk of respiratory depression. Continuous epidural infusion techniques may be better suited for patients with a risk of respiratory depression or sedation. The initial loading dose of opioid may then be reduced and analgesia maintained by a low-rate continuous infusion. Local anesthetics, such as bupivacaine, may also be added to opioids using the continuous epidural catheter infusion technique. An epidural infusion of an opioid and local anesthetic can provide excellent analgesia while decreasing the amount of opioid required. These catheters may be used for several days following surgery to provide prolonged analgesia.

Regional analgesia involves the blockade of impulse conduction in peripheral nerves by local anesthetics. Once again, a catheter is commonly placed to allow continuous infusion of medications in the immediate postoperative period. Details of these two modalities are described in Chapter 16.

## Above and Beyond the Standard Acute Pain Ladder

The basic ladder for acute pain (step one, foundational analgesics; step two, tramadol; step three, potent opioids) works well for the vast majority of patients. However, some patients will report inadequate pain control despite receiving foundational analgesics and significant doses of a potent opioid. In this setting, it is important to re-evaluate the patient to confirm that there hasn't been a complication of surgery that is causing the increased pain. Before escalating the opioid analgesic therapy, it is also important to consider the possibility of pronociceptive mechanisms at work creating a hyperalgesic state. Just as pain signals may be modulated down by antinociceptive mechanisms, they can also be facilitated by pronociceptive mechanisms. Chronic pain patients often have an imbalance with too much pronociceptive activity. Increasing the antinociceptive drug (e.g., morphine) may actually increase the compensatory pronociceptive mechanisms, potentially leading to even more pain (i.e., opioid-induced hyperalgesia). In these settings, it is more logical to wind down the pronociceptive mechanisms with anti-pronociceptive (or antihyperalgesic) drugs (e.g., ketamine, pregabalin, gabapentin). To view an analogy of this concept see http:www.anesthesiaprimer.com/AP/Ch17AcutePain/Analogy.png.

The appreciation of the existence of pronociceptive mechanisms that can counter or even dominate the antinociceptive mechanisms has been a major breakthrough in our understanding of how different patients with similar injuries have vastly different pain experiences. It also helps to explain how the experience of pain can change over time in the same patient. It has led to an important change in pain management.

Many drugs classically referred to as analgesic adjuncts or co-analgesics act as antihyperalgesic medications. Examples are NMDA antagonists, such as ketamine, dextromethorphan, and memantine. Gabapentinoids, systemic lidocaine, and clonidine may also primarily mediate their analgesic effects via

223

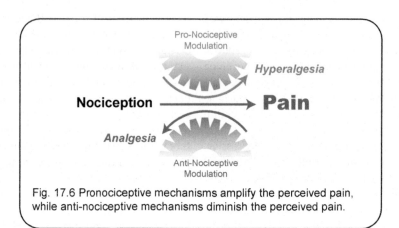

Fig. 17.6 Pronociceptive mechanisms amplify the perceived pain, while anti-nociceptive mechanisms diminish the perceived pain.

antihyperalgesic mechanisms. Herein lies an important principle. For these drugs to have any analgesic benefit, pronociceptive mechanisms that respond to the agent administered must be involved in the patient's pain. These agents don't work uniformly as analgesics in all patients.

Where do these anti-pronociceptive agents fit into the acute pain ladder? Once it has been determined that a medication is effective in treating a particular patient's pain, the medication should be administered regularly to provide a continuous support role to the foundational analgesics. For example, a patient with sciatica resulting from a prolapsed intervertebral disc could receive an anti-pronociceptive agent, such as pregabalin, along with acetaminophen and an NSAID for foundational analgesia. Tramadol could be added (step two in the analgesic ladder), and hydromorphone could then be administered if required (step three of the analgesic ladder).

## N-Methyl-D-Aspartate (NMDA) Receptor Antagonists

NMDA receptors are located peripherally and centrally in the central nervous system.

Activation of NMDA receptors by glutamate release augments the propagation of nociceptive information (nociceptive facilitation). At the spinal level, NMDA receptor activation results in central sensitization, leading to hyperalgesia and allodynia. Ketamine is one of the most commonly used NMDA-receptor antagonists. It is effective as an adjuvant in the treatment of pain associated with central sensitization, such as severe acute pain, neuropathic pain, and opioid-resistant pain. Ketamine can also be very helpful in treating acute pain in opioid-tolerant patients. These patients are frequently taking high doses of opioids and may have developed opioid-induced hyperalgesia. It is important to appreciate that the dose of ketamine required to mediate its antihyperalgesic effects is very low compared with the dose of ketamine required to produce sedation and analgesia on its own. A single IV bolus dose of 2 mg each time, or infusions of 5 mg·hr$^{-1}$ are generally effective. Psychomimetric side effects are generally not a problem at this low dose. Other examples of NMDA receptor antagonists include dextromethorphan, amantadine, and memantine.[4]

## Anticonvulsants

One method to facilitate nociceptive mechanisms is via excitatory neurotransmitter-induced elevation of intraneuronal calcium in the region of the presynapse. This is analogous to stuffing extra gunpowder into a shotgun shell. When a nociceptive action potential comes down the neuron, the extra calcium results in a more powerful depolarization and a more vigorous expulsion of nociceptive neurotransmitter across the synapse. Gabapentin and its newer analogue, pregabalin, were initially developed as anticonvulsants. They bind to the alpha-2-delta subunit of the voltage-dependent calcium channel located presynaptically on nociceptive neurons within the central nervous system (CNS). This action leads to a normalization of calcium levels in the pre-synaptic region of nociceptive neurons, thereby restoring the wound up nociceptive neuron to its normal neutral state of excitability. In meta-analyses, gabapentinoids have been shown to improve analgesia and reduce postoperative opioid consumption.[5] Gabapentinoids can be very useful in patients who have pronociceptive mechanisms contributing to their pain. Examples of patients expected to have pain facilitated by pronociception include those scheduled to have surgery on an area of the body affected by chronic pain (e.g., spinal surgery, joint arthroplasty, vascular reconstruction for ischemia, intestinal surgery in patients with inflammatory bowel disease). Patients with generalized chronic pain, such as fibromyalgia and opioid-tolerance, may also benefit from gabapentinoids. They are not suitable for mild pain where simple analgesics, such as acetaminophen, NSAIDS, tramadol, and low-dose opioids, would suffice. One of the prominent side effects of these drugs is excessive sedation.

Special attention should be paid while using these drugs in sleep-deprived patients, the elderly, and patients who are receiving significant amounts of opioid medications. Drug dosing should be tailored to the individual patient as drug binding has considerable variability between patients and can result in unpredictable responses. The typical dose for pregabalin is 75 mg *po* 2 hr preoperatively and 50 mg *po* *q*8hr for 3 - 5 days postoperatively.

## Concept of Total Pain and Non-Pharmacological Approaches to Acute Pain

Our chapter has focused on pharmacologic mechanisms and interventions in the management of acute pain. Other alternative means of pain control can be employed alone or in conjunction with the pharmacologic interventions outlined in this chapter. Psychological interventions (e.g., stress reduction and cognitive-behavioral interventions) may influence a patient's pain experience.[5] Useful techniques in managing pain include imagery, music distraction, biofeedback, relaxation exercises, and laughter. Physical agents, such as acupuncture, transcutaneous electrical nerve stimulation, application of heat or cold compresses, and massage therapies, may also help to alleviate pain.

**Pain is always a shade of purple.** Pain is a complex fusion of the physical aspects of the body (shades of red) and non-physical aspects of the mind (shades of blue). As anesthesiologists, we are body focused; however, no pain management approach can be complete without attention to non-physical factors, such as psychological, social, cultural, and spiritual aspects, that comprise the concept of "total pain" together with the physical factors.

**References:**
1. Clinical Practice Guideline. Acute Pain Management: Operative or Medical Procedures and Trauma. U.S. Department of Health and Human Services. Agency for Health Care Policy and Research. 1992.
2. Gasche Y, Daali Y, Fathi M, et al. Codeine intoxication associated with ultrarapid CYP2D6 metabolism. NEJM 2004; 351:2827-31.
3. Caraco Y. Editorial. Genes and the response to drugs. NEJM 2004: 351; 2867-2869.
4. Acute pain management: Scientific evidence. Australian and New Zealand College of Anaesthetists and Faculty of Pain Medicine; 3rd Edition 2010.
5. Managing Pain. The Canadian Healthcare Professional's Reference. 2nd Edition 2008. Roman D. Jovey MD, Editor. Endorsed by The Canadian Pain Society.

## URL Resources:
1. Prospect procedure specific post-op pain management. http://www.postoppain.org/frameset.htm
2. The Canadian Pain Society. http://www.canadianpainsociety.ca/en
3. International Association for the Study of Pain.
4. http://www.iasp-pain.org//AM/Template.cfm?Section=Home
5. Practice Guidelines for Acute Pain Management in the Perioperative Setting. An Updated Report by the American Society of Anesthesiologist Task Force on Acute Pain Management. Anesthesiology 2012; 116:248 - 73.
6. The University of Ottawa web-based self learning pain module can be accessed at www.managingpaintogether.com/pathophysiology
7. An explanation of the "Purple House of Pain" describing an overview of factors contributing to the patients' total pain experience was developed at the University of Ottawa. A short video explaining the "Purple House of Pain" can be accessed through the additional resources section.

## Additional Resources
The Ottawa Hospital Acute Pain Service Opiod Conversion Chart
http://www.anesthesiaprimer.com/AP/Ch17AcutePain/APSOpioidConversion.pdf

# CHAPTER 18

# Chronic Pain

Alim Punja MD, George Evans MD and Shona Nair MD

## Learning Objectives

1. To gain an understanding of the terminology used in chronic pain.
2. To develop an approach to the evaluation of the chronic pain patient.
3. To acquire knowledge regarding the etiology and management of common chronic pain conditions, including chronic back pain, myofascial pain syndrome, fibromyalgia, diabetic neuropathy, post herpetic neuralgia, complex regional pain syndrome, and oncological pain.
4. To review recommendations for the management of the chronic pain patient in the perioperative period.

## Key Points

1. A multidisciplinary approach is a key component in the effective management of chronic pain. This includes psychological, social, physical, pharmacological, and interventional therapies.

2. Pain pathophysiology involves many different receptors and pathways. Rather than relying on monotherapy, different medications are used to target different pain receptors and pathways.

3. Taking time for the proper diagnosis of a patient's symptoms is a key component in the effective management of chronic pain conditions.

4. Chronic pain patients often have tolerance to opioids and an increase in pronociceptive neural activity.

5. Realistic goals for postoperative pain control in chronic pain patients may differ from that in other patients, as their baseline visual analogue scale (VAS) may be significantly elevated.

6. Whenever possible, patients should continue their regular long-acting opioids in the perioperative period. Regional techniques, adjuvants, and additional (oral or PCA) opioids are used to provide acute postoperative pain control.

7. Patients on buprenorphine and Suboxone® require a coordinated plan to manage their pain in the perioperative period (refer to the advanced supplementary discussion).

8. Cauda equina syndrome is a surgical emergency and should be suspected whenever a patient develops saddle anesthesia, bowel incontinence and difficulty voiding.

## Important Chronic Pain Definitions: (see www.iasp-pain.org)

**Pain:** An unpleasant sensory and emotional experience associated with actual or potential tissue damage or described in terms of such damage. Pain is always subjective.

**Allodynia:** Pain due to a stimulus that does not normally cause pain.

**Central Pain:** Pain initiated or caused by a primary lesion or dysfunction in the central nervous system.

**Dysesthesia:** An unpleasant abnormal sensation, whether spontaneous or evoked.

**Hyperalgesia:** Increased pain from a stimulus that normally provokes pain.

**Hypoalgesia:** Diminished pain in response to a normally painful stimulus.

**Neuralgia:** Pain in the distribution of a nerve or nerves.

**Neuropathic pain:** Pain caused by a lesion or disease of the somatosensory nervous system.

**Neuropathy:** A disturbance of function or pathological change in a nerve: mononeuropathy (in one nerve), mononeuropathy multiplex (in several nerves), and polyneuropathy (diffuse and bilateral).

**Nociceptive pain:** Pain that arises from actual or threatened damage to non-neural tissue and is due to the activation of nociceptors.

**Nociceptor:** A high-threshold sensory receptor of the peripheral somatosensory nervous system that is capable of transducing and encoding noxious stimuli.

**Pain threshold:** The minimum intensity of a stimulus that is perceived as painful.

**Sensitization:** Increased responsiveness of nociceptive neurons to a normal input and/or recruitment of a response to normally sub-threshold inputs.

**Central sensitization:** Increased responsiveness of nociceptive neurons in the central nervous system to their normal or sub-threshold afferent input.

**Peripheral sensitization:** Increased responsiveness and reduced threshold of nociceptive neurons in the periphery to the stimulation of their receptive fields.

## Introduction

Pain is "an unpleasant sensory and emotional experience associated with actual or potential tissue damage or described in terms of such damage." Chronic pain has been defined as "pain of a duration or intensity that adversely affects the function or well-being of the patient" and/or "pain without apparent biological value that has persisted beyond the normal tissue healing time."[1]

Inadequately treated pain may lead to significant consequences in the physiologic, psychological, social, and economic domains. Patients may experience reduced mobility, loss of strength, disturbed sleep, increased susceptibility to disease, and negative emotions related to the increased co-dependence on caregivers or family members. The multifaceted impact of pain on the individual warrants a multidisciplinary approach to management. In addition to being seen by a physician, other specialties are often required to optimize patient care, for example, psychiatry, psychology, physiotherapy, occupational therapy, and social work.

## Pathophysiology

The complexity and plasticity of the nervous system are at times advantageous, but the changes that occur with chronic pain are more disadvantageous. Physiologic pain produces a behavior modification to protect the organism from further injury. When this response becomes inappropriate, exaggerated, and persistent despite resolution of the original injury, the pain response becomes pathologic.

The sensation, transmission, and response to pain are complex processes that are susceptible to modulation at many levels. Altering these pathways can acutely decrease or even abolish the pain response (Chapter 17). Persistent stimulation or inappropriate neural reorganization may alter the nervous system, resulting in abnormal pain perception (e.g., hyperalgesia, allodynia, dysesthesia, paresthesia). Part of this abnormal signaling may be due to peripheral receptor up-/down-regulation, windup, decreased central inhibition, or central sensitization. The exact reason why some patients go on to experience chronic pain is not well understood, but it seems that some patients have a pre-existing genetic susceptibility.

Nociceptors are primary afferent nerves that communicate thermal, mechanical, or chemical injury. Nociceptive input leads to an alteration in the ion channels and a change in the membrane potential. If the stimulus exceeds a threshold, the primary afferent nerve depolarizes and communicates its message with spinal interneurons, which then communicate with ascending tracts to supraspinal areas.

We now know that there are nociceptive stimuli, antinociceptive and pronociceptive pathways, as well as methods to modulate these pathways (see Chapter 17).

Medical management focuses on targeting areas in the peripheral tissues, the peripheral nervous system, and the central nervous system. These areas include the cyclooxygenase pathways (COX-1, COX-2, and COX-3), as well as opioid, serotonin, norepinephrine, cannabinoid, gamma-aminobutyric acid (GABA), and N-methyl-D-aspartate (NMDA) receptors. Sodium, calcium, and potassium channels are also involved. Unfortunately, medications used to target these pathways, receptors, and channels all have significant side-effect profiles that frequently limit their use.

Non-pharmacologic therapies include heat, ice, vibration, transcutaneous electrical nerve stimulation, massage therapy, physiotherapy, exercise, psychotherapy, and spinal cord stimulation.

Interventional approaches to chronic pain management include regional nerve blocks, epidural injections, neurolysis, neuromodulation, radiofrequency ablation, intrathecal pumps, spinal cord stimulators, and peripheral nerve stimulators. As no one therapy or pharmacotherapy can be expected to cure or completely alleviate chronic pain, the goal of medical and interventional management is to minimize pain, improve functional ability, and allow for other therapies to be effectively instituted. Functional goals should be set before initiating therapy, and the intervention or pharmacotherapy should only be continued long term if it provides improved function and has minimal side effects.

Previously, it was thought that opioids did not have a significant ceiling; however, reliance on these drugs as monotherapy or primary therapy has led to an epidemic of tolerance, hyperalgesia, addiction, diversion, and misuse. In the United States, the number of overdose deaths from diversion and misuse of prescribed opioids is now greater than the number of deaths from heroin and cocaine combined.[2]

If patients are taking more than the equivalent of 200 mg of oral morphine, current Canadian guidelines recommend subspecialty consultation. Chronic use of high-dose opioids contributes to many opioid side effects, including variable degrees of tolerance, depression, decreased immunity, hormonal deficiencies (hypotestosteronism), constipation, and hyperalgesia.[3] Current recommendations stipulate that all patients on chronic opioid therapy should undergo regular random drug screening to ensure compliance and that each patient should receive opioid prescriptions from only one physician.

## Evaluation of the Chronic Pain Patient

When evaluating a patient with chronic pain, it is essential to complete a thorough history. Often these patients have experienced pain for many years, so it is important to cover both the course of their symptoms and any treatments they have received over this time.

When inquiring about a patient's pain, the mnemonic "OPQRST" can be used to assess their symptoms (*Onset* - When did the pain start and what was the patient doing at the time? *Provocation / Palliation, Quality* - of the pain, *Region / Radiation, Severity, Time* - How has the pain evolved since its onset?). In some cases, the quality of the pain can help distinguish nociceptive pain (i.e., pain that arises from actual or threatened damage to non-neural tissue and is due to the activation of nociceptors) from neuropathic pain (i.e., pain caused by a lesion or disease of the somatosensory nervous system).

Nociceptive pain is often categorized as thermal, mechanical, chemical, visceral, and deep somatic or superficial somatic. Visceral and deep somatic pain is usually poorly localized, non-dermatomal and described as dull, aching, or squeezing. Neuropathic pain is generally described as burning, tingling, electrical shocks, stabbing, or the sensation of pins and needles.

The impact of previous treatments, including medications, alternative therapies, and interventional and surgical procedures, should also be evaluated. It is important to assess a patient's coexisting medical problems as their comorbidities will impact on the use of certain medications and therapies.

A chronic pain history also examines the impact of the pain on other areas of the patient's life, such as activities of daily living (ADL), sleep, work, and personal relationships. The Brief Pain Inventory is one example of a number of available tools used to evaluate these factors: The Brief Pain Inventory is one example of a number of tools available through the painknowledge/org/physician-tools website.

Patients should be screened for addiction to alcohol and street drugs to help assess the patient's appropriateness for possibly addictive pain medications. An example of an opioid risk assessment tool can be found at: http://nationalpaincentre.mcmaster.ca/opioid/cgop_b_app_b02.html. Patients should be screened for depression and mood disorders as these disorders are common in patients with chronic pain. Examination begins with inspection of the affected area followed by palpation, range of motion, strength testing, sensory changes, and special tests. Investigations are focused on evaluation of the underlying cause of a patient's pain to aid in providing the most appropriate therapy. A relevant musculoskeletal and neurologic evaluation should be performed when a new patient is assessed and when there are significant changes in a patient's symptoms. Urine drug screening should likely be performed in all new patients and intermittently in patients on established opioid therapy.

## Low Back Pain

From 60 - 90% of adults will experience low back pain at some point in their lives. Fortunately, most cases are self-limited; however, up to 30% of patients will go on to develop chronic back pain. Back pain is classified as acute when it lasts < 4 weeks, subacute when it lasts 4 - 12 weeks, and chronic when it persists for > 12 weeks. Epidemiological studies have identified multiple risk factors for developing back pain. Common causes of low back pain include both mechanical and non-mechanical causes (Table 18.1).

## Table 18.1 Risk Factors and Causes of Back Pain

| Risk Factors | Mechanical Causes | Non Mechanical Causes |
|---|---|---|
| Smoking | Muscular strain | Cancer |
| Obesity | Disc herniation | Metastatic disease |
| Heavy lifting | Spinal stenosis | Infection |
| Scoliosis | Facet joint arthropathy | Shingles |
| Multiple pregnancies | Foraminal stenosis | Inflammatory arthritis |
| Stressful occupation | Spondyloarthropathies | Paget's disease |
| Anxiety | Sacroiliac joint pain | Kidney stones |
| Depression | Spinal fractures | Aortic aneurysm |
| | | Epidural hematoma |
| | | Pancreatitis |

## Table 18.2 Red Flags in Patients with Back Pain

| Red Flags for Back Pain | | |
|---|---|---|
| Recent trauma | History of cancer | Age > 70 |
| Unexplained weight loss | Intravenous drug use | Focal neurologic |
| Unexplained fever | Osteoporosis | deficit |
| Immunosuppression | Chronic steroid use | Disabling symptoms > 6 weeks |
| **Cauda Equina Syndrome Red Flags** | | |
| Saddle anesthesia | Leg pain (sciatica) or | Urinary retention or |
| Bowel incontinence | weakness | incontinence |

Cauda equina red flags require emergent surgical assessment.

**Evaluation of the Patient:**

In additional to the usual pain history, the clinician should look for other red flag features associated with back pain (Table 18.2). Clinicians should inquire about bladder or bowel dysfunction combined with saddle anesthesia, leg pain, or weakness as these are symptoms of a cauda equina syndrome. If a patient has cauda equina symptoms, they should be immediately referred to a surgeon as this is a surgical emergency.

If the patient has radicular pain, the exact location of their pain should be identified as it can help distinguish which nerve root(s) are involved. The pain associated with spinal stenosis tends to be worse with ambulation (neurogenic claudication) and is generally relieved by sitting or spinal flexion (e.g., walking while leaning forward on a shopping cart). Facet joint pain is characterized by axial back pain or buttock pain (it may radiate into the upper legs but should not extend below the knee), and it tends to present as stiffness or aching. This pain is generally aggravated by prolonged sitting or standing and relieved by lying down.

**Physical examination:**

Inspection, palpation, range of motion testing, and a detailed neuromuscular exam is performed to identify any motor or sensory deficits. The result of the straight leg raise test is considered positive for a herniated disc if the patient experiences sciatic pain radiating below the knee at 30-70 degrees of elevation.

**Investigations:**

Patients with red flag symptoms require urgent imaging with computerized tomography (CT), myelography, or magnetic resonance imaging (MRI) to rule out systemic causes of back pain or cauda equina syndrome. Plain *x-rays* will help identify fractures, tumors, infection, spondylolisthesis, and osteoporosis, loss of disc height, malalignments, and scoliosis. Compared with *x-rays*, CT scans show a more detailed evaluation of bony structures. This imaging modality shows some soft tissue changes, including disc abnormalities, but it does not show the same degree of soft tissue detail provided by MRI. The main advantages of MRI are a better evaluation of the soft tissues and discs and lack of exposure to radiation. The main disadvantages are a longer scan time, greater expense, and reduced access to MRI in some locations. Identified abnormalities, such as a disc herniation, may not correlate with the patient's symptoms. Studies have shown that many patients will have some degree of disc bulging and herniation without having any pain. Electromyography (EMG) may be indicated in selected patients to help distinguish muscular pain from radicular pain or other medical conditions, such as diabetic neuropathy.

**Treatment:**

Initial management of acute back pain involves conservative treatment, as the majority of patients suffering from acute low back pain will have resolution of their symptoms within 4 - 8 weeks. Patients should continue to keep active, as multiple studies have shown faster resolution of lower back pain (LBP) when patients continue low impact activities. Patients may benefit from information regarding appropriate stretching and strengthening exercises to maintain movement, strengthen core muscles, and prevent recurrence. Others will benefit from referral to a physical therapist for more hands-on instruction and therapy until an appropriate home exercise regimen is established. Obese patients should be encouraged to lose weight as this has been shown to decrease the rate of recurrence. Patients should be counseled regarding smoking cessation as smoking is associated with an increased incidence of chronic pain.

Local application of heat or cold may provide relief in some patients. There are multiple treatments available for LBP, including transcutaneous electrical nerve stimulation (TENS), acupuncture, prolotherapy, traction, corsets, back braces, or chiropractic manipulation; however, there is little consistent evidence for efficacy of any of these modalities.

Nonsteroidal anti-inflammatory drugs (NSAIDs) or acetaminophen should be used as a first-line pharmacological treatment. Medications classified as muscle relaxants have not consistently shown effectiveness in acute or chronic low back pain, and many patients have difficulty tolerating sedating side effects associated with many of these medications (e.g., methocarbamol, cyclobenzaprine, benzodiazepines or baclofen).

Tramadol or codeine-containing medications may be a useful second-line pharmacological option when initial therapy with NSAIDS and acetaminophen is inadequate. Adjuvants that are especially useful in patients with radicular pain include gabapentin, pregabalin or tricyclic antidepressants, such as nortriptyline and amitriptyline.

Opioids should be a third-line therapy considered in patients who continue to have inadequate pain relief despite using first or second-line medications. For prescribing guidelines, refer to the "Canadian Guideline for Safe and Effective Use of Opioids for Chronic Non-Cancer Pain". Evidence exists supporting the use of opioids in the treatment of acute LBP; however, there is no clear consistent evidence of efficacy for long-term usage. When a decision is made to treat chronic LBP with opioids, there should be clear functional goals and an opioid contract with the patient is highly recommended.

The lowest dose possible should be used to decrease long-term side effects, tolerance, and hyperalagesia. When a patient reports poor efficacy or is requesting increasing doses of opioids and they have reached the daily equivalent of 200 mg of oral morphine, the effectiveness of therapy must be re-evaluated. Lack of efficacy may signify opioid tolerance, hyperalagesia, pain that is poorly opioid responsive, misuse, or divergence.

Other medications to consider include serotonin-norepinephrine reuptake inhibitors (SNRIs) (e.g., duloxetine, venlafaxine), buprenorphine, extended-release tramadol, tapentadol, and cannabinoids. Care should be taken when combining tricyclic antidepressants (TCAs), tramadol, and tapentadol with selective serotonin reuptake inhibitors (SSRIs) or SNRIs, as serotonin syndrome is possible at higher doses or when combining multiple medications.

If after 4 - 8 weeks the patient continues to report difficulty with activities of daily living (ADLs) or their ability to work as a result of persistent radicular pain, referral to a pain specialist or spine surgeon should be considered. Interventions, such as epidural injections, have better efficacy when performed early. Epidural injections or spinal surgery can be effective in relieving radicular pain but may not resolve persistent axial LBP.

Interventional treatments for radicular pain, radiculopathy, spinal stenosis, and failed back syndrome include epidural steroid injections (transforaminal, caudal, or interlaminar) or epidurolysis (for failed back syndrome). Current evidence supports the use of fluoroscopic needle guidance when performing these injections. Contrast dye is used to ensure that the medication reaches the affected area and is not injected into a blood vessel or outside the epidural space. When these treatments fail to treat the patient's symptoms, other interventional therapies include surgery, pulsed radiofrequency nerve root stimulation, and spinal cord stimulation. Patients with facet joint pain may benefit from intra-articular injections or medial branch block followed by radiofrequency ablation.

## Myofascial Pain Syndrome

Myofascial pain is a chronic condition that affects the fascia (connective tissue that covers the muscles). This condition is considered distinct from fibromyalgia. It includes "trigger points" in the form of localized tender areas containing palpable taut muscle bands. Common locations of trigger points include the head, neck, shoulders, arms, legs, and lower back with each site having characteristic referral patterns. An illustration of common trigger points can be viewed at the "Trigger Point and Referred Pain Guide" (http://www.triggerpoints.net/).

Myofascial pain may be associated with trauma or surgery but can also occur without an apparent inciting event. Symptoms include painful or tight muscles and may be associated with a limited range of motion. Trigger points can be identified by palpating the muscle and identifying "knots" or fascial constrictions. When palpated, they elicit local and referred pain that does not follow a dermatomal distribution (e.g., trigger points in the trapezius or rhomboid muscles are often mistakenly diagnosed as radicular neck pain).

Treatment includes stretching exercises, physical therapy, massage, manual therapy, and pain psychology. Acupuncture or dry needling has been shown to be effective, as have trigger point injections using local anesthetic, steroid, or botulinum toxin. Botulinum toxin injections have been shown to provide a longer period of relief compared with placebo or steroid. Other treatments may include ultrasound, laser, or electrotherapy. Pharmacologic treatment may include NSAIDs, tramadol, TCAs, or SNRIs.

## Fibromyalgia

Fibromyalgia (FM) is a rheumatological syndrome characterized by chronic diffuse multifocal pain and tenderness persisting for more than three months. Pain is typically migratory and waxes and wanes over time. Associated symptoms include sleep disturbances, fatigue, and affective dysfunction. Allodynia to digital pressure at 11 or more of 18 anatomically defined tender points (see http://www.home-health-care-physical-therapy.com/Fibromyalgia-Tender-Points.html) has been used for diagnosis; however, not all patients with FM will have 11 of 18 tender points test positive. Fibromyalgia patients typically have diffuse tenderness when pressure is applied to a number of locations. The key feature of FM is increased sensitivity compared with normal controls, and FM is often associated with other chronic pain conditions, including migraines, idiopathic low back pain, irritable bowel syndrome (IBS), gastroesophageal reflux disease (GERD), interstitial cystitis, noncardiac chest pain, and chemical sensitivities.

Neurochemical imbalances in the central nervous system have been identified in FM, leading to a "central amplification" of pain perception manifested as allodynia and hyperesthesia. Psychiatric disorders are present in

up to 30 - 60% of patients with FM, and psychological stress often has a strong influence on the severity of symptoms.

Pharmacological therapies for FM include TCAs, SNRIs, gabapentin, and pregabalin. There is moderate evidence supporting the use of SSRIs, tramadol, and dopamine agonists. Therapies that have been shown to be ineffective include NSAIDs, corticosteroids, benzodiazepines, and opioids. Nonpharmacological therapies, such as cognitive behavioral therapy and low impact exercise, have been shown to be effective in FM. Studies have shown varying success with trigger point injections, acupuncture, and myofascial release.

## Diabetic Neuropathy

Diabetic neuropathy often presents as a distal, symmetric polyneuropathy in a "stocking and glove" distribution. This can result in both sensory deficits and neuropathic pain. Focal and multifocal neuropathies may also be present (e.g., median nerve mononeuropathy). The incidence of diabetic neuropathy varies directly with the duration of diabetes, age, and degree of hyperglycemia.

There are a number of proposed mechanisms that explain the pathophysiology of diabetic neuropathy. The common end pathway is nerve injury, either through chronic ischemia or a decreased capacity to repair structural injury. This nerve injury may cause any number of neuropathic symptoms, such as deep burning pain, electrical shock-like stabbing pain, paresthesia, allodynia, or hyperesthesia.

Treatment for diabetic neuropathy is similar to pharmacotherapy used in other neuropathic pain conditions and includes anticonvulsants, TCAs, SNRIs, and, in more severe pain, tramadol and opioids.

## Post-herpetic Neuralgia

Post-herpetic neuralgia (PHN) is a common complication of varicella-zoster reactivation resulting in chronic pain. Ten to fifteen percent of those in whom reactivation has occurred will develop PHN. In patients over the age of 60, the incidence increases to 30 - 50%. It is defined as a dermatomal chronic pain condition that persists 120 days after the onset of the zoster rash.

Post-herpetic neuralgia may produce neuropathic pain as a result of axonal inflammation or injury, loss, and scarring of ganglionic tissue. Both stimulus-independent and stimulus-dependent pain may be present as a result. Stimulus independent pain includes continuous or intermittent burning, throbbing, sharp, shooting, and electric shock-like pain. Stimulus-dependent pain includes allodynia, hyperalgesia, paresthesia, and dysesthesia.

Antiviral therapy is started ideally within 72 hr of appearance of the initial rash but may be beneficial even if initiated after 72 hr. Antiviral therapy reduces viral replication and hastens healing. It reduces the degree of neural damage, viral shedding, as well as the duration and severity of acute and chronic PHN pain. Common treatment regimens are 7-10 days of acyclovir (800 mg *po* 5 times daily) or 7 days of valacyclovir (1,000 mg *po tid*).

Acute herpes-zoster infection is often accompanied by a moderate degree of pain, which may be treated with acetaminophen, NSAIDS, tramadol, TCAs, pregabalin, Neurontin, topical capsaicin cream, or local anesthetics and opioid analgesics. Early and effective treatment of the pain associated with an acute outbreak may reduce both the incidence and severity of cases that progress to PHN. Other treatments may include the use of oral steroids, epidural or neuroforaminal steroid injection, peripheral nerve blocks, and sympathetic blocks. Spinal cord stimulation may be effective in patients with severe chronic PHN pain. Patients with severe catastrophic pain or poor coping skills may benefit from therapy with a pain psychologist.

## Complex Regional Pain Syndrome (CRPS)

Complex regional pain syndrome (CRPS) was previously known as "reflex sympathetic dystrophy" and "causalgia". The International Association for the Study of Pain (IASP) has renamed these two neuropathic pain syndromes Complex Regional Pain Syndrome 1(CRPS 1) and Complex Regional Pain Syndrome II (CRPS II), respectively. CRPS 1 occurs without an identifiable nerve lesion, while CRPS II results from an obvious nerve lesion.

Pain is the main feature of CRPS. It is often spontaneous and described as burning, sharp, lancinating, electric, shock-like, or aching in nature. Allodynia and hyperalgesia are generally present. Sensory changes, autonomic dysfunction, trophic changes, motor impairment, and psychological changes may also be present. Autonomic dysfunction may result in sympathetically mediated pain and vasomotor (skin blood flow) or sudomotor (sweating) disturbances. These disturbances result in changes in skin color, edema, and skin temperature differences. Trophic changes are often the result of disuse and include muscle weakness and atrophy, changes in nail growth, thinning or thickening of the overlying skin, hair loss, osteoporosis, and joint ankylosis.[4]

## Table 18.3 Criteria for Complex Regional Pain Syndrome

| IASP Diagnostic Criteria for CRPS I and II | |
|---|---|
| 1 | Continuing pain, which is disproportionate to any inciting event. |
| 2 | At least one symptom in three of the four following categories:<br>*Sensory:* Hyperesthesia and/or allodynia.<br>*Vasomotor:* Temperature asymmetry, and/or skin color changes, and/or skin color asymmetry.<br>*Sudomotor/Edema:* Edema, and/or sweating changes, and/or sweating asymmetry.<br>*Motor/Trophic:* Decreased range of motion, and/or motor dysfunction (weakness, tremor, dystonia), and/or trophic changes (hair, nail, skin). |
| 3 | At least one sign in two or more of the following categories:<br>*Sensory:* Hyperalgesia (to pinprick), and/or allodynia (to light touch and/or temperature sensation, and/or deep somatic pressure, and/or joint movement).<br>*Vasomotor:* Temperature asymmetry (>1°C), and/or skin color changes, and/or asymmetry.<br>*Sudomotor/Edema:* Edema, and/or sweating changes, and/or sweating asymmetry<br>*Motor/Trophic:* Decreased range of motion, and/or motor dysfunction (weakness, tremor, dystonia), and/or trophic changes (hair, nail, skin). |
| 4 | No other diagnosis can better explain the signs and symptoms. |

Adapted from: Objectification of the Diagnostic Criteria for CRPS, R. Norman Harden, MD Pain Medicine 2010; 11: 1212–1215 Wiley Periodicals, Inc.

The goal of treatment is alleviation of symptoms and restoration of function. This mandates early and aggressive physiotherapy, which itself will reduce pain and the complications of disuse. Pharmacologic and interventional pain management is often necessary for this early therapy to be possible.

The pain of CRPS is neuropathic in nature, and therefore, therapies discussed previously with post-herpetic neuralgia and diabetic neuropathy are indicated (i.e. TCAs, SNRIs, anticonvulsants, tramadol, tapentadol, and local anesthetics). If pain is not well controlled with these medications, other traditional opioids may be considered. Agents aimed at regulating bone metabolism, such as calcitonin and bisphosphonates, have also been advocated for osteopenia resulting from lack of use of the affected extremity. These medications may also decrease the synthesis of prostaglandins, lactic acid, and pro-inflammatory cytokines that stimulate pain pathways. Corticosteroids may also be efficacious in the early stages of CRPS.

The goal of interventional management is to decrease pain, restore function, and permit improved physiotherapy. Interventions employed include sympathetic blockade (stellate ganglion or lumbar sympathetic block), intravenous regional blockade, or epidural blockade. Neuromodulation or neuroablation techniques have also been used with the best long-term results obtained with spinal cord stimulation.

Coping with this devastating condition is often very difficult. Depression and other mood disorders are common and referral to a pain psychologist, social worker, or psychiatrist should be considered.

## Oncologic Pain

Cancer related pain is common and may be due either to the malignancy itself or secondary to treatment. Malignancies can stretch, compress, or invade surrounding tissues, as well as produce mediators that alter the body's complex pain physiology. Treatment of an underlying malignancy with chemotherapy, radiation, and surgery may cause pain (mucositis, tissue damage) but can also be one of the most effective ways of reducing cancer-related pain. Treatment should include attempts at eradication of the malignancy as well as management of the somatic, visceral, and neuropathic components of cancer-related pain. Acetaminophen, NSAIDs, and opioids are effective at dealing with somatic and visceral pain. The addition of anticonvulsants, antidepressants, NMDA receptor antagonists, and interventional techniques can all be used in an escalating manner.

As introduced in Chapter 17, the World Health Organization (WHO) has devised a "pain relief ladder", providing a simple framework for the management of cancer-related pain. The ladder begins and escalates therapy in a structured fashion, starting with early oral administration of non-opioids (acetaminophen and a NSAID or COX-2 inhibitor) and followed by opioids and adjuvant medications as needed to treat additional pain and coexisting anxiety. Medications are given "by the clock" (i.e., straight scheduling) rather than on demand. According to the WHO, this approach is 80-90% effective (see http://www.who.int/cancer/palliative/painladder/en/). This ladder has been extended to include more invasive techniques, such as neurolysis, regional anesthesia, intrathecal pumps, and spinal cord stimulators.

## Suggestions for management of chronic pain patients presenting for surgery:

1. Continue the patient's normal pain medications and adjuvants.
2. Consider adding acetaminophen and a NSAID or COX-2 inhibitor and adjuvants, such as gabapentin, pregabalin and tramadol.
3. Consider regional or neuraxial anesthetic techniques (see Chapter 16).
4. Consider a preoperative sympathetic block for patients with CRPS who are scheduled to have surgery on the affected limb.
5. Consider the addition of intraoperative intravenous lidocaine. Intravenous lidocaine infusions of $2 - 3$ mg·kg$^{-1}$·hr$^{-1}$ have been used to reduce opioid requirements and improve analgesia.
6. Consider intravenous ketamine. The suggested intravenous infusion range is $0.15 - 0.5$ mg·kg$^{-1}$·hr$^{-1}$ with $0.15 - 0.3$ mg·kg$^{-1}$·hr$^{-1}$ being adequate for most procedures when used alone or in combination with intravenous lidocaine.
7. Consider dexmedetomidine ($1$ µg·kg$^{-1}$ bolus then $0.4 - 0.5$ µg·kg$^{-1}$·hr$^{-1}$) To avoid significant hypotension and excessive postoperative sedation, consider omitting the bolus dose.
8. Whenever possible, titrate the opioid dose to the patient's respiratory rate (RR) at the end of the case. Aim for a RR of $8 - 10$ breaths·min$^{-1}$ in patients with a normal respiratory status or for a baseline RR in patient's with significant respiratory disease.
9. Liquid methadone is available and can be administered by a gastric tube. Conversion calculations for converting

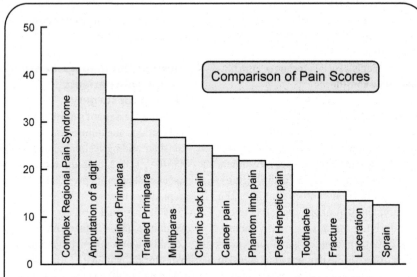

Fig. 18.1 Comparison of pain scores of common pain conditions using the McGill Pain Questionnaire. Adapted from Melzack R. Psychological aspects of pain: implications for neural blockade. In Neural blockade. Cousins MJ, Bridenbaugh PO. (eds) 2nd edit. J.B. Lippincott Co. 1988.

methadone to other opioids are complicated. The University of Michigan offers a conversion tool for methodone dosing.

The following electronic link provides an advanced discussion of additional suggestions to manage difficult chronic pain patients presenting for surgery. (http://www.anesthesiaprimer.com/AP/Ch18ChronicPain/Ch18Supplement.pdf)

Finally, realistic attainable perioperative analgesic goals should be discussed with the patient and the surgical team. If a chronic pain patient's baseline pain score is 8/10 before surgery, aiming to attain a VAS score of 5/10 in the postoperative period may be unrealistic. Educating the patient, surgeon, nursing staff, and family members about the analgesic plan and the patient's available options will assist the acute pain service (APS) team in providing safe and effective analgesic care. Chronic pain patients frequently have opioid tolerance, hyperalgesia, and central sensitization, making delivery of effective and safe analgesic care a challenge for the APS and surgical teams.

**Resources:**

Canadian Pain Society http://www.canadianpainsociety.ca/en/
National Pain Centre (opioid prescribing guidelines) http://nationalpaincentre.mcmaster.ca/opioid/index.html
National Pain Foundation http://www.nationalpainfoundation.org/
The American Chronic Pain Association http://www.theacpa.org/default.aspx
The American Academy of Pain Medicine http://www.painmed.org/
IASP (International Association for the Study of Pain) http://www.iasp-pain.org/AM/Template.cfm?Section=General_Resource_Links

AFSA (The American Fibromyalgia Syndrome Association) http://www.afsafund.org/resource.htm
For further explanation and information on the validity of the Brief Pain Inventory:
http://www.ottawa-anesthesia.org/lido/00002508_200409000_00011.pdf
Pain and Disability Assessment Tools: http://pain-topics.org/clinical_concepts/assess.php
Depression Screening Tool: http://patienteducation.stanford.edu/research/phq.pdf
Canadian Guideline for Safe and Effective Use of Opioids for Chronic Non-Cancer Pain
http://nationalpaincentre.mcmaster.ca/opioid/
Opioid Conversion Chart / Guides: see Chapter 14, Opioids

**References:**
1. Part III: Pain Terms, A Current List with Definitions and Notes on Usage (pp. 209 - 214) Classification of Chronic Pain, Second Edition, IASP Task Force on Taxonomy, edited by H. Merskey and N. Bogduk, IASP Press, Seattle, 1994.
   http://www.iasp-pain.org/Content/NavigationMenu/GeneralResourceLinks/PainDefinitions/default.htm
2. Centers for disease control and prevention,
   http://www.cdc.gov/vitalsigns/PainkillerOverdoses/index.html (November 2011)
3. Prevalence of Side Effects of Prolonged Low or Moderate Dose Opioid Therapy with Concomitant Benzodiazepine and/or Antidepressant Therapy in Chronic Non-Cancer Pain, Laxmaiah Manchikanti, MD,et al, Pain Physician 2009; 12:259-267 • ISSN 1533-3159
4. Massachusetts General Hospital Handbook of Pain Management, Third Edition. 2006 Lippincott Williams & Wilkins, Philadelphia 530 Walnut Street, Philadelphia, PA
5. Bonica's Management of Pain, 4th Edition. Fishman, Ballantyne and Rathmell. Chapters 24, 27, 35, 36, 71, 72.
6. Barash 6th ed. Ch 58.
7. The Science of Fibromyalgia, Clauw D; Arnold LM; McCarber BH, Mayo Clinic Proceedings September 2011 vol. 86 no. 9 907-911

# CHAPTER 19

# Obstetrical Anesthesia

Janie Des Rosiers MD, Catherine Gallant MD

## Learning Objectives

1. To review the physiological changes associated with pregnancy.
2. To gain an understanding of the supine hypotensive syndrome and interventions for its prevention and treatment.
3. To gain an understanding of factors influencing maternal pain during labour and delivery.
4. To review analgesic options for labour and delivery as well as the anesthetic options for Cesarean delivery.
5. To gain an appreciation of the risks and benefits of epidural analgesia for labour and delivery.

## Key Points

1. A lateral decubitus position or left lateral uterine tilt with a right hip wedge can be used to decrease the risk of the supine hypotensive syndrome.

2. When general anesthesia is induced for emergent Cesarean delivery, the physiologic changes associated with pregnancy can result in a rapid desaturation, an increase in difficulty with direct laryngoscopy and tracheal intubation, and an increase in the risk of aspiration pneumonitis.

3. Epidural analgesia is generally safe for both the mother and infant and can provide the best form of continuous pain relief during labour and delivery.

4. Uterine atony may result in significant postpartum bleeding. Identification of risk factors and specific interventions is key to the successful management of uterine atony.

Profound physiological changes occur with pregnancy and increase the parturient's risk of anesthesia-related morbidity and mortality. Complications related to pregnancy may influence the options for labour analgesia and the anesthetic technique for operative delivery. In addition to a basic history and physical examination, anesthesiologists must direct their attention to the mother's parity, the fetal gestational age, coexisting maternal comorbidities, and the identification of pregnancy-related complications (e.g., pregnancy-induced hypertension, HELLP syndrome, preeclampsia, gestational diabetes, and coagulopathies). Anesthetic medications are important considerations for both the mother and infant.

## Table 19.1 Physiological changes of pregnancy

### Nervous System

| Variable | Change | Cause | Importance |
|---|---|---|---|
| General anesthesia | Minimum alveolar concentration (MAC) requirements decreased by 25 – 40%. | Central nervous system (CNS) effect of progesterone and (or) beta-endorphin. | General anesthesia drug requirements are decreased. |
| Regional anesthesia | Local anesthesia (LA) dose requirements are decreased by about 40%. | Decrease in size of epidural space due to engorged epidural veins and hormonal changes. | Increased epidural spread of LA may occur, esp. if aortocaval compression is not prevented. |

### Cardiovascular System

| Variable | Change | Cause | Importance |
|---|---|---|---|
| Blood volume (BV) | Total BV increased by 35%. Plasma volume increased by 45%. Red blood cell (RBC) BV increased by 20%. | Hormonal effect | An increase of approx. 1L compensates for the 400 – 600 mL of blood loss with delivery. |
| Cardiac Output (CO) | Increased by 40% at 10 weeks. Labour increases CO by 45% above pre-labour values. After delivery, CO increases 60% above pre-labour values. | Increases in CO are in response to increased metabolic demands (Stroke volume increases more than heart rate). | Patients with pre-existing heart disease may decompensate (e.g., pulmonary edema may occur during labour or after delivery in the patient with significant mitral stenosis). |

### Respiratory System

| Variable | Change | Cause | Importance |
|---|---|---|---|
| Upper airway | Mucosal edema makes the parturient prone to upper airway obstruction, difficulty with tracheal intubation, and bleeding with airway instrumentation. | Capillary engorgement | Trauma may occur with suctioning and placement of nasal and oral airways. Choose a smaller endotracheal tube (ETT). |

| Respiratory System | | |
|---|---|---|
| Ventilation | Minute ventilation increases by 50%. Tidal volume increases by 40%. Respiratory rate increases by 10%. | Normal resting maternal PaCO2 drops to approx. 30 mmHg in the first trimester. Pain from labour and delivery result in further hyperventilation. Labour may increase O2 consumption > 100%. |
| Lung Volumes | Functional reserve capacity (FRC) decreases 20%. No change in vital capacity. | By fifth month, the rising uterus begins to force up the diaphragm. |
| Arterial oxygenation (PaO2) | Increased by 10 mmHg. | Due to hyperventilation. |
| | An increase in oxygen consumption begins in the first trimester. | Faster uptake of inhaled anesthetics due to an increased minute ventilation with a smaller FRC. |
| | | Decreased FRC with increased O2 consumption results in very rapid decreases in PaO2 during apnea (e.g., induction of general anesthesia). |
| Gastrointestinal System | | |
| Gastric fluid volume | Increased | Enlarged uterus displaces pylorus and delays gastric emptying. |
| | | N.B. All parturients are considered to have a "full stomach". Pain, anxiety, and opioids (e.g., morphine, hydromorphone) all delay gastric emptying and increase gastric volume. |
| Gastric fluid acidity | Increased | Gastrin secreted by placenta (stimulates H+ secretion). |
| | | Use of H2 receptor antagonists (e.g., ranitidine 150 mg orally [po] or 50 mg iv) will decrease gastric volume and increase gastric pH. 0.3 M Na citrate 30 mL will increase gastric pH. |

Complications during labour and delivery can threaten the well-being of both the mother and infant; consequently, the anesthesiologist must be able to respond quickly and work closely with the obstetric, neonatal, and nursing teams. The anesthesiologist must have an intimate knowledge of pharmacology, pathophysiology, and available anesthetic options and must possess a skill set to facilitate safe and quality care for both the mother and infant.

## Physiological Changes

Profound physiological changes occur during pregnancy. Table 19.1 summarizes the changes in the nervous, cardiorespiratory, and gastrointestinal systems, and the resulting implications with respect to anesthesia management.

## Supine Hypotensive Syndrome

The gravid uterus may compress the inferior vena cava (IVC) and or the aorta when the parturient lies in the supine position. This occurs in approximately 15% of patients as early as the 20th week and increases in frequency in the third trimester.

When IVC compression results from uterine compression, there is a decrease in venous return to the heart. The parturient may experience signs and symptoms of shock, including hypotension, pallor, sweating, nausea, vomiting, and changes in mentation. Venous pressure increases in the lower extremities and in the uterus. Blood flow to the uterus is not autoregulated but is dependent on the difference between the uterine artery and venous pressures. Hence, an increase in uterine venous pressure will decrease the uterine blood flow to the placenta and fetus.

Compression of the aorta by itself is not associated with maternal hypotension but may result in arterial hypotension in the uterus. This decrease in uterine blood flow may result in fetal distress or asphyxia. It is important to appreciate that a lack of maternal symptoms does not exclude decreased placental perfusion.

The term parturient should never be placed in the supine position. Abnormal fetal heart rate patterns indicating insufficient uterine blood flow are frequently observed when patients are placed in the supine position (Fig. 19.1). Positioning the parturient on her side or using a right hip wedge is usually sufficient to move the weight of the uterus off the IVC and aorta. A minimum left lateral tilt of 15 degrees should be employed. If the parturient is symptomatic, increasing the tilt may be beneficial as individual susceptibility to this syndrome varies.

Lumbar regional anesthetic techniques (epidural or spinal anesthesia) block the sympathetic nerves and decrease vascular tone in the lower body. This may result in an exaggeration of the hypotensive effects of aortocaval compression.

## Analgesia: Labour and Delivery

The pain of labour is generally described as being more intense than any other previous pain experience, and the pain is generally more intense in primiparous compared with multiparous women.

## The American Society of Anesthesiology (ASA) state:

"There is no other circumstance where it is considered acceptable for an individual to experience untreated severe pain, amenable to safe intervention, while under a physician's care. In the absence of a medical contraindication, maternal request is a sufficient medical indication for pain relief during labour."

Pain varies depending on the stage of labour. During the first stage, pain is mostly visceral due to uterine contractions (latent phase) and cervical dilatation (active phase). Nociceptive impulses are transmitted from nerve fibres entering the spinal cord at T10 to L1. During the second stage of labour (delivery), the baby's descent stretches and compresses the pelvic floor leading to somatic perineal pain. New nociceptive impulses enter the spinal cord at S2 to S4 (Fig. 19.2). Table 19.2 lists some of the factors that influence the degree and intensity of the pain experience during labour.

## Table 19.2 Factors influencing the pain of labour and delivery

| | |
|---|---|
| • Parturient's psychological state | • Mental preparation |
| • Family support | • Medical support |
| • Cultural background | • Primipara *vs* multiparous |
| • Size and presentation of the fetus | • Size and anatomy of the pelvis |
| • Use of medications to augment labour (oxytocin) | • Duration of labour |

### Psychoprophylaxis

The Lamaze method postulates that the parturient's pain can be replaced with conditioned "positive" reflexes. With this method, a partner or friend functions as a coach to help the parturient concentrate on breathing techniques and on releasing muscle tension. Nevertheless, studies have shown that two-thirds of Lamaze mothers will require some kind of analgesic therapy.

In fact, excessive pain may result in more harm to the fetus than the judicious use of pharmacologic analgesia. Psychological stress during labour may cause hypoxia and acidosis in the fetus. This is believed to result from decreased uterine blood flow secondary to elevated levels of blood catecholamines and (or) decreased carbon dioxide tensions caused by hyperventilation. With adequate pain relief, epidural anesthesia can minimize the stress of labour and facilitate patient participation during labour and delivery. It is important to recognize differences in pain tolerance and analgesic requirements in order to promote maternal self-esteem and bonding with the newborn.

Table 19.3 lists some of the options currently available for pain management during labour.

## Table 19.3 Labour analgesic options

| | |
|---|---|
| • Nothing | • Massage, walking |
| • Hypnotherapy (relaxation exercises practiced in prenatal classes) | • Psychological support (Lamaze technique), labour coach, husband etc. |
| • Entonox® (gas and air) | • Intramuscular opioids |
| Nalbuphine | Intravenous opioids (e.g., fentanyl, patient-controlled analgesia [PCA]) |
| Epidural analgesia (local anesthetics +/- opioids) | Combined spinal-epidural analgesia |

Table 19.4 Opioid analgesics in labour

| Opioid | Dose | Peak effect | Duration | Comments |
|---|---|---|---|---|
| Fentanyl | 25 – 50 µg iv<br>50 – 100 µg IM | 2 – 3 min iv<br>10 min IM | 30 – 60 min | Short action, potent respiratory depressant; can be used in PCA modality – see Chapter 17 (e.g., PCA bolus = 25 µg, lockout = 5 min, infusion = 25 µg·hr$^{-1}$, 1 hr max. = 200 µg). |
| Meperidine | 25 – 50 mg iv<br>50 – 100 mg IM every 2 – 4 hr | 5 – 10 min<br>40 – 45 min | 2 – 3 hr | Active metabolite is normeperidine; neonatal depression can occur if administered 1 – 4 hr prior to delivery: less neonatal depression compared with morphine. |
| Nalbuphine | 10 – 20 mg iv<br>10 – 20 mg IM, SQ | 2 – 3 min<br>15 min | 3 – 6 hr | Has both agonist and antagonist opioid properties. Less nausea and vomiting compared with meperidine. |

*iv* = intravenous; *IM* = intramuscular; *SQ* = subcutaneous; PCA = patient controlled analgesia.

## Parenteral Opioids

All parenteral opioids readily cross the placenta. This can potentially cause an issue both in the early and late stages of labour. Opioids will depress the fetal central nervous system and cause sedation. This can lead to a combination of decreased beat-to-beat fetal heart variability and decreased fetal movements, which makes fetal monitoring challenging during the early stage of labour. During the late stage, parenteral opioid use may result in neonatal respiratory depression at birth. It is therefore important to consider the pharmacokinetic properties of an opioid prior to administering it during the later stage.

Fentanyl is the most common opioid used to manage pain during labour and delivery (Table 19.4)

Fentanyl is transferred to the fetus extremely rapidly and redistributes back to the mother. With doses of 1 µg·kg⁻¹, fentanyl does not produce adverse effects on the neonate. It is eliminated from the fetus more quickly than other opioids, such as meperidine or morphine. Our institution has a protocol where the obstetrical nurse may administer a bolus dose of 25 to 50 µg *iv* every 15 min for labour analgesia up to a maximum of 200 µg·hr⁻¹.

Nalbuphine is a mixed mu-opioid receptor agonist-antagonist that can be a good choice for labour analgesia as it provides pain relief without fetal respiratory depression. A dose of 10-20 mg *iv/IM*/SQ is usually sufficient.

Although meperidine was once used frequently, it has fallen out of favor in the past several years (see Chapter 14). Peak levels are reached in the fetus 2 - 3 hr after administration, and elimination of the drug takes 2 to 3 days.

Morphine is not commonly used for labour analgesia as it causes more fetal respiratory depression than meperidine and fentanyl, especially when administered within 3 hr of delivery.

## Nitrous Oxide

Nitrous oxide ($N_2O$) is an odorless invisible gas with weak analgesic and amnestic properties (see Chapter 13). It is relatively insoluble in the blood, resulting in rapid onset (induction) and offset (recovery). For labour analgesia, it can be administered at a subanesthetic concentration in a 50:50 mixture of $N_2O$ and oxygen (supplied as Entonox®). At this concentration, it is unable to provide adequate pain relief for most mothers; however, it may be a useful adjuvant to epidural analgesia or opioid analgesia. Entonox® should be self-administered by instructing the mother to hold and breathe into the Entonox® mask. A health care provider should be present to ensure that it is used properly and that the patient has an adequate level of consciousness during the treatment. The peak effect occurs within 1 min of use; hence, the patient should be instructed to use the Entonox® as soon as the contraction begins and to discontinue its use as soon as the contraction begins to subside. Studies on its effectiveness have shown that $N_2O$ could provide a significant reduction in labour pain in most patients, but it could not provide complete analgesia. Common side effects include dizziness, nausea, inability to cooperate, and dysphoria. If these side effects become troublesome, the patient can simply remove the mask from her face. Entonox® is used infrequently although it is widely available and has a good safety profile for both the mother and baby.

## Epidural Analgesia

In Chapter 17, the recommended doses for epidural analgesia and anesthesia were summarized and its complications and contraindications were reviewed. Table 19.5 reviews some of the potential maternal and neonatal advantages of epidural analgesia.

## Table 19.5 Maternal and neonatal advantages of epidural labour analgesia

| Maternal advantages | Neonatal advantages |
|---|---|
| Excellent pain relief possible compared with opioid analgesia alone. | Less drug transfer to the infant. Reduced neonatal depression. |
| Normal progress of labour is not impeded. | Improved uterine blood flow and fetal well-being as a result of a decreased maternal stress response during labour and delivery. |
| General anesthesia can be avoided (epidural anesthesia can be provided for Cesarean delivery). | May reduce neonatal trauma when an instrumented delivery is required. |
| Improved maternal participation and bonding during delivery. | |

In addition to the contraindications to regional anesthesia identified in Chapter 16, a number of conditions associated with pregnancy may contraindicate the use of a regional anesthesia technique. One of the most common conditions is termed HELLP syndrome (frequency 1:1000 pregnancies or 10 – 20% of pregnancies associated with severe preeclampsia or eclampsia). HELLP is characterized by hemolysis, elevated liver enzymes, and low platelets. It can affect parturients with preeclampsia as well as parturients without hypertension. Clinical signs may include the presence of right upper quadrant pain with or without signs of preeclampsia (headache, blurred vision). Laboratory findings include an increase in aspartate transaminase (AST), lactate dehydrogenase (LDH), and total bilirubin and a decrease in platelet count. The platelet count trend is very important when considering a regional anesthesia technique (whether for a labour epidural or for a spinal for Cesarean delivery).

Lidocaine, bupivacaine, and ropivacaine are the most common local anesthesia agents used for managing epidural analgesia - anesthesia. Low concentrations of bupivacaine or ropivacaine can provide a differential nerve block, resulting in only a minor motor nerve block. As a consequence, the patient maintains her motor strength, permitting her to move during labour. During the second stage of labour, the differential nerve block facilitates her efforts to push by minimizing the motor block while maintaining an adequate sensory block.

The combination of a local anesthetic agent with an opioid is commonly used for epidural analgesia. This combination is superior to the use of a local anesthetic or opioid alone due to the synergy between the two classes of drugs. Morphine and fentanyl are the two most popular opioids used for epidural analgesia and anesthesia. Commonly used solutions are bupivacaine 0.0625% - 0.125% with fentanyl 2-3 $\mu g \cdot mL^{-1}$ or 0.08% - 0.1% ropivacaine with fentanyl 2-3 $\mu g \cdot mL^{-1}$. Ropivacaine causes less motor blockade and cardiac toxicity compared with bupivacaine. Epinephrine may be added to epidural solutions to prolong the block and decrease systemic absorption; however, the addition of epinephrine may not be necessary and must be weighed against its potential side effects, which may include a significant increase in motor block, accentuation of hypertension in preeclamptic patients, and diminished uterine activity due to its beta agonist activity.

Controversy exists as to whether a mixture of dilute local anesthetic and opioid has any significant effect on the progress of labour. Some studies have shown a slightly longer second stage of labour (15 minutes), while others report no difference. Some clinicians prefer to ensure labour is well established (i.e., regular contractions, 3 cm dilatation, engagement of fetal head) prior to placing an epidural for labour analgesia, while others believe that placing an epidural early once labour is established is both easier and safer when the patient is still relatively comfortable and cooperative. Waiting for specific labour criteria to be met prior to placing an epidural may not be warranted.

Epidural labour analgesia may be provided with intermittent boluses administered by a nurse or anesthesiologist or by using a continuous infusion technique with or without supplementary bolus doses. An increasingly popular method of providing epidural labour analgesia is patient-controlled epidural analgesia (PCEA). With PCEA, the patient initiates the administration of a bolus after a set minimum time interval. PCEA also permits the use of a continuous basal infusion. Studies have shown better patient satisfaction with PCEA.

While epidurals are commonly performed for labour analgesia, they can be associated with significant risks and complications. These should be discussed with the patient prior to the administration of the epidural in order to obtain an informed consent (see patient information sheet. Postpartum women commonly report local pain and soreness at the needle insertion site. Furthermore, up to 50% of patients will suffer from back pain following delivery; however, there is no evidence that epidurals increase this risk. Variations in epidural insertion technique, epidural anatomy, and epidural catheter positioning may result in epidural failure, a "one-sided" block, or a "patchy" block. Occasionally, the epidural catheter will need to be adjusted or replaced. When the catheter is properly placed, administration of local anesthetics will decrease the patient's sympathetic tone, which may result in hypotension. Maternal hypotension following epidural local anesthetic administration may require treatment with an intravenous fluid bolus, left uterine displacement, and (or) small boluses of vasopressors, such as ephedrine or phenylephrine. Hypotension is less commonly seen with the use of dilute local anesthetic solutions. If the epidural catheter is inadvertently placed in an epidural vein, rapid intravenous absorption of the local anesthetic solution may result in systemic toxicity (see Chapter 15). If the epidural catheter is inadvertently placed into the cerebrospinal fluid space a high spinal block with cardiorespiratory collapse may result following the administration of local anesthetic medications. If the epidural needle is advanced past the epidural space through the dura, an inadvertent dural puncture can result. There is a 1% risk of an epidural dural puncture, which may result in a postdural puncture headache (PDPH). A discussion of PDPH and its management is discussed later in this chapter. Very rare complications associated with epidural techniques include an epidural infection or abscess formation, epidural hematoma formation, and temporary or permanent nerve injury.

The use of ultrasound for neuraxial anesthesia is increasingly used to improve the success of spinal and epidural techniques. The University of Toronto has developed a free web-based interactive 3-D model to facilitate teaching clinicians the skills to use ultrasound for neuraxial anesthesia. Their website can be accessed at http://pie.med.utoronto.ca/vspine.

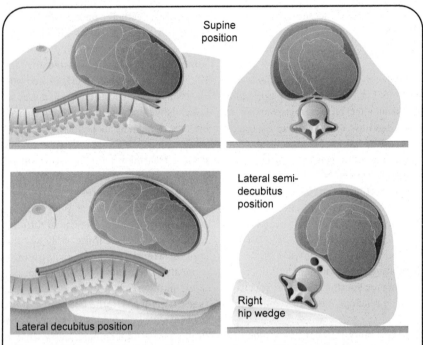

Fig. 19.1 The supine hypotensive syndrome. The top images illustrate dynamic compression of the aorta and vena cava by the gravid uterus in the supine position. In the lateral or wedged position, (bottom images) aorto-caval compression is resolved with displacement of the gravid uterus off the vascular structures.

## Combined Spinal Epidural Analgesia (CSE)

This technique can be used to provide a rapid onset of spinal analgesia with minimal risk of toxicity or motor block. It involves the placement of a spinal needle into the cerebrospinal fluid (CSF) space as well as placement of an epidural catheter. The most common technique involves the following steps: identification of the epidural space with an epidural Tuohy needle; passage of a long fine (25 – 27G) pencil point spinal needle through the epidural needle into the CSF space; administration of the spinal medications; and removal of the spinal needle to permit placement of an

epidural catheter 4 – 5 cm into the epidural space. Alternatively, an epidural catheter can be inserted followed by a spinal injection at a lower lumbar interspace. The spinal medication administered typically combines a low dose of opioid and local anesthetic (e.g., fentanyl 15 mg with bupivacaine 2.0 mg and can provide analgesia for 60 – 90 minutes. At the same time, the epidural catheter placement allows the anesthesiologist to administer local anesthetic and opioid medications into the epidural space to provide prolonged analgesia or surgical anesthesia should a Cesarean delivery be required.

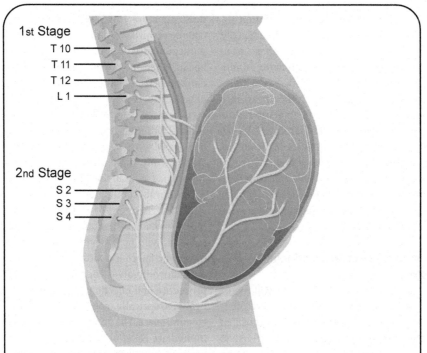

Fig. 19.2 Labour pain. In the first stage of labour, pain is primarily from uterine contractions as a result of cervical dilation and stretching of the lower uterine segment. Sympathetic visceral afferent C fibers transmit the pain impulses with pain experienced primarily in the T-10 to L-1 dermatomes. In the second stage of labour, pain is primarily a result of pressure of the presenting part on the pelvic structures and is mediated through the parasympathetic pudendal nerves and experienced as pain primarily in the S-2 to S-4 dermatomes. Somatic pain is experienced from the L-2 to S-5 dermatomes. The ilioinguinal, genitofemoral and posterior nerve of the thigh may also be involved in the transmission of pain during labour.

Side effects include nausea, vomiting, pruritis, and urinary retention. Occasionally, fetal bradycardia may result in a "non-reassuring fetal heart rate" following administration of the spinal anesthetic medications. This usually resolves within 5 to 10 min and is thought to be due to an acute reduction in maternal catecholamines and an increase in alpha agonist effects on the uterus. Retrospective studies have shown this technique to provide rapid reliable analgesia with no increase in the risk of Cesarean delivery or the need for emergent Cesarean delivery due to fetal bradycardia.

## Postdural Puncture Headache (PDPH)

Approximately 1 in 7 women will report having a headache in the immediate postpartum period. The differential diagnosis of a headache in this population is extensive; however, common causes include tension headaches, migraines, preeclampsia, postdural puncture headache, and caffeine withdrawal.[3] Uncommon serious causes of headache in the postpartum patient include meningitis, cerebral hemorrhage, or thrombosis and sinusitis. The pathophysiology of a postdural puncture headache (PDPH) is not well understood. It has been postulated that the CSF leak resulting from the "wet tap" creates a change in CSF pressure around the brain resulting in pain when a patient assumes an upright position. Others have proposed that the loss of CSF volume results in a compensatory cerebral vasodilation that is perceived as a headache. There is a paucity of evidence to support either theory. The headache is typically described as a dull, non-throbbing, frontal occipital discomfort of variable severity. A classic characteristic of a PDPH is the aggravation and relief of symptoms in an upright and supine position, respectively. The typical onset of a PDPH is usually within 24 hr following the inadvertent dural puncture. Untreated, the headache will usually resolve within 1 - 6 wk following the dural puncture. The severity of headache may be such that the mother is unable to perform daily tasks with her newborn (e.g., getting out of bed and breastfeeding). Conservative treatment options can provide symptom relief and include hydration, bed rest, and a combination of oral analgesics, such as acetaminophen, non-steroidal anti-inflammatory drugs (NSAIDS) +/- opioids and caffeine (300 – 500 mg·day⁻¹). An epidural blood patch provides the most effective treatment of a PDPH. An epidural blood patch (EBP) should be considered in patients who have severe symptoms or in those who fail conservative management. The procedure involves repeating the epidural procedure and injecting 15 – 20 mL of blood drawn aseptically from the patient into the epidural space. The procedure provides almost immediate relief of symptoms in almost all patients. Initial studies reported a 95% cure rate with the initial EBP and a 97% cure rate if a second EBP was required.[4] More recent studies suggest the cure rate is more likely in the range of 50 – 75% with the initial EBP.[5,6] The patient should be instructed to rest in bed for 30 min after the blood patch and should avoid strenuous activity for the next 48 hr.

## Cesarean Delivery

General anesthesia for Cesarean delivery is associated with an increase in maternal morbidity and mortality. The increase in risk is primarily related to the management of the airway (i.e., inability to intubate the trachea, inability to ventilate the lungs, and aspiration pneumonitis). Complications associated with general anesthesia may occur during the induction, maintenance, or emergence phase of anesthesia. For these and other reasons, neuraxial anesthesia is preferred for Cesarean delivery. Spinal anesthesia is typically regarded as the anesthetic of choice for Cesarean delivery due to its reliability, rapid onset, and intense block. Advantages associated with regional anesthesia for an operative delivery include a decrease in the neonate's exposure to anesthetic drugs, a decrease in the risk of maternal aspiration of gastric contents, early maternal bonding with the infant at the time of birth, and improved postoperative analgesia with the use of neuraxial opioid administration. The neuraxial technique (epidural or spinal anesthesia) requires a T4 sensory block as the fundus of the uterus is innervated by T6.

## Spinal Anesthesia for Cesarean Delivery

Spinal anesthesia for operative delivery is typically performed using a strict aseptic technique in the operating room. Standard monitors (oximetry, blood pressure) are established, resuscitation equipment and medications are prepared, and a functional intravenous catheter is secured for the co-administration of a 10 mL·kg$^{-1}$ intravenous bolus of crystalloid fluid (e.g., Ringer's lactate). The patient is typically placed in a curled sitting position and the lumbar skin area is exposed and cleansed using an antiseptic solution (e.g., 2% chlorhexidine gluconate with 70% isopropyl alcohol). Local anesthesia (1 – 2% lidocaine with or without epinephrine) is administered to the skin overlying the site of the spinal needle insertion. A fine (24 – 27G) pencil point spinal needle (e.g., Whitacre®, Pencan®, or Sprotte®) is used to minimize the risk of a PDPH (see Chapter 16).

A combination of local anesthetic and opioid is commonly used to provide surgical anesthesia. A common combination for Cesarean delivery is 0.75% hyperbaric bupivacaine 9 – 12 mg with fentanyl 10 – 15 µg and preservative-free morphine 100 – 150 µg (0.1 µg - 0.15 µg). The spinal fentanyl may be used to intensify and prolong the local anesthetic block. Preservative-free spinal

morphine is commonly administered to provide postoperative pain relief for up to 24 hr. Once the spinal anesthetic medication is administered, the patient is placed in a supine position with a right hip wedge to create left uterine displacement and minimize aortocaval compression. An electrocardiogram (ECG) monitor is attached, and the patient's blood pressure and heart rate are closely monitored. Hypotension following spinal anesthesia is common in the parturient and may require an increase in left uterine displacement, an intravenous fluid bolus, or administration of a vasopressor. Significant hypotension is commonly associated with maternal nausea and vomiting. While both ephedrine and phenylephrine are effective in treating maternal hypotension, phenylephrine is associated with a more favorable neonatal acid base status at delivery. Ephedrine has been shown to cross the placenta rapidly causing a release of fetal catecholamines, an increase in fetal heart rate, and fetal acidosis. A growing body of evidence supports the prophylactic administration of a continuous infusion of phenylephrine for spinal anesthesia for Cesarean delivery to minimize maternal hypotension and nausea and vomiting and to improve fetal well-being.[7,8,9] The phenylephrine infusion is typically initiated as soon as the spinal anesthetic medication is administered (starting at 40 mg·min$^{-1}$) and gradually titrated off over the next 30 – 40 min.

## Epidural Anesthesia for Cesarean Delivery

Although the spinal is usually the primary choice of regional anesthesia for a Cesarean delivery given its reliability, rapidity, and intense block, an epidural may be used if the patient already has one in place (previously placed for labour analgesia) or has contraindications to a spinal. A common solution for top up is 2% lidocaine 15 – 20 mL +/- epinephrine with fentanyl 5 μg/mL⁻¹, providing adequate analgesia for surgical delivery. Once the infant is delivered, preservative free morphine 2 – 3 μg may be injected into the epidural space for postoperative pain control.

## General Anesthesia for Cesarean Delivery

When regional anesthesia is contra-indicated (see Chapter 16) or when there is insufficient time to establish regional anesthesia (e.g., severe sustained fetal bradycardia, umbilical cord prolapse, or severe peripartum hemorrhage), general anesthesia for operative delivery may be required.

The anesthesiologist faced with providing general anesthesia for emergent Cesarean delivery must consider the physiological changes of pregnancy and be prepared to provide care for a compromised neonate. All parturients are considered to have a "full stomach", and gastric precautions, including a rapid sequence induction (RSI) with cricoid pressure, are indicated (see Chapter 9 RSI). Parturients have a potentially difficult airway with associated upper airway edema related to pregnancy and large breasts that may impede positioning the laryngoscope. All parturients have a propensity to rapid desaturation on induction of general anesthesia, thus pre-oxygenation prior to induction of anesthesia is especially important. Maternal anesthetic drug transfer to the neonate must also be considered as this may contribute to neonatal depression and increase the need for neonatal resuscitation. The use of a volatile anesthetic gas promotes uterine relaxation and may increase intraoperative blood loss.

A thorough evaluation of the airway (Chapter 6) is especially important in the pregnant patient prior to a rapid sequence induction. On rare occasions, the anesthesiologist may be unable to intubate the patient's trachea on the first attempt. A difficult tracheal intubation in the pregnant patient increases the risk of pulmonary aspiration, which is associated with a high mortality rate. Every anesthesiologist must have a clear backup plan to manage a failed tracheal intubation. Persistent attempts without alterations in technique will rapidly result in airway edema, trauma, and subsequent maternal and fetal hypoxemia. Significant hypoxemia can occur after 1 min of apnea despite preoxygenation. Rescue airway tools to manage an unexpected difficult tracheal intubation must be immediately available for use. Rescue insertion of a LMA Proseal™ has been reported to be an effective tool in the management of the unexpected difficult and failed tracheal intubation in the parturient.[11,12] A review of the LMA Proseal™ as a primary airway for Cesarean delivery suggests it is a safe and effective airway tool for parturients undergoing Cesarean delivery.[12] Immediate alternate rescue tools might include a videolaryngoscope (e.g., Glidescope®), an intubating laryngeal mask airway device, a gum elastic bougie, a McCoy blade, or a lighted stylet (see Chapters 6 and 7).

Induction of anesthesia in the obstetrical patient is administered only when the patient is prepared and draped for surgery to minimize the drug exposure time to the fetus. A right hip wedge should be placed to create left uterine displacement, and the patient should be placed in an optimal position for tracheal intubation. A RSI technique (see Chapter 9) is employed after anesthesia equipment and rescue emergency medications and airway tools have been prepared. A reduced induction dose of propofol (1.5 – 2 mg·kg⁻¹) is typically administered to induce anesthesia and minimize neonatal depression. Alternatively, ketamine (1 mg·kg⁻¹) or thiopental (2 - 3 mg·kg⁻¹) may be used (see induction agents, Chapter 11). Muscle relaxation for tracheal intubation is provided using succinylcholine (1 - 1.5 mg·kg⁻¹). Following tracheal intubation, anesthesia is maintained with a volatile anesthetic agent, such as sevoflurane or desflurane, at a dose of 0.5 MAC to minimize neonatal depression and uterine atony. A 50:50 combination of nitrous oxide and oxygen is administered to supplement the volatile anesthetic agent. An intermediate duration muscle relaxant, such as rocuronium, may be used for relaxation if required. The use of narcotics and other agents are usually withheld until the infant is delivered to minimize drug transfer and neonatal depression. Once the infant is delivered, narcotics and other agents may be used to deepen the level of anesthesia. The volatile anesthetic agent is reduced to minimize uterine relaxation and the potential for increased maternal blood loss. Prophylactic antiemetics should be considered (see Chapter 22) as well as an agent to augment uterine tone (e.g., oxytocin, Duratocin®). Reversal of any residual neuromuscular blockade is considered if a depolarizing neuromuscular relaxant has been used. Tracheal extubation is performed after the patient has regained her protective airway reflexes and is responding to commands.

## Intrapartum hemorrhage vs Postpartum hemorrhage

Intrapartum hemorrhage is usually associated with conditions (e.g., placenta previa, abruptio placenta, and uterine rupture) that predispose the parturient to abnormal bleeding.

**Placenta previa** describes the position of the placenta next to the cervical opening. Placenta previa may be marginal (adjacent to the cervical opening), partial (partially covering the cervical opening), or complete (completely covering the cervical opening). It occurs in 1 in 200 pregnancies and is associated with a risk of severe hemorrhage that may present at any time during the pregnancy, typically as painless vaginal bleeding.

**Placenta accreta** is a condition in which there is an abnormal attachment of the placenta to the myometrium. More severe degrees of invasion of the chorionic villi into the myometrium (**placenta increta**) and through the uterus and into adjacent structures (**placenta percreta**) can also occur. Prior to the 1960s, the incidence of accreta was estimated to be 1 in 30,000 deliveries. The most common risk factor associated with accreta is a previous Cesarean delivery. With the increased frequency of operative delivery, the current incidence of placenta accreta is estimated to be 1:500 to 1:2500 deliveries. These conditions impede the separation of the placenta from the uterus and significantly increase the risk of life-threatening maternal hemorrhage. An emergency postpartum hysterectomy may be required to control the bleeding. When identified by ultrasound prior to delivery, a team approach (obstetrical, neonatology, anesthesia, blood bank, and interventional radiology) is required to minimize the risks of life-threatening hemorrhage and reduce the maternal and fetal risks. The planned Cesarean delivery should be coordinated in an operating room (OR) environment where additional equipment, such as a Level 1 infuser, cell saver, and additional assistance is available. The patient should be crossed-matched for blood products, and the blood should be in the OR, checked, and ready for use. In addition to standard anesthesia monitoring, an arterial line, two large-bore intravenous catheters, and a central line catheter (i.e., cordis) or a rapid infusion catheter should be considered. Interventional radiology consultation should be considered for placement of uterine artery balloon catheters prior to operative delivery. These catheters can then be inflated during the operation to occlude the internal iliac arteries temporarily should uncontrolled bleeding occur. Expert surgical assistance and clear communication between the anesthesia and obstetrical teams is especially important to achieve a good outcome.

**Abruptio placenta** is defined as an early separation of the placenta from the uterine wall. The condition can range from mild to severe depending on the size and degree of separation. It is the most common cause of intrapartum fetal death and usually presents as painful vaginal bleeding. Some cases can be managed with vaginal delivery while others will require an emergency Cesarean delivery. The urgency of the Cesarean delivery and thus the decision between a regional (neuraxial) and general anesthetic is determined by the hemodynamic stability of the mother as well as the degree of fetal distress. Some of the bleeding from the abruption may be concealed in the uterus making it difficult to estimate the degree of bleeding. This can result in an underestimation of the actual blood loss. Abruption also increases the risk of coagulopathy. Intrauterine fetal death may result in a disseminated intravascular coagulopathy (DIC). Special attention should be directed at the maternal coagulation factors, and repeated measurements of coagulation as well as supportive blood product treatment may be required.

**Uterine rupture** is a rare but potentially catastrophic complication associated with labour and has a high incidence of maternal and fetal morbidity. When the uterus does not have a previous surgical scar, the incidence of uterine rupture is less than 1 in 8,500 pregnancies. In the presence of a previous uterine scar (e.g., Cesarean delivery) the risk of rupture is approximately 1 in 1,500 deliveries. In the presence of multiple risk factors, such as a history of multiple previous operative deliveries, a large baby, previous failed vaginal delivery, and use of oxytocin to augment labour, the risk of rupture increases to more than 1 in 200. The most consistent sign of uterine rupture is the sudden onset of a deep, prolonged, and persistent fetal bradycardia. This may be accompanied by the sudden onset of constant abdominal pain (even with epidural analgesia) and maternal hypotension. The definitive treatment is urgent operative delivery within 20 – 30 min of fetal distress. Even when performed within this time period, it may not be possible to save the fetus, and significant blood loss may threaten the life of the mother. In addition to providing general anesthesia and fluid resuscitation with blood products, emergency ligation of the internal iliac arteries and or hysterectomy may be required to save the mother.

**Postpartum hemorrhage** (PPH) is a serious complication following a vaginal delivery or Cesarean delivery. Certain conditions, such as placenta previa, placenta accreta, placental abruption, and vaginal birth after Cesarean (VBAC) increase the parturient's risk of hemorrhage. It is characterised by the loss of > 500 mL of blood with a vaginal delivery or > 1,000 mL of blood with a Cesarean delivery. Postpartum hemorrhage is classified as early, when it occurs within 24 hr of delivery, or late, when it occurs up to 6 wk postpartum. The causes of PPH involve one or more of the following four categories:

### A decrease in uterine tone

Prolonged labour may prevent the uterus from contracting normally. A reduced uterine tone is also associated with multiple gestation, grand multiparous women, and volatile anesthetic agents.

### Retained placental tissue

Retained fragments of placenta predispose the parturient to postpartum bleeding and may require operative removal of the fragments.

### Tissue trauma

Trauma to the vagina, cervix, or uterus following delivery may result in PPH. This can

## EPIDURAL INFORMATION CARD

This card is for information only.

### *What is an Epidural?*

Epidural medication temporarily numbs the nerves carrying pain signals during labour and delivery. You should still be able to move your legs and push but the goal is to minimize pain.

An anesthesiologist will insert a special needle into your lower back that will be used to thread a small plastic tube (epidural catheter) into your *Epidural Space* (the area that contains nerves just outside the spinal cord). The needle is removed once the catheter is in the right spot.

Freezing medication (local anesthetic) and pain medication may be given through the epidural catheter.

Not every woman can have an epidural; some medical conditions may make the epidural insertion impossible or risky.

### *What is needed for an Epidural?*

A detailed history and physical examination by an anesthesia physician.

Consent for the procedure.

An intravenous (IV) to give you fluid or medications.

The ability to sit in the proper position during the procedure.

Time: It usually takes 15 - 20 minutes to place the epidural, then an additional 15 - 20 minutes for the medications to take full effect.

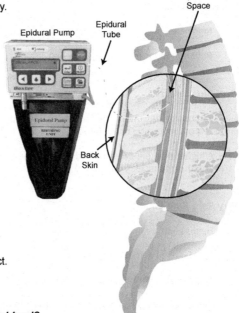

Epidural Pump

Epidural Tube

Epidural Space

Back Skin

### *What are the advantages of an Epidural?*

It can provide the best form of continuous pain relief during labour.

It is safe for you and your baby.

If an epidural is already in place, stronger medications can be put through it should you need to have a cesarean section.

## Patient Information Sheet
## RISKS OF EPIDURAL ANALGESIA

No anesthetic or analgesic is risk free. Most patients however do not suffer any serious complications. It is important to review the information below and please ask a member of the anesthesia team if you have any questions.

### Common Side Effects

- Local discomfort and bruising where the epidural was inserted.

- Temporary difficulty in passing urine; in some cases a urinary catheter is required.

- Insufficient pain control that may need extra medication through the epidural, removing and re-inserting the epidural in a different location, or extra intravenous medications.

### Uncommon Side Effects

- Significant drop in blood pressure (1 in 50 patients)

- Severe headache (1 in 100 patients)

### Rare Side Effects

- Temporary nerve damage (such as leg weakness or a numb patch on your leg or foot lasting more than 24 hours; 1 in 1000 patients).

- A higher than expected spread of medication which can affect your breathing muscles (1 in 13,000 patients).

### Very Rare Side Effects

- Epidural abscess (1 in 50,000 patients)

- Meningitis (1 in 100,000 patients)

- Accidental unconsciousness (1 in 100,000 patients)

- Blood clot with spinal cord damage (1 in 170,000 patients)

- Permanent nerve damage with possible paralysis (1 in 250,000 patients)

Comparison: Risk of death from a motor vehicle collision (1 in 10,000)

Sources: (1) Lobato, E., Graenstein, N., Kirby, R. Complications in Anesthesiology. (2) Obstetric Anaesthetetists' Association. (3) Statistics Canada.

result from an episiotomy, forceps delivery, or from complications such as an unrecognized cervical laceration. On rare occasions, a significant PPH may result from uterine inversion or rupture.

## Coagulation disorders

Preexisting coagulopathy disorders (e.g., hemophilia, von Willebrand disease (vWD), idiopathic thrombocytopenic purpura (ITP), thrombotic thrombocytopenic purpura (TTP), and thrombocytopenia) as well as antiplatelet agents and anticoagulation medications may result in a PPH.

The treatment for PPH is dependent and specific to the cause of the bleeding. Therapeutic interventions may include one or more of local, medical, or surgical interventions. Local measures may include bimanual uterine massage, uterine packing, and repair of lacerations (e.g., cervical laceration). Medical therapy may include the use of oxytocin, duratocin, methylergonovine maleate (ergotamine), carboprost (Hemabate), and administration of fluids and blood products. Surgical interventions may include removal of retained products (dilation and curettage), interventional radiology (to embolize the uterine arteries), or an emergency hysterectomy.

## Test your knowledge:
1. What is the supine hypotensive syndrome? How can it be prevented?
2. What factors may influence a patient's experience of pain during labour and delivery?
3. What options are available for dealing with the pain of labour and delivery?
4. What are the major risks involved with general anesthesia in the parturient undergoing a Cesarean delivery?

## References:
1. Miller RD et al. Editors Miller's Anesthesia. Seventh Edition. Churchill Livingston 2009
2. Chestnut DH. Obstetric Anesthesia: Principles and Practice. Third Edition. Elsevier Mosby 2004
3. Stella CI et al. Postpartum headache: Is your workup complete? Am J Obstet Gynecol 2007;196:318e1-7.
4. Brodsky JB. Epidural blood patch. A safe, effective treatment for postlumbar-puncture headaches. West J Med 1978;129:85-87.
5. Safa-Tisseront V. et al. Effectiveness of epidural blood patch in the management of post-dural puncture headaches. Anesthesiology 2001;95:334-9.
6. Campbell NJ. Effective management of the post dural puncture headache. Anaesthesia tutorial of the week 181. May 2010.
7. Ngan Kee WD, Khaw KS, Ng FF. Prevention of hypotension during spinal anesthesia for cesarean section delivery. Anesthesiology 200;103:744-750.
8. Dyer RA, Reed AR. Spinal anesthesia during elective cesarean delivery: closer to a solution. Anesth Analg 2010;111:1093-1095.
9. Ngan Kee WD. Prevention of maternal hypotension after regional anesthesia for cesarean section. Curr Opin Anaesthesiol 2010;23:304-309.
10. Awan R, Nolan JP, Cook TM. Use of a Proseal™ laryngeal mask airway for airway maintenance during emergency caesarean section after failed tracheal intubation. BJA 2004;92:144-146.
11. Keller C et al. Failed obstetric tracheal intubation and postoperative respiratory support with the Proseal™ laryngeal mask airway. Anesth Analg 2004;98:1467-1470.
12. Halaseh BK et al. The use of Proseal laryngeal mask airway in caesarean section – experience in 3000 cases. Anaesth Int Care 2010;38:1023-1028.

# CHAPTER 20

# Neonatal Resuscitation

Jennifer Mihill MD, Catherine Gallant MD

## Learning Objectives

1. To identify neonates in need of resuscitation.
2. To learn the basic ABCs of neonatal resuscitation.
3. To gain an understanding of the equipment and medication used in neonatal resuscitation.
4. To gain an appreciation for basic neonatal resuscitation and an interest in attending a formal neonatal resuscitation workshop.

## Key Points

| | |
|---|---|
| 1 | Effective ventilation of an infant's lungs is the most important element of neonatal resuscitation. |
| 2 | Only 10% of neonates require resuscitation at birth, and only 1% will require advanced measures, such as chest compressions or tracheal intubation. The majority of neonates are born vigorous. |
| 3 | Pulse oximetry is highly recommended whenever supplemental oxygen is provided. Pulse oximetry should be measured from the newborn's right hand or wrist. |
| 4 | Oximetry targets were developed based on the normal transition of the healthy term newborn after birth. The administration of 100% oxygen may be detrimental, especially in the preterm infant. |
| 5 | Antepartum and intrapartum risk factors can be used to identify which infants are likely to require resuscitation. |
| 6 | A care provider trained in neonatal resuscitation should be present for all deliveries, and personnel with advanced neonatal resuscitation skills should be present at preterm deliveries. |
| 7 | Evaluation of the neonate should proceed quickly. No more than 30 seconds should be required to achieve a response before proceeding to the next step. |

## Introduction

Approximately 10% of newborns will require resuscitation in the delivery room, and approximately 1% will require advanced resuscitation techniques. This chapter summarizes the basic principles of neonatal resuscitation and reviews the basic skills required to perform neonatal resuscitation, including the use of specific equipment and medication. For comprehensive training in neonatal resuscitation, students are encouraged to enrol in a neonatal resuscitation course offered by the Canadian Pediatrics Association (http://www.cps.ca/).

The most important concept to grasp in this chapter is how to identify when a neonate is in need of resuscitation. Once the need is identified, assistance should be requested from personnel trained in neonatal resuscitation. After reviewing this chapter, students should be able to provide basic resuscitation skills, such as warming, drying, positioning, suctioning, and providing oxygen to the infant. Medications and advanced airway techniques will be discussed, but these are skills that are generally acquired during residency training or from a formal neonatal resuscitation course.

## Overview: Neonatal Resuscitation Basics

Interventions following delivery of an infant should include:

1. Airway: Position and clear the airway.
2. Dry and warm the infant.
3. Breathing: Gently stimulate the infant to breathe.
4. Circulation: Assess heart rate and oxygenation.
5. Assess the need for help or advanced intervention.

## Normal Fetal Heart Rate (FHR)

The normal FHR in an infant at least 37 weeks gestation varies from 120 - 160 beats·min$^{-1}$; however, heart rates ranging from 100 - 180 beats·min$^{-1}$ may still be considered normal. Preterm infants (less than 37 weeks) have an average heart rate that is slightly higher, ranging from 130 - 170 beats·min$^{-1}$. The normal fetal heart rate variability ranges from 5 to 25 beats·min$^{-1}$.

## APGAR Score

In the late 1950s, Dr. Virginia Apgar, an American anesthesiologist, devised a simple system to assess an infant's viability at birth. The Apgar score is commonly used as an objective way to assess and convey information about a newborn. The score is based on five clinical criteria that are assigned a score of 0 to 2 for a maximum score of 10. Dr. Apgar's name has been used as a simple mnemonic for the scoring criteria.

| APGAR Scoring System | |
|---|---|
| A | Appearance (Color) |
| P | Pulse (Heart rate) |
| G | Grimace (Reflex irritability) |
| A | Activity (Muscle tone) |
| R | Respirations |

The criteria are typically evaluated at 1 and 5 min of age. An additional score at 10 min is frequently performed if the infant's score is < 7 at 5 min. The latest neonatal resuscitation guidelines have de-emphasized the use of the APGAR score, and no longer recommend evaluation of the infant's color.

### Clinical Pearl:

*When measured, the APGAR scoring system should NOT be used to determine the need for resuscitation and should not delay or interrupt resuscitation of the infant.*

## Table 20.1 APGAR Scoring

| APGAR Score | 0 | 1 | 2 |
|---|---|---|---|
| Heart Rate | Absent | < 100 beats·min$^{-1}$ | > 100 beats·min$^{-1}$ |
| Respiratory effort | Absent | Weak, irregular, or gasping | Good, crying |
| Muscle tone | Flaccid | Some flexion of arms and legs | Well flexed, active movement of extremities |
| Reflex/irritability | No response | Grimace or weak cry | Good cry, cough, sneeze |
| Color | Blue all over or pale | Body pink, hands and feet blue | Pink all over |

### Primary vs Secondary Apnea

Deficiencies in blood flow or oxygen supply in utero may result in asphyxia of the newborn. The first sign that the newborn has experienced compromise in utero is a cessation of respiratory efforts. Initially, asphyxia results in rapid respirations. The respirations eventually cease with continued asphyxia resulting in what is termed primary apnea. During primary apnea, the infant will generally breathe again when stimulated. When asphyxia persists for a longer period, the infant develops irregular gasping respirations, which then decrease in frequency and eventually cease. Apnea resulting from prolonged asphyxia is termed secondary apnea. Secondary apnea is assumed to be present when an infant does not start to breathe at birth with physical stimulation. In this setting, positive pressure ventilation must be initiated, and additional help should be requested.

### Fetal Circulation

Fetal hemoglobin has a higher affinity for oxygen than that of adults. This results in a diffusion of oxygen from the mother's circulatory system to the fetus. The placenta acts as the infant's lungs in utero providing oxygen and removing carbon dioxide from the neonatal circulation. It also provides nutrients to the fetus and removes waste products of metabolism.

In the fetal circulation, oxygenated placental blood passes from the right to left heart bypassing the fetal lungs via two channels. The first channel is the ductus arteriosus, which connects the pulmonary artery directly to the aorta. The second channel is the foramen ovale, which is a small hole in the heart allowing blood to pass from the right atrium into the left atrium.

Prior to birth, only a small amount of oxygenated blood flows through the fetal lungs due to the small lung volume and high vascular resistance. The infant's lungs are filled with fluid in utero as blood flows preferentially to the lower resistance placenta.

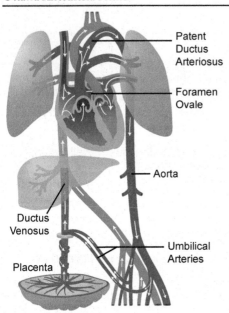

**Patent Ductus Arteriosus**

**Foramen Ovale**

**Aorta**

**Ductus Venosus**

**Umbilical Arteries**

**Placenta**

Fig. 20.1 Neonatal circulation. Oxygenated blood from the uterine artery passes through the ductus venosus, foramen ovale and ductus arteriosus to the systemic circulation.

## What happens immediately after delivery?

At term, the fetal lungs contain approximately 90 mL of plasma ultrafiltrate. During normal vaginal delivery, this fluid is squeezed from the lungs as the infant passes through the birth canal. The extrusion of fluid from the lungs immediately prior to birth helps with lung expansion and oxygenation at the time of delivery. Infants delivered via Cesarean delivery do not get this squeeze and may develop laboured respiratory efforts. This respiratory distress has been termed "transient tachypnea of the newborn", and it typically resolves within 24 hr with observation and oxygen therapy.

Immediately following birth, mild hypoxia and acidosis in concert with the clamping of the umbilical cord help to initiate respirations. When the umbilical cord is clamped, the low resistance placenta is removed from the circulation. This causes an increase in vascular resistance on the left side of the heart, resulting in a functional closure of the foramen ovale and diversion of blood into the lungs. Fresh oxygen in the infant's alveoli and the newly expanded lung volume further decrease the resistance of blood flow into the lungs.

Hypoxia, hypothermia, acidosis, hypovolemia, and hypocarbia are factors that increase pulmonary vascular resistance and force blood through the foramen ovale and ductus arteriosus. These factors tend to cause a "persistent fetal circulation" impeding the newborn's oxygenation and ventilation.

## Which infants require resuscitation?

Risk factors can be used to predict which infants may be in need of resuscitation at delivery. Most neonates will transition from neonatal to newborn blood flow with no complications; however, even neonates with no risk factors occasionally require resuscitation, so care providers should remain vigilant at all times. Immediately following delivery, all neonates require a basic assessment by a health care provider trained in basic neonatal resuscitation.

Several conditions may place a neonate at greater risk for requiring advanced resuscitation at delivery. Common antepartum and intrapartum risk factors predicting a heightened need for resuscitation at birth are listed in Table 20.2. Personnel with advanced neonatal resuscitation skills should be immediately available at the time of delivery of these infants.

## Table 20.2 Risk factors predicting a heightened risk for neonatal resuscitation at delivery

| ANTEPARTUM | INTRAPARTUM |
| --- | --- |
| Maternal age > 35 | Breech or any abnormal presentation |
| Diabetes | Cesarean delivery, especially emergent |
| Gestational hypertension | Forceps or vacuum-assisted delivery |
| Chronic hypertension | Prolonged rupture of membranes (> 18hr) |
| Fetal anemia | Precipitous labour |
| Previous neonatal death | Choriamionitis |
| Bleeding in 2nd or 3rd trimester | Macrosomia |
| Maternal infection | Abnormal fetal heart rate tracing |
| No prenatal care | Use of general anesthetic |
| Maternal substance abuse | Maternal opioids within 4 hr of delivery |
| Rh sensitization | Presence of meconium |
| Maternal drug therapy (i.e., magnesium, lithium, adrenergic drugs) | Prolapsed umbilical cord |
| Maternal cardiac, renal, respiratory, thyroid, or neurologic disorders | Placental abruption |
| Polyhydramnios and olihydramnios | Placenta previa |
| Multiple gestation | Uterine tetany |
| Pre or post term | Prolonged labour (> 24 hours) |
| Fetal abnormalities | |
| Fetus small for dates | |

**Fetal Heart Rate Patterns**

Fetal heart rate (FHR) decelerations may indicate a change in the baby's well-being in utero and are most significant if the rate drops below 100 beats·min$^{-1}$. Early decelerations occurring with contractions and then returning to baseline are probably a reflex response to head compression during the contraction and are usually benign. Late decelerations are more ominous, usually occurring with contractions and having a delayed return to the baseline FHR. They often signify fetal hypoxia and acidosis. Variable decelerations are not associated with contractions and have a quick onset and recovery. They are due to transient cord compression and are usually benign. Sustained bradycardia with a FHR < 100 beats·min$^{-1}$ indicates serious fetal distress and requires urgent intervention. Sustained tachycardia is often associated with fever or sepsis, but may be observed as a response to maternal drug administration (e.g., atropine or ephedrine).

## What should be done if the infant appears distressed?

1. If the fetus is showing signs of distress, the following measures should be taken
2. Call for help.
3. Ensure the mother's abdomen is tilted to the left (left uterine displacement).
4. Provide supplemental oxygen to the mother.
5. Discontinue oxytocin infusion if it is being administered.
6. Consider changing maternal position for variable decelerations.
7. Evaluate and correct maternal hypotension.
8. Ensure accurate FHR monitoring and consider more invasive fetal monitoring, such as a scalp probe.

## What is meconium?

Meconium is the earliest stools of an infant. Unlike later feces, meconium is composed of materials ingested during the time the infant spends in the uterus: intestinal epithelial cells, lanugo, mucus, amniotic fluid, bile, and water. When meconium is passed by the infant in utero, it colors the amniotic fluid and indicates that the infant has been subjected to a stress. Meconium excretion in utero is observed more frequently in the term or post-term infant. A thick "pea-soup" meconium may suggest a recent episode of hypoxia and prompt more aggressive fetal monitoring or management of the labour and delivery.

When the neonate initiates respirations at birth, the meconium can move from the trachea and larger airways down into the periphery of the lung. Meconium can obstruct the lungs and may cause difficulty with oxygenation and ventilation. The resuscitation guidelines support the use of tracheal intubation and tracheal suctioning when the infant with meconium is not vigorous (a vigorous infant is crying, has good tone, and a heart rate > 100 beats·min⁻¹).

## Equipment Needed for Neonatal Resuscitation

Table 20.3 lists the basic equipment needed for neonatal resuscitation. In the case of preterm deliveries or special medical conditions, more specialized equipment and personnel may be required.

## Table 20.3 Basic Neonatal Resuscitation Equipment

| | |
|---|---|
| Trained personnel | Suction and meconium aspirator |
| Radiant heater | Monitors – electrocardiogram (ECG), pulse oximeter, noninvasive blood pressure (NIBP) |
| Pediatric stethoscope | Neonatal laryngoscope and several different blades |
| Oxygen source and appropriate tubing | Stylet for endotracheal tube |
| Towel for drying infant | Endotracheal tubes (2.5 mm, 3.0 mm, 3.5 mm internal diameter) |
| Neonate resuscitation bag | Medications as described in chapter |
| Airway pressure monitor | Umbilical catheter kits |
| Facemask, oral airways (various sizes) | Needles and syringes |

## The Basics of Neonatal Resuscitation

### Airway

Position the infant supine with the neck either in a neutral position or slightly extended. Avoid overextension or flexion, which may produce airway obstruction. A folded towel under the infant's shoulders may be useful as infants often have a large occiput.

Routine suctioning of the infant is no longer recommended due to an increased risk of vagal stimulation and fetal bradycardia. When the infant has absent, slow, or laboured respirations, apply suction first to the mouth and then the nose. If the nose is cleared first, the infant may gasp and aspirate secretions into the pharynx. If mechanical suctioning with an 8F or 10F catheter is used, make sure the vacuum does not exceed 100 mmHg. Limit suctioning to 5 sec at a time, and monitor heart rate for bradycardia, which may occur with deep oropharyngeal suctioning due to vagal stimulation.

If meconium is present in the amniotic fluid, special endotracheal suctioning may be required in the depressed infant.

### Provide warmth

Place the infant under an overhead radiant heater, and dry the infant's body and head to remove amniotic fluid and prevent heat loss. Gentle stimulation will also help initiate and maintain breathing.

### Physical stimulation

If drying and suctioning do not induce effective breathing, gently slapping or flicking the soles of the feet or rubbing the infants back may be useful. Do not waste time continuing tactile stimulation if there is no response after 10 – 15 sec.

### Evaluate the infant

**Respirations:** Infants who are apneic or gasping despite brief stimulation attempts are likely in secondary apnea and should receive positive pressure ventilation with an AMBU type of bag and mask.

**Heart Rate:** Monitor either by auscultating the apical beat or by palpating the base of the umbilical cord. If the heart rate is <100 beats·min⁻¹, begin positive pressure ventilation even if the infant is making some respiratory efforts.

**Color:** The latest neonatal resuscitation guidelines (2010) no longer recommend evaluation of the infant's color at birth. The normal saturation at birth is 60%. Supplemental oxygen is titrated to meet the target saturation levels of a healthy newborn (Table 20.4).

## Table 20.4 Target Newborn Oxygen Saturation Levels

| Targeted Preductal* SpO$_2$ Levels after Birth | |
|---|---|
| 1 min | 60 – 65% |
| 2 min | 65 – 70% |
| 3 min | 70 – 75% |
| 4 min | 75 – 80% |
| 5 min | 80 – 85% |
| 10 min | 85 – 95% |
| *measured in the right hand or wrist | |

## Technique of Positive Pressure Ventilation (PPV)

### Positive Pressure Ventilation is required when:

1. Apnea or gasping respirations are present.
2. The heart rate is <100 beats·min⁻¹.

Most neonates can be adequately ventilated with a bag and mask. The assisted ventilatory rate should be between 40 - 60 breaths·min⁻¹. Usually ventilation can be achieved with airway pressures of 15 - 20 cmH$_2$O, although higher pressures of 30 – 40 cmH$_2$O may occasionally be transiently required to open the airways. Adequate ventilation is best assessed by heart rate response. The presence of bilateral breath sounds and expired $CO_2$ on a $CO_2$ detector are also helpful.

Watching for chest movement may result in excessive ventilation.

**When chest expansion is inadequate, use the mnemonic MR SOPA**

| Table 20.5 | | Inadequate Mask Ventilation: MR SOPA |
|---|---|---|
| **M** | **M**ask | Reapply the face**m**ask and attempt to get a better seal. |
| **R** | **R**eposition | **R**eposition the infant's head; consider extending the head a bit further and repositioning the shoulder towel. |
| **S** | **S**uction | **S**uction any secretions. |
| **O** | **O**ral Airway **O**pen mouth | Consider an **o**ral airway and ventilating with the infant's mouth slightly **o**pen. |
| **P** | **P**ressure | Increase ventilation **p**ressures to 20 - 40 cmH$_2$0. |
| **A** | **A**irway | If unsuccessful, abandon the bag and mask technique and intubate the trachea or place a size 1 laryngeal mask **a**irway device. |

After 15 - 30 sec of effective ventilation, the neonate's heart rate should be re-evaluated. The neonate's heart rate is counted over a 6-sec period and then multiplied by 10 to give an approximation of the 1 min heart rate (e.g., 8 beats in 6 sec = 80 beats·min$^{-1}$).

Positive pressure ventilation can be withdrawn gradually if the heart rate remains > 100 beats·min$^{-1}$ and spontaneous breathing efforts are present. The care provider should continue to provide physical stimulation and supplemental oxygen to the infant if needed.

If the neonate's heart rate is < 100 beats·min$^{-1}$, ventilation should continue. If the heart rate is < 60 beats·min$^{-1}$ after 30 seconds of effective ventilation, chest compressions are initiated and ventilation of the neonate's lungs with 100% oxygen is introduced.

**Chest Compressions:**

Compression of the sternum results in compression of the heart and increases intrathoracic pressure. During compression, blood is pumped into the arterial circulation, and the release of the sternum results in an increase

in venous return to the heart. Chest compressions must be accompanied by ventilation with 100% oxygen. Asphyxia in the neonate not only slows the heart rate but decreases myocardial contractility, resulting in diminished blood flow and oxygen delivery to vital organs.

**When should I start chest compressions?**

You should begin chest compressions when the heart rate remains < 60 beats·min$^{-1}$ after 30 sec of effective ventilation. Chest compressions can be discontinued when the heart rate is ≥ 60 beats·min$^{-1}$; however, PPV should continue until the heart rate is > 100 beats·min$^{-1}$.

**What is the proper technique for administering chest compressions to an infant?**

There are two methods of administering chest compressions in infants. With the two-thumb method, both hands encircle the infant's torso, while the fingers support the infant's

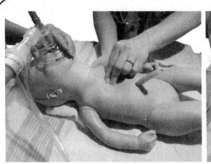 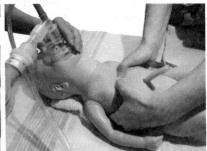

| Two-finger Technique | Thumb Technique |

Fig. 20.2 Neonatal chest compressions.

back and the two thumbs are positioned side by side over the sternum as they create chest compressions by downward displacement of the sternum. With the two-finger approach, the middle and ring fingers of one hand are held perpendicular to the chest as the finger tips apply pressure to the sternum. The other hand is used to support the infants back from below. The two-thumb technique is the preferred method as it results in a higher cardiac output.

The amount of pressure for chest compressions is adjusted to achieve a compression of the chest equal to 1/3 of the anterior-posterior diameter of the chest. A full cycle consists of both a compression and a release phase, and the rate is adjusted to achieve 2 cycles per second.

Once the fingers (thumbs) have been correctly positioned over the infant's sternum, care should be taken to ensure that the hands are not moved from this position. Valuable time may be wasted attempting to relocate the correct hand position. Complications of incorrect hand placement and chest compressions include fractured ribs, lacerated spleen, and pneumothorax.

Every three chest compressions are followed by a pause to insert an effective breath. The resulting 90 compressions with 30 ventilations yield a combined rate of compression and ventilation of 120 per minute. Coordination of ventilation with chest compressions is important to avoid compromising the tidal volume with chest compressions and gastric insufflation with ventilation (when the infant's trachea is not intubated).

Compressions are interrupted after 45 – 60 sec to take a 6-sec heart rate count. Compressions are stopped once the heart rate is > 60 beats·min$^{-1}$, and ventilation is stopped when the heart rate is > 100 beats·min$^{-1}$.

## Endotracheal intubation is indicated when:

1. Prolonged PPV is required (to minimize gastric distension).
2. Ventilation with a bag and mask is ineffective (poor chest expansion, persistent low heart rate).
3. Tracheal suctioning is required (thick or particulate meconium).
4. Diaphragmatic hernia is suspected (to prevent bowel distension in the chest).

5. Delivery of medications is required before intravenous access is obtained.

While endotracheal intubation may play an essential part of an infant's resuscitation, it is not within the scope of this chapter.

## Commonly used Medications
### Oxygen

One of the most significant changes in the 2010 American Heart Association's guidelines for neonatal resuscitation concerns the delivery of oxygen. The new guidelines recommend the use of a pulse oximeter and blended oxygen in any delivery area. Pulse oximetry is highly recommended for use whenever supplemental oxygen, PPV, or continuous positive airway pressure (CPAP) is provided. Evidence suggests that it may be detrimental to the infant to increase a newborn's oxygen level as fast as possible with 100% supplemental oxygen. When supplemental oxygen is administered, the oximeter sensor should be placed on the newborn's right hand or wrist. Regardless of gestation, the goal of oxygen administration is an oxygen saturation resembling that of a healthy term newborn (see Table 20.4). The administration of supplemental oxygen should be reduced or removed if the oxygen saturation is > 90% at any time in the first 10 min. Oxygen saturation levels > 90% in healthy newborns breathing room air are both acceptable and normal. The priority is to ensure adequate lung inflation, increasing inspired oxygen concentration only if PPV or CPAP fail to achieve the target peripheral oxygen saturation ($SpO_2$). A blended concentration of air and oxygen that provides a 30 – 50% oxygen concentration should be introduced in infants < 32 wk gestation who do not meet the targeted oxygen level. Resuscitation should be initiated with air when an appropriate blender is not available. Oximetry is recommended when:

1. The need for resuscitation is anticipated;

2. Positive pressure ventilation (PPV) is administered for more than a few breaths; or

3. Whenever persistent cyanosis is suspected during resuscitation or any time after birth.

For the majority of infants who require resuscitation, the only medication they may require is oxygen. Typically, oxygen is delivered starting with an inspired concentration of 21% (room air). If the neonate continues to have difficulty with oxygenation after 30 sec, then supplemental oxygen with positive pressure ventilation may be introduced. Neonates very rarely require other medications. In fact, it is much more important to ensure effective ventilation than to administer other medications.

### Naloxone

Naloxone is a pure opioid antagonist without intrinsic respiratory depression activity. Naloxone is indicated for the reversal of respiratory depression when the mother has received opioids within 4 hr of delivery and the infant is observed to have depressed respirations. While naloxone works very rapidly, adequate ventilatory assistance should always be provided first. Naloxone has a shorter duration than some opioids; consequently, the infant's respiration must be monitored for a further 4 - 6 hr.

Naloxone can be given either intravenously or via an endotracheal tube (ETT). Subcutaneous or intramuscular routes can also be used if the infant's perfusion is adequate; however, there may be a slower onset of action with these routes. If maternal opioid addiction is suspected, it is probably prudent not to give naloxone, but rather, to support ventilation until the infant's respiratory drive is adequate. Administering naloxone to infants of opioid-dependent mothers may result in a withdrawal reaction and seizures in the infant. Naloxone is supplied in a 0.4 mg·mL$^{-1}$ concentration for

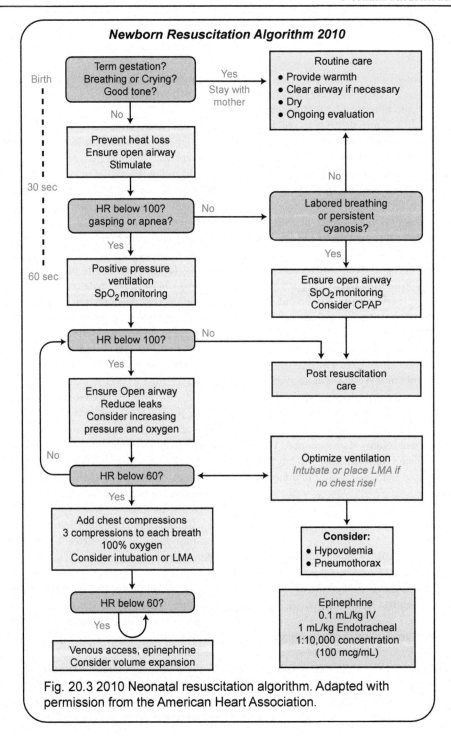

Fig. 20.3 2010 Neonatal resuscitation algorithm. Adapted with permission from the American Heart Association.

neonatal resuscitation. The dose is 0.1 mg·kg⁻¹ for infant resuscitation.

### Epinephrine

Epinephrine (adrenaline) is an alpha and beta-adrenergic stimulant. The alpha effect causes vasoconstriction that raises the perfusion pressure during chest compressions and augments oxygen delivery to both the heart and brain. The beta effect enhances cardiac contractility, stimulates spontaneous contractions, and increases the heart rate.

Epinephrine can be given either intravenously or through the ETT every 3 - 5 min as required. The epinephrine concentration used in neonatal resuscitation is supplied as a 1:10,000 dilution (i.e., 0.1 mg or 100 µg·mL⁻¹). The intravenous dose is 0.1 mL·kg⁻¹ of a 1:10,000 concentration. If the infant does not have intravenous access, the epinephrine can also be given via the ETT. The ETT dose of epinephrine is 1 mL·kg⁻¹ (0.1 mg·kg⁻¹) of 1:10,000 concentration every 3 - 5 min. The intravenous route of epinephrine delivery is preferable to the endotracheal route. Neonatal resuscitation can be a stressful situation; recalling the recommended volume of the neonatal (1:10,000) epinephrine concentration and not the µg is associated with less chance of a medication error.

*Clinical Pearl:*

*The neonatal epinephrine dose (1:10,000 concentration) for a term infant is 0.3 mL intravenously or 3 mL through the ETT every 3 - 5 min as required.*

### When should I give epinephrine?

Epinephrine is indicated when the infant's heart rate remains < 60 beats·min⁻¹ following 30 sec of effective assisted ventilation plus 45 - 60 sec of effective chest compressions along with coordinated assisted ventilation with100% oxygen.

## Intravenous Fluids and Red Blood Cells

### How will I know if the infant is hypovolemic?

Conditions that result in acute maternal hypovolemia prior to delivery of the infant should make the clinician suspect that the infant may also suffer from the effects of hypovolemia. Maternal hemorrhage prior to delivery is one such condition. A few of the causes of maternal hemorrhage prior to delivery include placental abruption, placenta previa, transection of the placenta during Cesarean delivery, and maternal trauma. Other conditions that may result in neonatal hypovolemia include multiple gestation pregnancies, umbilical cord tear during delivery, and a strangulating umbilical cord requiring umbilical cord transection prior to delivery.

Hypovolemia occurs more frequently in the newborn than is commonly recognized. Blood loss is often not obvious, and initial tests of hemoglobin and hematocrit are usually misleading. Initial fluid resuscitation with normal saline or Ringer's lactate can be used to increase the vascular volume, improve tissue perfusion, and reduce the development of metabolic acidosis.

Clinical signs of hypovolemia resulting from an acute loss of > 20% of the blood volume include:
1. Pallor persisting after oxygenation.
2. A weak pulse despite a good heart rate.
3. A poor response to resuscitative efforts.
4. A decreased blood pressure (< 55/30).

### Red Blood Cells

In addition to crystalloid resuscitation, type O Rh-negative packed red blood cells (PRBCs) should be considered for volume replacement when severe fetal anemia or bleeding has occurred or is expected. If time permits, the donor unit can be cross-matched to the mother to identify any maternal antibodies. When blood is required immediately, uncross-matched type O Rh-negative PRBCs should be used. A volume of 10 mL·kg$^{-1}$ (approximately 35 mL in a term infant) should be administered as an infusion over 5 – 10 min. The amount and rate of fluid must be carefully controlled to avoid volume overload and heart failure (see Chapter 26).

## Special Considerations

### Preterm Neonates

A comprehensive discussion of the many considerations for the preterm infant is beyond the scope of this chapter. When anticipating a preterm delivery, it is important to ensure that trained personnel are present and equipment has been prepared for use. One of the great challenges in preterm deliveries is temperature regulation in the neonate. These neonates are at high risk for hypothermia, and students can help by ensuring that the ambient temperature in the delivery room is turned up to approximately 26°C. A polyethylene plastic bag should be immediately available for neonates that are < 29 wk gestational age. Once delivered, the neonate is immediately placed in the polyethylene bag and placed under a radiant warmer. Trained personnel will then initiate resuscitation as required.

### Blockage of the Nasal Passages

Infants are "obligate nasal breathers". Blockage of the nasal passages by mucous or meconium may result in respiratory distress. On rare occasions, a congenital abnormality called choanal atresia may be the cause of a blockage of the nasal passages. A small suction catheter can be passed through the nasal passages into the nasopharynx to ensure there is no nasal obstruction. If bilateral choanal atresia is present, the infant will develop an upper airway obstruction unless stimulated to cry and breathe through the mouth. An oral airway can be used to open a passage through which the baby can breathe. Consultation with a pediatrician will initiate the steps for definitive management.

### Congenital Airway Malformation: Pierre Robin Syndrome

Pierre Robin syndrome is a condition in which the infant is born with a very small mandible, reducing the size of the pharyngeal space and creating an upper airway obstruction. The tracheas of these babies are very difficult to intubate, and tracheal intubation should be considered only if an airway expert is present. Two simple maneuvers can be used to relieve the upper airway obstruction. The first maneuver is to place the infant in the prone position, which helps bring the soft airway structures forward and allows the infant to breathe. If this maneuver is not successful, a short small ETT tube can be used as a nasopharyngeal airway (NPA) by inserting it into the infant's nose towards the back of the pharynx and behind the tongue without entering the trachea. This will generally relieve the obstruction and allow the infant to breathe through the NPA. Consultation with a pediatrician is required to initiate the care required for the ultimate management of this problem.

A full discussion of the considerations of neonatal resuscitation for the term and preterm infant is beyond the scope of this chapter. Investigative procedures are frequently performed to support the clinical diagnosis and direct management, including measurements of glucose, electrolytes, complete blood count, calcium, blood gases, and a chest X-ray. Students are encouraged to learn more about neonatal resuscitation by enrolling in one of the many neonatal resuscitation workshops offered by the Canadian Pediatric Association.

**Test your knowledge:**

1. Describe the basic steps in neonatal resuscitation.
2. Identify 3 antepartum and 3 intrapartum risk factors for requiring neonatal resuscitation.
3. A newborn is still not breathing after you have provided gentle stimulation and warmth. What is your next step?
4. What are the signs that positive pressure ventilation has been effective and may be stopped?
5. What criteria do you use to decide if a neonate requires chest compressions?
6. When should you ask for help when resuscitating a newborn?

**Recommended Web Links:**

1. Canadian Pediatrics Association http://www.cps.ca/
2. American Academy of Pediatrics http://www.aap.org/
3. Neonatal resuscitation Program http://www.aap.org/nrp/default.html
4. Canadian Pediatric Anesthesia Society http://www.cpas-sapc.ca/

**Resources:**

Neonatal Resuscitation Textbook- 6th Edition. American Academy of Pediatrics and American Heart Association; Editor John Kattwinkel, MD, FAAP. Published May 17th, 2011.

Miller's Anesthesia, 7th Edition. Ronald D. Miller, MD, Lars I. Eriksson, Lee A. Fleisher, MD, Jeanine P. Wiener-Kronish, MD and William L. Young. Churchill Livingstone, 2010.

Clinical Anesthesia (6th Edition). Paul G. Barash, Bruce F. Cullen, Robert K. Stoelting, Michael Cahalan, M. Christine Stock. Philadelphia, PA: Lippincott Williams & Wilkins, 2009.

Kattwinkel J, Perlman JM, Aziz K, et al. Part 15: Neonatal resuscitation: 2010 American heart association guidelines for cardiopulmonary resuscitation and emergency cardiovascular care. Circulation 2010;122:S909-S919.

# CHAPTER 21

# Intravenous Fluids and Blood Component Therapy

Sandra Bromley MD, Dennis Reid MD

## Learning Objectives

1. To prescribe and administer appropriate intravenous crystalloids, colloids, and blood products commonly used in the perioperative period.
2. To monitor the clinical and hematological effects of these treatments.
3. To recognize and prevent potential complications of intravenous fluid and blood component therapy.
4. To acquire an understanding of current blood conservation strategies.

## Key Points

1  An understanding of fluid physiology and normal perioperative requirements is essential to the proper administration of fluids and can have a major influence on the well-being of patients following surgery.

2  Current evidence does not support the routine replacement of theoretical third space fluid losses.

3  Balanced salt solutions, such as Ringer's lactate, are preferable to 0.9% saline for routine crystalloid replacement and resuscitation.

4  In 2013 Health Canada released a new box warning concerning an increase in mortality and severe renal injury associated with the administration of intravenous synthetic starch solutions (e.g., Voluven, Volulyte). Current evidence dose not support the administration of these solutions in the setting of sepsis, severe liver disease and or renal impairment requiring emergent care.

5  Hyperchloremic acidosis associated with 0.9% saline administration results in renal vasoconstriction and a reduction in the glomerular filtration rate (GFR), impairing the ability of the kidneys to excrete sodium and water even in the presence of fluid overload.

6    Patients who do not have disorders in gastric emptying should continue clear oral fluids up to 3 hr prior to surgery. Oral intake of carbohydrate beverages should be encouraged up to 3 hr prior to surgery in patients who do not have diabetes. A return to oral fluids should be achieved as soon as possible following surgery.

7    The decision to transfuse in the perioperative period should be made only after a careful patient-specific risk-benefit analysis.

8    Preoperative anemia of unknown etiology requires investigation prior to elective surgery when there is a risk for significant (> 500 mL) blood loss.

9    Intraoperative blood conservation strategies are an effective means of decreasing a patient's exposure to blood products.

Optimal perioperative fluid therapy requires an understanding of the volume and composition of the body's fluid compartments. Intravenous fluids are routinely administered to replenish existing fluid deficits as well as losses resulting from surgery. Many factors influence the type and amount of fluid that is given to a patient. Common factors include the type of surgery, preexisting comorbidities (e.g., heart failure, renal dysfunction), the amount of blood lost, and the patient's personal beliefs and wishes. Evidence from clinical trials suggests that perioperative fluid management can influence morbidity and mortality,[1] and both inadequate and excessive fluid therapy can be detrimental. Serial evaluations of a patient's fluid status are essential to optimize oxygenation and organ perfusion.

**Body fluid distribution**

Total body water (TBW) constitutes approximately 60% of body weight. In a 70 kg adult, this equates to 42 L, but TBW will also vary by sex, age, and body type. Total body water is typically decreased in the elderly and obese and increased in neonates and lean individuals. Two-thirds of the TBW (representing 40% of the body weight) is contained within cells as intracellular fluid (ICF). The remaining one-third (20% of the body weight) is in the extracellular fluid (ECF). Plasma and the cellular components of blood comprise approximately 7% of the total body weight or 5 L in a 70 kg adult (0.07 x 70 kg = 4.9 L).

The distribution of body fluid into its various compartments is determined by capillary permeability, hydrostatic pressure, and oncotic pressure (recall the Starling equation). Normal serum osmolarity is 290 ± 10 mOsm·L$^{-1}$. Sodium, the predominant extracellular cation, is found in equal concentrations in plasma and interstitial fluid (140 mEq·L$^{-1}$). When sodium is administered intravenously, it redistributes itself within the ECF. Potassium is the predominant cation found in the ICF (K$^+$ = 150 mEq·L$^{-1}$). Albumin is located mainly in the plasma and exerts the majority of oncotic pressure. Intravascular volume is tightly regulated by antidiuretic hormone, aldosterone, and atrial natriuretic peptide.[2]

**Fluid requirements**

The human body requires approximately 1.5 - 2.5 L of water as well as 50 - 100 mEq of sodium and 40 - 80 mEq of potassium per day to balance out losses from the gastrointestinal, respiratory, cutaneous, and urinary systems.[2,21] In a person with normal renal and cardiac function, excess water is excreted in the urine. Fluid requirements for short periods of

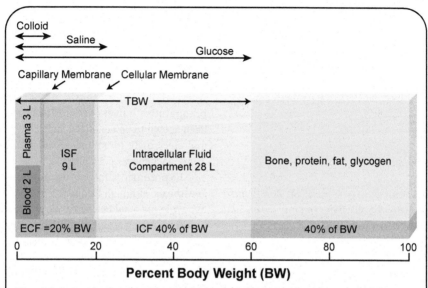

**Fig. 21.1** Approximate distribution and volume of fluids in a 70 kg adult. Water and glucose solutions distribute across the extracellular and intracellular compartments. Colloids are restricted to the intravascular (blood and plasma) compartment. ECF = Extracellular fluid, ISF = Interstitial fluid, ICF = Intracellular fluid, TBW = Total body water.

time (< 1 wk) can be met with water, sodium, and potassium. Any additional amount should only be given to replace deficits or ongoing losses. For prolonged periods of fasting, additional electrolyte and mineral supplementation are also required. Hyperglycemia is a normal response to the stress of surgery, and most patients do not require supplemental glucose in the perioperative period. An exception to this is the diabetic patient who is at risk of hypoglycemia.[2]

### Maintenance

If surgery is planned within 24 hr and the patient is to receive nothing by mouth (NPO), maintenance fluids, 0.9% saline (NS) or Ringer's lactate (RL) are appropriate. If the patient is able to drink, it is preferable to give clear carbohydrate fluids orally up to 3 hr prior to surgery rather than to administer fluids intravenously. For periods > 24 hr but < 1 wk, maintenance requirements can be met by administering IV fluids (i.e., ⅔ of 5% dextrose [D5W] with ⅓ NS or ½ NS with D5W). Potassium (15 - 20 mEq·L⁻¹) is also often added to these solutions.

Hourly maintenance fluid requirements for children and adults can be calculated using the "4-2-1 rule" with the patient's weight. First, 4 mL·hr⁻¹ are administered for the first 10 kg of the patient's body weight, then 2 mL·hr⁻¹ for the next 10 kg, and 1 mL·hr⁻¹ for each kg > 20 kg (see example below). Alternatively, for adults, adding 40 to the patient's weight in kg can be used to quickly calculate the maintenance fluid rate in mL·hr⁻¹.

Example: The maintenance fluid requirement for a 75 kg adult is 115 mL·hr⁻¹.

$$4 \text{ mL·hr}^{-1} \text{ x } 10 \text{ kg} = 40 \text{ mL·hr}^{-1}$$
$$+ \quad 2 \text{ mL·kg}^{-1} \text{ x } 10 \text{ kg} = 20 \text{ mL·hr}^{-1}$$
$$+ \quad 1 \text{ mL·hr-1 x } 55 \text{ kg} = 55 \text{ mL·hr}^{-1}$$
$$\underline{115 \text{ mL·hr}^{-1}}$$

Alternatively, wt (kg) + 40 = maintenance fluids in mL·hr⁻¹, i.e.,

75 + 40 = 115 mL·hr⁻¹

*Clinical pearl:*

*A quick way to calculate the hourly intravenous maintenance fluids (mL·hr⁻¹) in an adult is to add 40 to the patient's weight in kg.*

## Deficit

A fluid deficit may develop as a result of prolonged fasting or from a pathological process. The fluid deficit from fasting can be roughly calculated by multiplying the patient's hourly maintenance requirements by the number of hours fasted. Fluid deficits from a pathological process are much more difficult to quantify. Table 21.1 lists clinical conditions frequently associated with fluid deficits as well as associated common physical and laboratory findings. When significant fluid deficits are not corrected prior to surgery, severe hemodynamic instability may occur with induction of anesthesia. This is more common during emergency surgery. Preoperative bowel preparations in elective abdominal surgery can worsen fluid deficits considerably.[2] Routine preoperative bowel preparations have not been shown to be beneficial, may create fluid and electrolyte imbalances, and should be avoided whenever possible.[21]

Hypotension following induction of anesthesia, although frequently attributed to hypovolemia, may be the result of a number of causes acting alone or together. Common causes include vasodilation secondary to volatile anesthetic agents, decreased preload and increased right ventricular afterload secondary to positive pressure ventilation, direct myocardial depression secondary to intravenous anesthetic medications, a decrease in sympathetic tone associated with neuraxial anesthesia, and the presence of a pre-existing intravascular volume deficit. Vasopressors, such as ephedrine and phenylephrine, adjusting the anesthetic depth, and a fluid challenge are commonly used to mitigate the decrease in blood pressure.

## Table 21.1 Clinical conditions associated with fluid deficits and common associated physical and laboratory findings.

| Conditions | Physical findings | Laboratory findings |
|---|---|---|
| Bowel obstruction<br>Bowel preparation<br>Fractured hip / femur / pelvis<br>Trauma<br>Vomiting, diarrhea<br>Burns<br>Sepsis<br>Pancreatitis<br>Diuretic use | Tachycardia<br>Orthostatic or supine hypotension<br>Oliguria<br>Tachycardia<br>Low jugular venous pressure<br>Dry mucous membranes<br>Decreased skin turgor | Elevated urea<br>Elevated creatinine<br>Elevated urine osmolarity<br>Low urine sodium<br>Elevated hematocrit<br>Metabolic alkalosis (mild)<br>Metabolic acidosis (severe) |

## Ongoing losses

Historically, fluid losses occurring during surgery were believed to be the result of blood loss during surgery as well as fluid movement into a "third space" compartment. This "third space" fluid loss was believed to result from fluids being sequestered in other body compartments, such as the bowel and lung, as a result of surgical manipulation and capillary leakage. A "4-6-8 mL·kg$^{-1}$·hr$^{-1}$" rule was used as a simplistic estimation of this third space loss, where the third space fluid losses were replaced with 4, 6, or 8 mL·kg$^{-1}$·hr$^{-1}$ for minor, moderate, and major surgical trauma, respectively.[2] Predetermined fluid replacement therapy using these calculations resulted in large amounts of crystalloids being administered to patients undergoing surgery.

Approximately 72 hr after surgery, fluids mobilize back into the circulatory system and may result in circulatory overload in patients with compromised cardiac or renal function. Excessive intravenous salt and fluid administration is now recognized as a major cause of postoperative morbidity and a major contributor to organ failure, increased hospital length of stay, and mortality.[3,21,22] Both inadequate fluid resuscitation and excessive fluid administration has been shown to increase morbidity in the perioperative period.[21] In major abdominal surgery, evidence suggests that goal-directed fluid regimens are associated with a lower rate of postoperative complications.[1,23] One litre of 0.9% saline contains 9 g of salt, which is more than double the daily required salt intake. Human physiology has not adapted well to eliminate salt efficiently from the body. In illness, adaptive mechanisms are even less capable of eliminating a salt load. Refer to the additional resources for an advanced discussion on optimizing perioperative fluid therapy.

## Crystalloids and colloids

Fluid and blood loss replacement is usually initiated with intravenous (IV) crystalloid or colloid solutions to replenish the intravascular volume. Table 21.2 lists commonly used IV solutions and their components. Intense debate continues over perioperative fluid therapy and both the type and quantity of fluid that should be administered for major surgery. Recent consensus guidelines recommend the use of a balanced crystalloid, e.g., Ringer's lactate, for routine crystalloid replacement and resuscitation rather than the use of 0.9% saline (evidence level 1b).[21] Currently, only saline is recommended for administration with blood products.[6]

The debate continues as research has yet to demonstrate clearly whether crystalloids or colloids are superior for resuscitation.[4] A recent (2011) Cochrane summary review found that colloids were no more effective than crystalloids in reducing mortality in people who are critically ill or injured. To complicate matters further, the distribution ratio of fluids in acutely ill patients may be shifted by alterations in membrane permeability. In practice, clinicians often use a combination of crystalloids and colloids for patients requiring large amounts of resuscitation fluids in an attempt to limit excessive interstitial edema from crystalloids. The administration of colloids is moderated by its increased cost and special considerations discussed later in this chapter.

Crystalloid solutions include NS, RL, and various concentrations of saline, with or without D5W. They contain salts that are semipermeable to cellular membranes, and thus, only a portion of these fluids stay in the intravascular space. For NS and RL (isotonic crystalloids), a mere 20 – 25% of the infused IV solution will remain in the intravascular compartment.[21] The remaining 75 - 80% will redistribute itself into the interstitial space. In

Table 21.2 Common intravenous solutions and their components.

| Solution | dextrose (g·dL⁻¹) | Na (mEq·L⁻¹) | Cl (mEq·L⁻¹) | K (mEq·L⁻¹) | pH | Osm | Other |
|---|---|---|---|---|---|---|---|
| NS | - | 154 | 154 | - | 5.5 | 308 | |
| Ringer's lactate | - | 130 | 109 | 4 | 6.5 | 272 | Ca 1.4, lactate 28 mEq·L⁻¹ |
| D5W | 5 | - | - | - | 4.0 | 252 | |
| "2/3" D5W 1/3NS | 3.3 | 51 | 51 | - | 4.0 | 269 | |
| ½ NS | - | 77 | 77 | - | 5.5 | 154 | |
| ½ NS + D5W | 5 | 77 | 77 | - | 4.0 | 406 | |
| NS + D5W | 5 | 154 | 154 | - | 4.0 | 560 | |
| 3% saline | - | 513 | 513 | - | 5.8 | 1,026 | |
| Pentaspan® | - | 154 | 154 | - | 5.0 | 326 | Pentastarch 10 g·dL⁻¹ |
| Voluven® | - | 154 | 154 | - | 4.0-5.5 | 308 | tetrastarch 6 g·dL⁻¹ |
| Volulyte® | - | 137 | 110 | 4 | 5.7 – 6.5 | 287 | Magnesium 1.5 mmol·L⁻¹, Acetate 34 mmol·L⁻¹ |

NS = normal saline; D5W = 5% dextrose in water; Osm = osmolality.

an attempt to maintain intravascular volume, crystalloid replacement of blood loss is generally replaced in a ratio of at least 3:1 (i.e., 500 mL of blood loss will require at least 1.5 L of NS or RL to maintain the intravascular volume). Crystalloids containing D5W and saline distribute themselves partially like water and partially like saline.

In contrast, colloid solutions contain large molecules that resist diffusion across capillary membranes and tend to stay in the intravascular space. They can replace blood loss on a 1:1 volume basis and have the advantage of requiring a smaller infused volume with less expansion into the interstitium. Colloids can be synthetic (Pentaspan®, Voluven®, Volulyte®) or collected from donor blood (albumin).

## Normal saline

Normal saline (0.9% NaCl) is commonly used to replace minimal to moderate blood loss and in the initial resuscitation of patients in shock. Saline contains supra normal amounts of both $Na^+$ and $Cl^-$ (154 $mEq·L^{-1}$) and is in fact not "normal". Rapid administration of NS or RL is followed by redistribution from the intravascular space to other fluid compartments over the next 10 – 15 min, with only 25% of the crystalloid remaining in the intravascular compartment. Administration of large amounts of NS may be accompanied by a hyperchloremic hypernatremic non-anion gap metabolic acidosis and is associated with a reduction in the GFR. The surgical stress response increases endogenous vasopressin, catecholamines, and activates the renin-angiotensin aldosterone system (RAAS). The result is an antidiuretic effect, retention of water, and oliguria, even in the presence of fluid overload. When NS is infused, both sodium and chloride serum concentrations increase resulting in hyperchloremia, which results in renal vasoconstriction, reduced GFR, and a reduced ability to excrete sodium and water.[21] Normal saline is indicated for the treatment of hypochloremia.

A hypochloremic metabolic alkalosis caused by chronic gastric losses (vomiting, nasogastric (NG) suction) is ideally treated with NS.[2] The osmolarity of a solution can also influence the choice of fluids. In patients with brain injury, for example, the administration of hypotonic solutions may contribute to brain swelling. As NS is more hypertonic than RL, it is generally the preferred crystalloid for these patients.

## Ringer's lactate

Ringer's lactate is also commonly used for resuscitation and redistributes in a similar manner to NS. It is slightly more hypotonic; it has less NaCl and a higher pH, and it contains $K^+$, $Ca^{2+}$, and lactate. Historically, RL was considered contraindicated in patients with renal failure due to its potassium content. The potassium concentration in RL is 4 $mEq·L^{-1}$, which pales in comparison with the body's vast intracellular $K^+$ stores (150 $mEq·L^{-1}$). The administration of NS (which contains no potassium) to patients with renal failure is paradoxically associated with a larger increase in serum $K^+$ when compared with RL. The more acidotic NS is believed to promote a shift in intracellular $K^+$ to the extracellular compartment. Consensus guidelines now recommend administration of electrolyte solutions containing potassium to patients with acute kidney injury in preference to NS.[21] Patients with chronic diarrhea may present with a hyperchloremic metabolic acidosis that may be corrected with RL as it contains the bicarbonate substrate, lactate.[2]

## 5% Dextrose in Water (D5W)

D5W results in a minimal expansion of the intravascular volume space because it distributes itself like water into all body fluid compartments (2/3 ICF, 1/3 ECF). Less than 10% of the fluid stays in the intravascular compartment, hence, D5W is not recommended for fluid resuscitation. If large volumes of D5W are infused, hyponatremia, hyperglycemia, and a decrease in serum osmolarity can occur. Water intoxication manifesting as severe hyponatremia can occur when D5W solutions are administered in patients on oxytocin (due to oxytocin's antidiuretic hormone [ADH] effect) and in patients with cerebrovascular pathology or undergoing neurosurgical procedures. Hyperglycemia is a common response to surgical stress, and perioperative dextrose-containing solutions are generally reserved for patients at high risk of hypoglycemia, such as diabetics and infants.[2]

**"2/3, 1/3" and ½ NS with D5W**

Normal saline mixed with 5% dextrose in water is commonly used as a maintenance fluid in fasting patients, and two common solutions include ⅔ D5W ⅓ NS and ½ NS + D5W. The more D5W a solution contains, the more it will distribute itself to the intracellular compartment. These solutions should not be used for resuscitation purposes as they have little effect on the circulating blood volume and can cause hyponatremia.

**Hypertonic saline**

Hypertonic saline has shown potential as a resuscitative solution due to its ability to draw fluid from the extravascular space via osmosis. Two concentrations are available (3% and 7.5% NaCl), but they have yet to become commonplace in the perioperative setting.

**Synthetic starches**

Hydroxyethyl starch (HES) solutions are plasma volume expanders derived artificially from amylopectine[5], and they are the most commonly used synthetic colloids. These solutions are more advantageous than crystalloid solutions because the intravascular volume is increased to equal to or slightly more than the volume of the solution administered[2] (1 to 1.6:1 ratio). This increase in volume is due to the large molecules in colloids that do not easily cross capillary membranes as well as exertion of higher oncotic pressure.

Two commonly used synthetic starches are Pentaspan® and Voluven®. They are more expensive than crystalloid solutions but less expensive than other blood substitutes, such as albumin. Both starches are mixed in 0.9% NaCl and are supplied in 250 mL and 500 mL bags. Recommended dosages are 33 mL·kg⁻¹ daily for Voluven® and 28 mL·kg⁻¹ daily for Pentaspan® (about 2L daily). Their effects on blood volume are thought to last 6 hr for Voluven® and 18 - 24 hr for Pentaspan®. Side effects may include circulatory overload, altered coagulation, and hypersensitivity reactions. They are contraindicated in patients with bleeding disorders, renal disease, and circulatory overload. In severe sepsis, they may also increase the risk of acute kidney injury.[5] Volulyte® is a relatively new colloid that is prepared in a crystalloid solution that more closely reflects normal physiologic electrolyte concentrations when compared to colloids that are prepared in saline.

In 2013 Health Canada issued an advisory based on recent literature concerning the association of Hydroxyethyl starch (HES) solutions with increased mortality and severe liver injury [26,27,28,29].

I.   An increase in mortality, renal injury and liver failure have been associated with the use of HES solutions.

II.  In patients requiring intensive or emergent care, the use of crystalloid solutions in preference to HES solutions should be considered.

III. HES solutions are now contraindicated in patients with a) sepsis, b) severe liver disease and c) with renal impairment with oliguria and anuria, not related to hypovolemia.

**Albumin**

Albumin is a plasma protein produced by the liver. It is extracted from donor blood and available as a 5% (500 mL) and 25%

(100 mL) solution. Like other blood products, consent should be obtained prior to administration. It is heat-treated at 60°C for 10 hr to eliminate bacterial and viral contamination. Administration of 5% albumin (which exerts a similar oncotic pressure as plasma) will increase intravascular volume by a factor of 1 to 1.5 times the volume administered. Administration of the 25% solution will draw interstitial fluid from the extravascular space and result in about a fourfold increase in the intravascular volume.[6] Albumin stays in the intravascular space for approximately 4 to 6 hr, no crossmatch is necessary, and it doesn't require a special filter for administration. Nevertheless, albumin is infrequently used perioperatively due to its high cost. Risks of albumin include anaphylaxis and circulatory overload. Albumin has not shown an advantage over crystalloids for resuscitation of the critically ill patient and may lead to an increased mortality in trauma patients with brain injury.[7,8]

### Blood components

While crystalloids and colloids are often used as initial replacement of blood loss, they have no oxygen-carrying capacity and may worsen coagulation due to dilution of platelets and coagulation factors. They are therefore not a substitute for blood products. During the initial resuscitation of a patient with acute blood loss, the need for transfusion should be assessed. When possible, informed consent for blood product administration should be obtained and documented.

A patient at risk of requiring a blood transfusion (preoperative anemia, anticipated significant blood loss) should have a type and screen or a type and crossmatch. If time permits, investigation and treatment of anemia is recommended. A type and screen confirms the patient's ABO and Rh (D) blood groups and screens the patient's blood for the presence of

antibodies. This process takes approximately 5 - 10 min. A type and crossmatch mixes the patient's blood with the donor's blood to determine if there is any untoward reaction. The type and crossmatch can be performed in approximately 45 min. If matched blood is unavailable, O negative blood should be given to all children and women of childbearing age, and O positive blood should be given to adult men.[10]

The ABO-Rh identification as well as an antibody screen is performed prior to elective surgical procedures that may require blood products. Most patients will not have identified antibodies to blood products. Rather than performing a traditional crossmatch that requires 45 minutes, the majority of patients having elective surgery in large modern hospitals are issued blood products using a much more rapid (5 minute) electronic crossmatch. The electronic crossmatch requires that two previously obtained independent specimens of blood from the patient have confirmed their blood type and lack of antibodies. The electronic crossmatch does not require the physical mixing of the donor and recipients blood.

Donors with group O blood are universal donors as they can donate blood to people with blood groups O, A, B, or AB (universal recipient). For plasma, the reverse is true. Patients with blood group O are universal recipients from donors with blood groups O, A, B, or AB (universal donor).

When the risk of requiring an intraoperative transfusion is high, blood products may be ordered and put on hold by the transfusionist for expedited release when needed. In some cases, blood is brought directly to the operating room (OR) even before the surgery has begun. Prior to administering blood products, the patient's identity must be verified and checked by two individuals against the identification on the blood product label. Omitting this simple but important step is the leading cause of acute hemolytic reactions.[6]

**Blood products**

Most blood transfusions are allogeneic, meaning they come from unrelated donors. In Canada, all donated units are tested for ABO and Rh (D) type red blood cell (RBC) alloantibodies, human immunodeficiency virus (HIV)-1, HIV-2, hepatitis B virus (HBV), hepatitis C virus (HCV), human T-lymphotropic virus (HTLV) I and II, West Nile virus, and syphilis.[6] Approximately 500 mL of whole blood is collected from the donor, and it is divided into RBCs, plasma, and a buffy coat. White cells are then removed from RBCs and platelets via leukoreduction.[6] Selected units are irradiated to prevent transfusion-associated graft *vs* host disease in at-risk patients. Current (2011) Ontario Transfusion recommendations state that all blood products should be transfused through a 170 - 260 micron filter to capture fibrin debris and should only be infused with NS.[6] A recent study challenging this practice examined the transfusion of RBCs with RL. In this study, there was no increase in clotting when RBCs were transfused with RL.[9] Table 21.3 lists the cost of various fluids, blood products, and tests.[6]

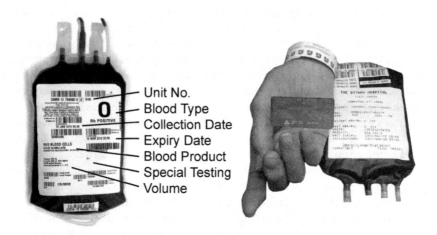

Unit No.
Blood Type
Collection Date
Expiry Date
Blood Product
Special Testing
Volume

Fig. 21.2 Blood product labelling information and verification. Blood products should be checked by two health care providers using the patient's name, medical record number (MRN), blood product number, blood type and the expiry date.

Table 21.3　　Cost of various fluids, blood products, and tests[A]

| Product | Cost | | |
|---|---|---|---|
| Albumin 5% (per 500 mL) | $65 | Normal saline (per litre)* | $1.40 |
| PRBCs (1 unit) | $419 | Ringer's lactate (per litre)* | $2.03 |
| Autologous whole blood | $419 | Pentaspan (per 500 mL) | $55 |
| Platelets (4 units buffy coat) | $286 | Voluven (per 500 mL) | $55 |
| Frozen plasma (4 units) | $156 | Blood group | $10 |
| Cryoprecipitate (8 units) | $1,080 | Antibody screen | $30 |
| Tranexamic acid (1 g)* | $9 | Crossmatch | $12 |
| Recombinant factor VIIa per mg | $1,163 | Crossmatch (antibody present) | $30 |
| Octaplex® (1,000 IU) | $720 | | |

*Ottawa Hospital cost quote. PRBCs = packed red blood cells.

[A] Costs are listed in the 2011 Ontario Transfusion Medicine Guide "Bloody Easy 3".

### Packed Red Blood Cells (PRBCs)

Forty to 70% of all PRBCs are transfused in the perioperative setting.[11] Additives of citrate-phosphate-dextrose (CPD) and saline-adenine-glucose-mannitol (SAGM) provide energy to red cells, anticoagulate the blood, and prolong shelf life to a maximum of 42 days. Red cells are stored at 1 - 6°C and can be kept at room temperature for up to 4 hr prior to administration.[10] The volume of each unit is 280 mL on average, with the exact volume of a specific unit indicated on the unit's label. One unit of PRBCs or 3 mL·kg$^{-1}$ will typically raise hemoglobin by approximately 10 g·L$^{-1}$.[6] Although PRBCs improve oxygen delivery, they do not have adequate amounts of coagulation factors and can contribute to dilutional coagulopathy when given in large amounts.

### Plasma

Plasma comes in two forms, random donor plasma (250 mL) and apheresis donor plasma (500 mL). Plasma from female donors is fractionated to make albumin and intravenous immunoglobulin (IVIg), whereas plasma from male donors is used for plasma and cryoprecipitate.[6] Plasma that is frozen within 8 hr of collection is referred to as fresh frozen plasma (FFP), while frozen plasma (FP) is frozen within 24 hours. Plasma contains coagulation factors II, V, VII, VIII, IX, X, XI, protein C, protein S, antithrombin III, and fibrinogen (400-900 mg per unit).[6] The half-life of the different coagulation factors varies from hours to days, but plasma can be kept for up to one year when stored at -18°C. It is indicated preoperatively in patients with multiple coagulation factor deficiencies (i.e., advanced liver disease), during massive transfusion, and for urgent reversal of warfarin anticoagulation. The dose is 10 - 15 mL·kg$^{-1}$ or approximately 3 - 4 units for an adult. Prothrombin time (PT), international normalized ratio (INR), and *activated partial thromboplastin time* (aPTT) can be measured to monitor the recovery of the coagulation factors. Prothrombin complex concentrate (Octaplex®) with vitamin K$_1$ is currently the preferred treatment to urgently reverse coumadin anticoagulation. Octaplex carries no transfusion risks and does not expose the patient to the risk of volume overload associated with FFP.

## Platelets

Random donor platelets consist of a pool of 4 units of buffy coat-derived platelets (350 mL) mixed with 1 unit of plasma. Platelets can also come from a single donor (collected by apheresis) and can be human leukocyte antigen (HLA)-matched to the recipient if necessary. One pool of donor platelets (4 units) typically raises the serum platelet count by about $15 - 25 \times 10^9 \cdot L^{-1}$. Platelets are stored at room temperature, and they have a very short shelf life of only 5 days.[6] They also carry a higher risk of sepsis than PRBCs and are checked for bacterial contamination. Although ABO and Rh identical platelets are preferred, unmatched platelets can be used if necessary. If Rh (+) platelets are given to an Rh (-) woman of childbearing age, Rh-immunoglobulin should also be administered.[6]

The risk of spontaneous hemorrhage is low in non-bleeding patients when the platelet count is greater than $10 \times 10^9 \cdot L^{-1}$. Platelets may be indicated for mild thrombocytopenia ($20 - 50 \times 10^9 \cdot L^{-1}$) with bleeding or when clinical signs of platelet dysfunction occur with bleeding. They are contraindicated in thrombotic thrombocytopenic purpura (TTP) and heparin-induced thrombocytopenia (HIT). For surgical procedures with an anticipated blood loss > 500 mL, platelets are indicated when the count is $< 50 \times 10^9 \cdot L^{-1}$. Platelets may also be indicated when the platelet count is $< 100 \times 10^9 \cdot L^{-1}$ for patients with head injuries or prior to neurosurgical procedures. Platelets may be indicated irrespective of the platelet count when there is platelet dysfunction and massive bleeding (e.g., acetylsalicylic acid, antiplatelet agents, trauma, post-cardiopulmonary bypass).[6]

## Cryoprecipitate

Cryoprecipitate contains coagulation factors II, VIII, XIII, fibrinogen, and von Willebrand's factor. Each unit of cryoprecipitate contains 150 mg of fibrinogen. A dose of 1 unit per 10 kg of body weight (i.e., 8 – 12 units per adult) will increase the fibrinogen level by $0.5$ g·L$^{-1}$. Cryoprecipitate can be stored for up to one year when frozen.[6] It is indicated in the treatment of disseminated intravascular coagulation (DIC) and for massive bleeding when fibrinogen levels are suspected or documented to be $< 1.0$ g·L$^{-1}$.

## Autologous blood

This involves the collection of a patient's own blood prior to surgery. Although this practice may seem appealing, it is not cost-effective and is infrequently performed. Autologous blood donation is reserved for cases where the chance of requiring a blood transfusion perioperatively is $> 10\%$.[6] Surgeries in which autologous blood donation may be considered include cardiac, major vascular, revision hip, major spine, radical prostatectomy, and hepatic resection.

A common misconception by patients is that autologous blood is safer because it eliminates the risk of transmission of infectious diseases and ABO incompatibility. However, the possibility of a clerical error is always present. About 10% of autologous blood donors will still require allogeneic blood products.[6] Potential advantages of autologous blood include a decrease in postoperative infection and prevention of alloimmunization and some adverse transfusion reactions.[12] It may also be useful in a patient who has a rare blood group or who is difficult to crossmatch due to the presence of antibodies.

The process should begin at least 4 wk prior to surgery, and suitable candidates typically donate 1 - 3 units. The ideal time to donate is 21 - 34 days prior to the procedure. Patients with anemia, unstable angina, recent myocardial infarction (MI), severe stenotic valvular disease, and bacterial or viral infections are not eligible.[6] Oral iron and recombinant erythropoietin therapy may be used to increase red cell production. The storage limit for autologous whole blood is 35 days (42 days for red cells if separated), and it is discarded if it is not administered to the donor (up to 50% of units are not used).[12] Transfusion triggers for autologous blood should be the same as those for transfusing allogeneic blood.

**Acceptable blood loss**

Estimating blood loss (EBL) associated with surgical procedures is an inexact science. Clinicians typically rely on visual estimates, and therefore, blood loss may be under or overestimated. The quantity of blood collected in the suction containers should be noted regularly. These containers are also used to collect fluids used for irrigation of the wound. The amount of irrigation fluid used should be subtracted from the total volume to estimate the true blood loss. The weight of surgical pads and sponges that are used to absorb blood from the surgical field can also be measured to estimate the blood loss. An approximate volume of the amount of blood absorbed by the sponges can be estimated by subtracting the "dry" sponge weight from the "wet'" sponge weight. The difference in grams provides an estimate of the blood loss in mL (the actual specific gravity of blood is 1.06). Close examination of the floor, surgical drains, and drapes may reveal hidden additional losses of blood. The estimation of blood loss is repeated several times during the operation and again at the end.

There is no universal answer to the question, "What is the minimal acceptable hemoglobin?" Normal circulating blood volume can be reduced by as much as 30% with little stress on the patient provided the intravascular volume is maintained.[2] However, patients with atherosclerotic disease who have a restriction in blood flow to vital organs have a limited ability to adapt to acute anemia. A patient who has received inadequate crystalloid and colloid replacement can have a relatively high hemoglobin value due to a concentration effect. Alternatively, a patient who has received more crystalloid and colloids than necessary may have a low hemoglobin level due to a dilution effect from these fluids. Sampling blood near the site of an IV infusion may result in a falsely low hemoglobin level secondary to dilution.

When deciding to transfuse blood products, the risks and benefits must be individualized for each patient. Questions to consider include:

1. Does the patient consent to receiving blood products?
2. Is the anemia acute or chronic?
3. Is there active uncontrolled bleeding or is the patient likely to need blood in the immediate future?
4. Does the patient have coronary artery disease or cerebrovascular disease?
5. Is there evidence of ischemia or coagulopathy?
6. Does blood loss exceed your estimate of acceptable blood loss?
7. Is the patient hemodynamically unstable despite other fluid resuscitation or showing clinical signs and symptoms of anemia?

Postoperative hemoglobin levels of 60 - 80 g·L$^{-1}$ may be acceptable in certain patients. A young healthy person will be able to compensate for acute anemia and meet the body's oxygen requirements with an increase in heart rate and stroke volume. A patient with cardiovascular disease, however, may not be able to tolerate this additional stress and will require a higher hemoglobin level to prevent ischemia (80 - 100 g·L⁻¹).

A recent randomized study of over 2,000 patients comparing a restrictive (hemoglobin < 80 g·dL⁻¹) vs a liberal (hemoglobin < 100 g·dL⁻¹) transfusion protocol for patients undergoing noncardiac surgery found no difference in death or ability to walk without assistance at 60 days and no difference in other complications.[24] In a recent retrospective review of over one million patients undergoing noncardiac surgery, transfusion of even one unit of PRBCs was associated with a significant increase in mortality, pulmonary complications, renal dysfunction, wound problems, sepsis, and a longer hospitalization.[25] The TRICC trial[13] looking at transfusion triggers in critically ill intensive care unit (ICU) patients found that a more restrictive transfusion strategy (70 g·L⁻¹ trigger) may decrease mortality and lower the incidence of myocardial infarctions and pulmonary edema compared with a higher trigger

level of 100 g·L⁻¹. In the perioperative setting, maintaining the intravascular volume while the patient is actively bleeding may necessitate transfusion at a higher hemoglobin level. However, it is rarely necessary to transfuse a patient with a hemoglobin level of > 100 g·L⁻¹.

A simple formula can be used to calculate the acceptable blood loss (ABL) for a given patient. It requires a preoperative hemoglobin value ($Hb_i$), identification of a transfusion trigger hemoglobin value ($Hb_f$), and the patient's estimated blood volume (EBV) based on their weight (usually 70 mL·kg⁻¹ for males and 60 mL·kg⁻¹ for females).

$$ABL = EBV \times ([Hb_i - Hb_f] / Hb_i)$$

For example:

A 70 kg adult male has an EBV of 70 mL·kg⁻¹ for a total of 4,900 mL. If his initial preoperative Hb is 150 g·L⁻¹ and the decision is made to allow his Hb to drop to 90 g·L⁻¹ before transfusing blood products, his ABL is ([150 – 90] / 150) x 4,900 = 1,960 mL.

## Table 21.4 Transfusion recommendations as per 2011 Ontario Transfusion Medicine Guidelines.[6]

| HEMOGLOBIN | RECOMMENDATION |
|---|---|
| > 100 g·L-1 | Likely inappropriate aside from exceptional circumstances |
| 70 - 100 g·L⁻¹ | Likely to be appropriate if there are signs or symptoms of impaired oxygen delivery |
| < 70 g·L⁻¹ | Likely to be appropriate |
| < 60 g·L⁻¹ | Transfusion highly recommended.[6] Young patients at low risk of ischemic cardiovascular disease may tolerate lower levels of hemoglobin |

### Massive transfusion

Massive blood loss is usually defined as the loss of a patient's entire blood volume within a 24 hr period. The most important determinant of adequate blood volume replacement is a patient's vital signs. Other hemodynamic parameters, such as central venous pressure (CVP), pulmonary capillary wedge pressure (PCWP), and urine production, can also provide additional information. Refer to the additional resources to view an advanced discussion on optimizing perioperative fluid therapy. Frequent monitoring of hemoglobin, electrolytes (especially calcium and potassium), and coagulation (platelets, INR, fibrinogen) is useful to assess the adequacy of transfusion and also to monitor for potential complications. Target serum levels are listed in Table 21.5.

It makes all the difference to have the right equipment available when rapid blood administration is required. The Level 1 Rapid Infuser warms blood products and infuses them under pressure. It can be found in some ORs and emergency departments that manage trauma. Evidence from the military and other trauma situations also suggests that earlier, more aggressive use of blood component therapy results in a marked reduction in mortality from bleeding.[14] Current practice is to administer 4 units of plasma for each blood volume lost, resulting in a PRBC to FP ratio of about 3:1. However, ratios of 2:1 and 1:1 are being used more frequently. Recent data also suggest a higher target fibrinogen level (> 2.0 $g \cdot L^{-1}$) over the previous target of > 1.0 $g \cdot L^{-1}$.[15]

## Table 21.5 Target serum levels during massive transfusion

| Test | Target |
|------|--------|
| Hemoglobin | 80 - 100 $g \cdot L^{-1}$ |
| Platelets | 50 - 100 x $10^9 \cdot L^{-1}$ |
| INR | < 1.5 |
| PTT | < 40 sec |
| Fibrinogen | > 2.0 $g \cdot L^{-1}$ |

INR = international normalized ratio; PTT = partial thromboplastin time.

## Complications of transfusion

Complications of blood transfusion are rare but can be life-threatening. Some complications of transfusion can occur after a single unit of blood, whereas others are more related to massive transfusion. Table 21.6 lists consequences of these complications as well as preventative measures. Table 21.7 lists the incidence of these complications. The most common cause of major morbidity and mortality from blood product transfusion is transfusion-related acute lung injury (TRALI). Mortality from TRALI is 5 - 10%, and about ¾ of patients will require mechanical ventilation.[16] It is more common with plasma and platelets transfusions and typically begins within 6 hr following the transfusion.[6]

Table 21.6 Risks of blood transfusion (per unit of component, unless specified).[6]

## Blood conservation strategies

Blood conservation strategies should be considered perioperatively if the patient has a > 10% chance of requiring a blood transfusion.[6]

Anemia has been identified as a major determinant of postoperative complications. Patients with preoperative hemoglobin levels of < 120 $g \cdot L^{-1}$ and deficiencies in serum ferritin, folate, or vitamin $B_{12}$ may benefit from replacement therapy.[11] If target hemoglobin levels are still not achieved, the patient may be a candidate for erythropoietin therapy.

Preoperative discontinuation of antiplatelet agents and anticoagulants is often indicated. For example, some medications are held when they are prescribed for primary prevention of cardiovascular or cerebrovascular disease or for elective surgery with a higher risk of bleeding. Commonly prescribed antiplatelet drugs like clopidogrel and acetylsalicylic acid (ASA) are typically discontinued 5 - 7 days preoperatively (some sources recommend up to 10 days).[18] For NSAIDs, the stop date varies according to the drug's half-life (5 half-lives should be adequate to ensure the drug's elimination in the body, usually 4 - 7 days).[6] Celecoxib is not usually held because it does not affect platelet function. Coumadin

Table 21.6 Consequences and prevention of transfusion-related complications. [2, 16, 17]

| Complications | Consequences | Prevention |
|---|---|---|
| Infection | Viral (most common), bacterial, and parasitic infections. May lead to sepsis (bacterial). | Screening of donated blood for certain viruses and platelets for bacterial contamination. |
| Hemolysis | Immediate reaction (ABO incompatibility): due to the interaction of a recipient's red cell antibodies and the surface antigens on donor RBCs; this complex binds complement and causes hemolysis of the transfused RBCs. May result in fever, chills, chest or flank pain, N/V, hypoxemia, hypotension, bleeding, hemoglobinuria, ARF, and DIC. *Delayed reaction:* occurs 7 - 21 days after the transfusion; usually due to trace antibodies formed after a previous transfusion or pregnancy; lysed cells are removed by the reticulo-endothelial system, and the usual course is benign. | Clerical error is the most common cause, thus checking blood and patient identification by two individuals prior to transfusion is recommended. If suspected, stop the transfusion immediately, notify blood bank, send remaining blood and patient samples to the lab, support the patient's hemodynamics, promote diuresis, and monitor for DIC. Delayed hemolytic reactions are often not preventable (undetectable antibody titres in the recipient's plasma during antibody screening). |
| Non-hemolytic febrile reactions | Fever, chills, N/V, headache, myalgias. Due to the reaction of donor leukocyte antigens and antibodies in the recipient's plasma which bind complement and release pyrogenic substances. In platelets, caused by cytokines released from leukocytes. | Leukoreduction Antipyretic administration (acetaminophen) More common with platelet transfusion. Stop or reduce the rate of transfusion. |

Table 21.6 Consequences and prevention of transfusion-related complications. [2, 16, 17]

| Complications | Consequences | Prevention |
|---|---|---|
| Allergy | Mild: urticaria, pruritus, flushing. Severe: anaphylaxis, shock. Usually an allergic reaction to proteins in the donor blood Some patients have elevated levels of IgA antibodies against IgA found in blood. | Monitor patient once transfusion started. For minor reaction, give diphenhydramine. For more severe reactions, consider steroids, epinephrine, fluids, vasopressor support, ventilatory support. |
| TRALI (transfusion-related acute lung injury) | Results in acute respiratory distress syndrome (ARDS). Symptoms include hypoxemia, dyspnea, fever, tachycardia, hypotension, noncardiogenic pulmonary edema. Immune (leukocyte antibodies in donor plasma reacting with the recipient's HLA antigens) and non-immune varieties (reactive lipid products in donor blood cells result in TRALI).[16] | Leukoreduction Treatment of blood products with solvent detergent. Avoiding blood products from multiparous women (high HLA antibody levels). Octaplas® (not yet available in Canada) |
| TACO* | TACO (Transfusion Associated Circulatory Overload) Congestive heart failure and acute pulmonary edema. May require oxygen and diuresis. | Avoid rapid volume administration in a patient with known cardiac dysfunction. Administer diuretics pre-transfusion. |

Table 21.6 Consequences and prevention of transfusion-related complications. [2,16,17]

| | | |
|---|---|---|
| **Immune System** | Immune suppression may lead to increased risk of postoperative infections and cancer recurrence. | If possible, avoid transfusion in immunocompromised patients or use irradiated blood products. |
| **Hypothermia*** | Coagulopathy<br>Cardiac dysrhythmias<br>Hypotension<br>Hypocalcemia<br>Reduction in tissue oxygen delivery (due to left shift of oxyhemoglobin dissociation curve). | Always warm blood products prior to transfusion by passing them through a blood warmer.<br>Warm other IV fluids.<br>Use warming blankets to reduce radiant heat loss, increase room temperature.<br>Monitor patient's temperature. |
| **Coagulopathy*** | Continued bleeding.<br>Often due to dilution of coagulation factors and platelets during massive transfusion of PRBCs.<br>If bleeding persists despite replacement of clotting factors, consider diagnosis of DIC. | Monitor for increased surgical bleeding.<br>Measurement of PTT, INR, platelets, and fibrinogen.<br>Replacement of clotting factors with plasma, platelets, and cryoprecipitate. |
| **Hyperkalemia*** | Peaked T waves on ECG, wide QRS, loss of P wave, cardiac dysrhythmias.<br>Due to increased potassium concentration of stored blood. | Monitor potassium and ECG changes.<br>Treat hyperkalemia.<br>Maintain normothermia and avoid acidosis. |
| **Hypocalcemia*** | Citrate (an anticoagulant added to blood products) binds calcium-producing hypocalcemia.<br>Results in decreased myocardial contractility, hypotension, widened QRS with a prolonged QT interval, and bleeding (calcium is an important co-factor in coagulation). | Monitor calcium frequently.<br>Administer calcium gluconate or calcium chloride (has 3x the calcium).<br>Ensure normothermia (hypothermia slows hepatic metabolism of citrate). |

Table 21.6 Consequences and prevention of transfusion-related complications. [2, 16, 17]

| | | |
|---|---|---|
| **Acid-base abnormalities*** | Metabolic acidosis: generated from citric acid and lactic acid within stored blood. <br><br> Metabolic alkalosis: due to hepatic metabolism of citrate into bicarbonate. | Maintain adequate tissue perfusion. |
| **Embolism** | Air embolism: from IV injection of air when blood is transfused under pressure. <br><br> Microembolism: small clots can lodge themselves into the pulmonary circulation. | Remove air from IV lines. <br><br> Ensure use of proper filter (170-260 microns) when transfusing blood products. |

* Complications associated with massive transfusion. ARF = acute renal failure; DIC = disseminated intravascular coagulation; ECG = electrocardiogram; HLA = human leukocyte antigens; INR = international normalized ratio; N/V = nausea and vomiting; PRBCs = packed red blood cells; PTT = *partial thromboplastin time.*

should be stopped 4 - 5 days preoperation,[18] with the INR repeated the day prior to surgery. Newer anticoagulants pose an additional challenge. Evidence for when to stop dabigatran is not yet available, but it is held for 4 days prior to surgery in our institution. Rivaroxaban should be held for 3 days prior to surgery.[6] Patients at high risk of thromboembolic events may require heparin bridging therapy. See also Chapters 3 and 16.

Other medications can be used intraoperatively to reduce blood loss. Antifibrinolytics, such as tranexamic acid, form a reversible complex that displaces plasminogen from fibrin and results in inhibition of fibrinolysis. Evidence suggests that tranexamic acid reduces allogeneic blood transfusion in the surgical population and can even reduce mortality from hemorrhage in trauma patients.[19] The recommended dose is 10 $mg \cdot kg^{-1}$ as an intravenous bolus over 5 min followed by an infusion of 2 - 4 $mg \cdot kg^{-1} \cdot hr^{-1}$. Tranexamic acid is contraindicated in patients with a history of thrombotic events and hematuria. Other adjunct medications used less frequently in major blood loss include desmopressin and recombinant factor VIIa. Desmopressin (DDAVP) may be used to improve platelet function by promoting the release of von Willebrand factor in patients with von Willebrand disease, hemophilia A, and thrombocytopenia. It may also improve platelet function in patients with uremia. Recombinant factor VIIa (rVIIa) has been used (off-label indication) in massive bleeding, but it is ineffective in the setting of hypothermia and acidosis. For the purposes of this book, these topics will not be discussed in detail.

Intraoperative cell salvage is a process by which a machine known as a "cell saver" collects blood from the surgical field. The cell saver filters the blood, washes it, and removes virtually all blood products, with the exception of the red blood cells which are then returned for infusion back to the patient. The cell saver is often used if > 1L of blood loss is anticipated. Advantages of this form of blood conservation is that there is no risk of ABO incompatibility; it may be useful in a patient with rare blood groups or antibodies; it reduces the need for allogeneic blood transfusion; and it may be an acceptable option for Jehovah's witnesses.[20] Contaminated surgical procedures (e.g., involving the gut) and sickle cell disease are contraindications to its use. Until recently, cell salvage was also contraindicated in patients with malignant disease (due to the risk of metastases with reinfusion of cancer cells) and in cases of obstetrical hemorrhage (due to the possibility of amniotic fluid embolism). Guidelines now advocate for its use in obstetrics and in certain malignancies, provided a leukocyte depletion filter is used to lower the amount of amniotic fluid or tumor cells in the salvaged blood.[20]

Acute normovolemic hemodilution (ANH) is a technique where approximately 30% of the patient's blood volume is removed and replaced with colloid or crystalloid following induction of anesthesia. The blood is stored until it is required and transfused back to the patient.[12] This technique is rarely performed and is contraindicated in patients with anemia or cardiovascular, cerebrovascular, or renal disease.[6] It may, however, be an acceptable option for Jehovah's witnesses, provided a continuous circuit is made between the blood and the patient. This technique may be suitable for a healthy patient undergoing major surgical procedures with an anticipated massive blood loss.

Other blood conservation strategies include controlling the blood pressure, meticulous surgical technique, topical hemostatic agents (e.g., fibrin sealants [Tisseel®] and topical thrombin), the use of regional anesthesia techniques, and minimizing blood sampling.[6] There is insufficient evidence to support the routine use of controlled hypotension, recombinant factor VIIa, and hypervolemic hemodilution.[6]

# References

1. Brandstrup B, Tonnesen H, Beier-Holgersen R, et al: Effects of intravenous fluid restriction on postoperative complications: Comparison of two perioperative fluid regimens – A randomized assessor-blinded multicenter trial. Ann Surg 2003; 238:641-648.
2. Barash PG, Cullen BF, Stoelting RK, et al. *Clinical anesthesia*. Lippincott Williams & Williams, Philadelphia, 2009.
3. Chappell D, Matthias J, Hofmann-Kiefer K, Conzen P, Rehm M: A rational approach to perioperative fluid management. Anesthesiology 2008; 109:723-7403.
4. Choi PT, Yip G, Quinonez LG, Cook DJ: Crystalloids vs. colloids in fluid resuscitation: A systematic review. Crit Care Med 1999; 27:200-10.
5. Westphal M, James MFM, Kozec-Langenecker S, et al. Hydroxyethyl starches: different products – different effects. Anesthesiology 2009;111:187-202.
6. Callum JL et al. *Bloody easy 3: Blood transfusions, blood alternatives ad transfusion reactions: A guide to transfusion medicine*. Ontario Regional Blood Coordinating Network, 2011.
7. Finfer S, Bellomo R, Boyce N, et al: A comparison of albumin and saline for fluid resuscitation in the intensive care unit. N Engl J Med 2004; 350: 2247-2256.
8. Myburgh J, Cooper, DJ, Finfer S, et al: Saline or albumin for fluid resuscitation in patients with traumatic brain injury. N Engl J Med 2007; 357: 874-884.
9. Albert K, van Vlymen J, James P, Parlow J: Ringer's lactate is compatible with the rapid infusion of AS-3 preserved packed red blood cells. Can J Anesth 2009; 56:352-356.
10. Stevenson H. *Clinical guide to transfusion*. Canadian Blood Services, Toronto, 2007.
11. Patel MS, Carson JL: Anemia in the preoperative patient. Anesthesiology Clin 2009;27:751-760.
12. Goodnough LT, Brecher ME, Kanter MH et al: Transfusion Medicine. Second of two parts. Blood conservation. N Engl J Med 1999;340:525-533.
13. Hebert PC, Wells G, Blajchman MA, et al: A multicenter, randomized, controlled clinical trial of transfusion requirements in critical care. N Engl J Med 1999;340:409-417.
14. Sperry JL, Ochoa JB, Gunn SR, Alarcon LH et al: An FFP:PRBC transfusion ratio >/=1:1.5 is associated with a lower risk of mortality after massive transfusion. J Trauma 2008;65:986-993.
15. Bolliger D, Szlam F, Molinaro RJ, Rahe-Meyer N, et al. Finding the optimal concentration range for fibrinogen replacement after severe haemodilution : an in vitro model. Br J Anaesth 2009;102:793-799.
16. Sachs UJH. Pathophysiology of TRALI: current concepts. Intensive Care Med 2007;33[Suppl 1]:S3-S11.
17. Maxwell MJ, Wilson MJA. Complications of blood transfusion. Contin Educ Anaesth Crit Care Pain 2006;6:225-229.
18. Hirsh J, Guyatt G, Albers GW, et al. Antithrombotic and thrombolytic therapy, 8th edition: ACCP guidelines. Chest 2008;133:6 suppl 71S-109S.
19. CRASH-2 trial collaborators. Effects of tranexamic acid on death, vascular occlusive events, and blood transfusion in trauma patients with significant hemorrhage (CRASH-2): a randomized, placebo-controlled trial. Lancet 2010;376:23-32.
20. Ashworth A, Klein AA. Cell salvage as part of a blood conservation strategy in anaesthesia. Br J Anaesth 2010;105:401-416.
21. Powell-Tuck J, Gosling P, Lobo D et al. The British Consensus Guidelines on Intravenous Fluid Therapy for Adult Surgical Patients (GIFTASUP); updated 2011.
22. Holte K, Sharrock NE, Kehlet H. Review article: Pathophysiology and clinical implications of perioperative fluid excess. Br J Anaesth 2002; 89: 622-632.
23. Joshi GP. Medical Intelligence: Intraoperative fluid restriction improves outcome after major elective gastrointestinal surgery. Anesth Analg 2005;101:601-605.
24. Carson JL, Terrin ML, Noveck H et al. Liberal or restrictive transfusion in high risk patients after surgery. NEJM 2011;365:2453-2462.
25. Ferraris VA, Davenport DL, Saha SP et al. Surgical outcomes and transfusion of minimal amounts of blood in the operating room. Arch Surg 2012;147:49-55.
26. Perner, A. et al. Hydroxyethyl Starch 130/0.42 versus Ringer's acetate in severe sepsis. N Engl J Med 2012; 367(2):124-134.
27. Myburgh, JA. et al. Hydroxyethyl starch or saline for fluid resuscitation in intensive care. N Engl J Med 2012; 367(20)1901-11.

28. Zarychanski R, Abou-Setta AM, Turgeon AF et al. Association of Hydroxyethyl starch administration with mortality and acute kidney injury in critically ill patients requiring volume resuscitation: A systematic review and meta-analysis. JAMA 2013; 309(7):678-688.

29. Perel P, Roberts I, Ker K. Colloids versus crystalloids for fluid resuscitation in critically ill patients. Cochrane database of systematic reviews (Online) 2013;2:000567.

# CHAPTER 22

# Common Perioperative Problems

Natalie Clavel MD, Jordan Hudson MD

## Learning Objectives

1. To recognize the differential diagnosis for common perioperative problems.
2. To develop an approach to the acute management of common perioperative problems.
3. To acquire an understanding of the different causes of postoperative nausea and vomiting and an approach to manage this problem.
4. To acquire knowledge of the risk factors for postoperative agitation and delirium and effective strategies that can be used to prevent and treat this problem.

## Key Points

1. A bag and mask (e.g., Ambu®) can be used to deliver 100% oxygen to a patient who is not breathing.

2. Hypovolemic shock is the most common type of shock.

3. Patient, anesthetic, and surgical risk factors have been identified for postoperative nausea and vomiting (PONV). Independent patient risk factors include female sex, non-smoking status, history of motion sickness, and a history of PONV.

4. Upper airway obstruction, residual paralysis, hypercarbia, hypoxemia, pain, and a distended bladder are common treatable causes of a postoperative agitated state.

5. Delirium occurs in up to two-thirds of critical care patients, typically occurring 2 to 7 days after surgery. Evidence-based effective strategies can be used to minimize the risk of delirium.

This chapter provides a general approach to common perioperative problems. For example, abnormalities in heart rate and blood pressure are common problems that require an organized approach for their initial management. Tables in this chapter provide a reference for common causes of hemodynamic disturbances and the treatments used to manage these problems.

Emergency situations that require intervention will undoubtedly occur during your years of medical training. The following discussion of common problems should help to prepare for these circumstances, which may occur on the ward, in the emergency department, or in a critical care setting, such as the operating room.

## A General Approach to Emergency Problems

For any perioperative problem, a stepped "ABC" (airway, breathing, circulation) approach can be used for simultaneous assessment, diagnosis, and treatment. The following is a 10-step ABC approach that can be used to manage perioperative problems.

*Clinical Pearl:*

*When in doubt, call for help and initiate resuscitation using a stepped ABC (airway, breathing, circulation) approach.*

1. **Evaluate the patient to ensure an adequate and unobstructed airway and consider recruiting additional help.**
2. **Evaluate the patient to ensure adequate ventilation.**
3. **Assess the patient's heart rate and rhythm.**
4. **Assess the patient's blood pressure and perfusion.**
5. **Assess the patient's volume status.**
6. **Check the patient's temperature.**
7. **Scan for obvious causes of the abnormality.**
8. **Establish additional monitors where appropriate.**
9. **Investigate.**
10. **Formulate a provisional diagnosis, a differential diagnosis, and a management plan.**

1. **Evaluate the patient to ensure an adequate and unobstructed airway.**

Maneuvers to resolve a partial or complete airway obstruction take precedence over any other interventions. The clinician must be able to recognize an airway obstruction as well as utilize maneuvers to resolve the problem.

When the patient's trachea is not intubated:

Quickly assess whether the airway obstruction prevents the patient from breathing. Maneuvers in the unconscious patient, such as a chin lift, jaw thrust, removal of foreign bodies, and insertion of oral or nasal airways, may be used to overcome an airway obstruction. Signs of an obstructed airway include lack of air movement despite respiratory efforts, noisy or stridorous respirations, intercostal indrawing, tracheal tugging, use of accessory muscles, and lack of air entry on auscultation of the chest.

When the patient's trachea is intubated:

If the patient's trachea is intubated, be quick to ensure that the endotracheal tube is in fact in the trachea. Immediate absolute proof that the tracheal tube is in the trachea can be obtained by observing continued return of end-tidal carbon dioxide ($ETCO_2$) with each exhalation and by visualizing (using direct laryngoscopy) the endotracheal tube (ETT) passing between the vocal cords (see Chapter 6). Indirect confirmation of tracheal intubation includes observing the rise and fall of the patient's chest with positive pressure ventilation, absence of air entry during auscultation of the epigastrium, and auscultation of breath sounds over the lung fields with ventilation and misting on the ETT. Tracheal intubation can also be confirmed using a fiberoptic scope passed through the ETT to visualize the tracheal lumen. A portable chest *x-ray* can be used to confirm that the tip of the ETT is mid-trachea.

If the ETT is positioned in the trachea and the patient is breathing spontaneously, the reservoir bag will empty with inspiration and fill with expiration. If awake, the patient will be unable to vocalize with the ETT positioned between the vocal cords.

In emergency situations, consider administration of supplemental oxygen. A bag and mask (e.g., Ambu®) can be used for rapid administration of 100% oxygen. It allows the patient to breathe 100% oxygen with the option of assisting their spontaneous efforts. Manual ventilation can be administered with a bag and mask when the patient is not breathing.

Examine the patient for evidence of cyanosis, and quickly scan any monitors attached to the patient. Ask for assistance in applying monitors, such as a blood pressure cuff, electrocardiograph (ECG) monitor, and pulse oximeter, and ensure that oxygen is being delivered from the source to the patient.

*Clinical Pearl:*

*The patient's inner lip is a reliable place to look for cyanosis.*

2. **Evaluate the patient to ensure adequate ventilation.**

There are many conditions that can result in respiratory insufficiency, and ventilation must be provided when a patient is not breathing. Vital signs, including the patient's heart rate (HR), blood pressure (BP), respiratory rate (RR), oxygen saturation ($SpO_2$), and temperature must be assessed after resolving any airway issues. Auscultation, palpation, and percussion of the patient's chest may also assist in formulating a differential diagnosis. Arterial blood gas analysis, chest *x-ray*, and pulmonary function tests may also be required to formulate a working diagnosis of the etiology of the respiratory insufficiency.

*Clinical pearl:*

*Aggressive bag and mask ventilation can result in gastric distension, regurgitation, and aspiration. Increased airway pressure in the thorax resulting from aggressive ventilation can impair cardiac function by increasing right ventricular afterload. This can impede venous return and result in a decrease in the systemic blood pressure.*

3. **Assess the patient's heart rate and rhythm.**

Quickly confirm or rule out an arrest situation. Severe bradycardia should be assumed to be secondary to hypoxemia until proven otherwise.

4. **Assess the patient's blood pressure and perfusion.**

Hypotension may result in decreased organ perfusion. Clinical findings associated with decreased organ perfusion may include signs of inadequate oxygen delivery to the patient's head, heart, and kidneys. Inadequate perfusion to the brain may result in anxiety, confusion, or unconsciousness. Inadequate delivery of oxygen to the patient's heart may result in dysrhythmias or ECG evidence of ischemia. Inadequate renal perfusion may result in decreased urine output.

A manual blood pressure cuff can be used if there are any questions concerning the blood pressure recordings. Arterial lines, automated blood pressure cuffs, and human error can all be responsible for factitious blood pressures.

5. **Assess the patient's volume status.**

Important changes in a patient's blood volume status may be clinically subtle and result in significant alterations to vital signs and mental status. Assess the patient's jugular venous pressure, recent fluid intake, fluid losses, and urine output. In the operating room, it would be appropriate to review the patient's duration of fasting and to examine the surgical wound, sponges, suction apparatus, and nasogastric drainage. An overall assessment of the blood losses and adequacy of fluid replacement should be performed (see Chapter 21: Intravenous and Blood Component Therapy).

### 6. Check the patient's temperature.

Alterations in temperature associated with anesthesia and surgery may result in important cardiorespiratory abnormalities, and hypothermia or hyperthermia may occur. Hypothermia is loss of body heat that is frequently the result of intraoperative temperature losses due to processes of evaporation, conduction, radiation, and convection. Patients undergoing surgery are exposed to a cold operating room with cold instruments, intravenous fluids, and an open wound through which heat loss occurs. The resulting hypothermia may result in postoperative shivering with a rise in heart rate, blood pressure, and a 5 to 6-fold increase in oxygen consumption. Increases in temperature in the perioperative period may result from drugs, such as atropine, or from the administration of blood products. Other causes of an increased temperature include fever, sepsis, active intraoperative warming efforts, and underlying disease states, such as thyrotoxicosis or malignant hyperthermia.

### 7. Scan for obvious causes of the abnormality.

Correct any obvious underlying abnormality. Common examples are hypotension and tachycardia with inadequate fluid replacement and hypertension and tachycardia with inadequate analgesia. Scan any monitors that are attached to the patient, and consider establishing a large-bore intravenous.

### 8. Establish additional monitors where appropriate.

Examples of additional monitors that may be appropriate include an ECG monitor, blood pressure cuff, pulse oximeter, and temperature probe. Invasive monitors may include a Foley catheter, arterial line, central venous pressure line, or pulmonary artery catheter.

### 9. Investigate.

Investigations may be used to aid in confirming the provisional diagnosis and to rule out other causes. Common investigations might include a complete blood count (CBC), international normalized ratio (INR), partial thromboplastin time (PTT), arterial blood gas (ABG), chest *x-ray* (CXR), ECG, glucose, electrolytes, and creatinine.

### 10. Formulate a provisional diagnosis, differential diagnosis, and a management plan.

In an emergency situation, you may not have the luxury of having an extensive history before you are required to act. Nevertheless, you can proceed with assessing the status of the patient's airway, oxygenation, ventilation, heart rate, rhythm, and blood pressure. Once the patient is hemodynamically stable and receiving adequate oxygen and ventilation, review the patient's history, recent lab data, and perioperative course (in the case of recent surgery), and formulate a provisional diagnosis, differential diagnosis, and management plan. Additional background information from family members or other health care providers involved in the patient's care can provide useful information. Remember to recruit help in any emergency.

Table 22.1 Differential diagnosis and treatment of perioperative bradycardia*

| Respiratory | Hypoxia, hypercarbia, acidosis | |
|---|---|---|
| Cardiovascular | **Decreased sympathetic tone** | |
| | Beta-blockers, high spinal or epidural anesthesia (> T1 – T4), neurogenic shock | |
| | **Increased parasympathetic tone** | |
| | Vagal reflexes (see CNS), drugs, pediatric patients | |
| | **Decreased conduction** | |
| | Sinus bradycardia, junctional bradycardia, ventricular escape rhythm, sick sinus syndrome, type II 2nd degree heart block, 3rd degree heart block | |
| Neurologic | **Baroreceptor reflex** | |
| | High intracranial pressure, hypertension | |
| | **Vagal reflex** | |
| | Vasovagal reflex, oculocardiac reflex, carotid sinus reflex, airway manipulation (especially important in pediatric patients) | |
| | **Drugs** | |
| | Anesthetic overdose, succinylcholine, opioids, neostigmine, beta-blockers | |
| Miscellaneous | **Hypothermia, hypothyroidism, athlete with low resting heart rate** | |
| Treatment | **Treatment options might include:** | |
| | Oxygen | Ephedrine |
| | Fluids | Dopamine |
| | Trendelenburg position | Epinephrine |
| | Removing the offending cause | Transcutaneous or transvenous pacing |
| | Atropine or glycopyrrolate | See Chapter 24 ACLS guidelines |

*Perioperative bradycardia is defined as a heart rate < 60 beats·min⁻¹.
ACLS = advanced cardiac life support; CNS = central nervous system.

Table 22.2 Differential diagnosis of perioperative tachycardia*

| Respiratory | Hypoxia, hypercarbia, acidosis |
|---|---|
| Cardiovascular | **Sinus tachycardia:**<br>A reflex sinus tachycardia may occur in shock states (see Table 22.6). Sinus tachycardia may arise due to decreases in preload, afterload, or contractility. Increased sympathetic stimulation resulting from anxiety, pain, surgical manipulation, and inadequate depth of anesthetic are common causes of sinus tachycardia.<br><br>**Other rhythms:**<br>Paroxysmal atrial tachycardia (PAT)          Atrial fibrillation<br>Accelerated junctional rhythm          Pre-excitation syndromes<br>Multifocal atrial tachycardia (e.g., patient with COPD)          Ventricular tachycardia<br>Atrial flutter |
| Neurologic | Inadequate anesthesia, anxiety, pain |
| Genitourinary | Bladder distension, renal colic, Foley catheter, urosepsis |
| Hematologic | Anemia, transfusion reaction |
| Endocrine | **Hypermetabolic states:**<br>Fever, sepsis, pheochromocytoma, thyrotoxicosis, malignant hyperthermia, malignant neuroleptic syndrome, serotonin syndrome<br><br>**Other:**<br>Hypoglycemia, hypercalcemia, Addisonian crisis, porphyria |
| Immune | Anaphylaxis |
| Medications | Atropine, cocaine, ephedrine, epinephrine, dopamine, dobutamine. Drug rebound (beta-blockers; naloxone) |
| | Treatment is directed at the underlying cause of the tachycardia. See Chapter 24 ACLS algorithms |

*Etiology of perioperative tachycardia is defined as a heart rate > 100 beats·min⁻¹

ACLS = advanced cardiac life support; COPD = Chronic obstructive pulmonary disease.

Table 22.3 Common causes and treatment options for perioperative hypertension

| Respiratory | Hypoxia | Hypercarbia |
|---|---|---|
| Cardiovascular | Essential hypertension<br>Volume overload | Post carotid endarterectomy (acute denervation of carotid baroreceptor) |
| Neurological | Pain<br>Anxiety<br>Shivering<br>Hypothermia<br>Inadequate anesthesia | Emergence delirium<br>Increased intracranial pressure (ICP)<br>Autonomic hyperreflexia (spinal cord injury) |
| Genitourinary | Bladder distension<br>Renal artery stenosis<br>Renal disease<br>Renal colic | Pregnancy-induced hypertension<br>Preeclampsia<br>Eclampsia |
| Endocrine | Hyperthyroidism<br>Cushing's syndrome<br>Pheochromocytoma<br>Carcinoid | Conn's syndrome (hyperaldosteronism)<br>Malignant hyperthermia<br>Malignant neuroleptic syndrome<br>Serotonin syndrome |
| Medications | Ephedrine<br>Epinephrine<br>Phenylephrine<br>Cocaine<br>Ketamine<br>Pain crisis following naloxone use | Withdrawal of medications (e.g., opioids, beta-blockers, clonidine, anti-hypertensive medications)<br>Drug interactions (e.g., TCA / MAO inhibitor / meperidine / ephedrine) |
| Treatment | Treatment options are directed at the cause of hypertension. Common treatment options include examination of the patient to exclude treatable causes (full bladder, raised ICP); optimize oxygenation and ventilation; sedation; increase depth of anesthesia; administration of opioids or local anesthesia; administration of beta-blockers (e.g., labetalol, esmolol), vasodilators (e.g., hydralazine, nitroglycerine), ACE-I (e.g., enalaprilat), or calcium channel blockers (e.g., Diltiazem). | |

*Etiology of hypertension is defined as a blood pressure > 140/90.
ACE-I = angiotensin-converting enzyme inhibitor; MAO = monoamine oxidase; TCA = tricyclic antidepressant.

**Bradycardia, Tachycardia, and Hypertension**

### Causes of Alterations in Heart Rate and Blood Pressure in the Perioperative Period

## Hypotension

The purpose of the cardiopulmonary circulation is to deliver oxygen and nutrients to body tissues. When tissue needs are not met, a state of shock will eventually ensue. The blood pressure is used as a gross indirect measurement of organ perfusion and assessment of the adequacy of the circulation. It represents a complex interaction between cardiac output, blood volume, and systemic vascular resistance (SVR). The cardiac output is determined by the heart rate, preload, contractility, and afterload (SVR).

## Table 22.4 Causes and treatment options for perioperative hypotension*

| Decreased Contractility | Decreased SVR | Impaired Venous Return |
|---|---|---|
| **Anesthetic agents** <br> Dose dependent depression with volatile anesthetic agents, propofol, benzodiazepines <br> **Cardiac medications** <br> Beta-blockers, calcium channel blockers <br> **Cardiac Dysfunction** <br> Ischemia, infarction, acidosis, alkalosis, hypothermia, impaired systolic or diastolic left ventricular function, cor pulmonale, hypothyroidism, vagal reflexes, local anesthetic toxicity | **Anesthetic agents** <br> Volatile anesthetic agents, opioids, benzodiazepines, nitrates, calcium channel blockers, angiotensin converting enzyme inhibitors, milrinone, alpha adrenergic antagonists <br> **Sympathetic block** <br> Neuraxial anesthesia <br> **Sepsis** <br> **Allergic reaction** <br> **Profound hypoxia** <br> **Adrenal suppression** | **Hypovolemia** <br> npo status, vomiting, NG drainage, bowel prep, diarrhea, diuresis <br> **Venous pooling** <br> Neuraxial anesthesia (sympathetic block), histamine release <br> **IVC obstruction** <br> Gravid uterus, surgical retraction, increased intra-abdominal pressure (insufflation, compartment syndrome) <br> **Elevated central venous and intrathoracic pressure** <br> High PEEP, hyper-inflation, auto-PEEP, tension pneumothorax, cardiac tamponade, pulmonary embolism |
| Treatment options are directed at the cause of hypotension. The BP measurement should be verified as correct, and the patient's normal BP and BP goals should be identified. Treatment options may include: | | |
| Decreased Contractility | Decreased SVR | Impaired Venous Return |
| Decrease anesthetic depth <br> Support contractility <br> Treat arrhythmias <br> Treat ischemia | Decrease anesthetic depth <br> Decrease epidural infusion rate <br> Vasopressor support <br> Volume expansion | Relieve mechanical obstruction <br> Volume expansion |

*Etiology of perioperative hypotension defined as a systolic blood pressure (SBP) < 90 mm Hg or a mean arterial pressure (MAP) < 60 mm Hg. IVC = inferior vena cava; NG = nasogastric; npo = nothing by mouth (*nil per os*); PEEP = positive end expiry pressure; SVR = systemic vascular resistance.

In a normal adult, hypotension is generally defined as a systolic blood pressure (SBP) of < 90 mm Hg or a mean arterial pressure (MAP) of < 60 mm Hg. The most common cause of a hypotensive state is a decrease in intravascular volume. This may result from an acute hemorrhage or from a loss of fluids and electrolytes. Acute hypovolemia reduces the venous return to the heart (preload) resulting in a decrease in cardiac output and systemic blood pressure. Carotid and aortic baroreceptors sense the decrease in arterial pressure and initiate a series of events resulting in an increase in sympathetic output from the central nervous system and adrenal gland. The resulting release of norepinephrine and epinephrine increase the heart rate, contractility, and SVR in an effort to redirect and maintain blood flow to vital organs.

***Clinical Pearl:***

*In the absence of medications or IV fluid, the fastest way to increase preload is to elevate the patient's legs and/ or place the patient in the Trendelenburg position*

### Hemorrhagic Shock Classification:

The normal response to increasing hemorrhage produces characteristic physiological signs. These signs have been used to classify hemorrhagic shock according to the quantity of blood loss. Table 22.5 defines four classes of hemorrhagic shock based on the patient's vital

## Table 22.5  Classification of hemorrhagic shock and common clinical findings in adults

| Hemorrhage | % BV Loss | Physiological changes | Treatment |
|---|---|---|---|
| **Class I** | < 15 | HR < 100 beats·min⁻¹, SBP normal, PP normal or increased, CR normal, RR 14 – 20 breaths·min⁻¹, CNS anxious | Rapidly infuse 10 - 20 mL·kg⁻¹ of a balanced salt solution (e.g., 1- 2 L in an adult) |
| **Class II** | 15 – 30 | HR > 100 beats·min⁻¹, SBP normal, DBP increased, postural hypotension, PP decreased, CR delayed, RR 20 – 30 breaths·min⁻¹, CNS more anxious | Rapidly infuse 2 L of a BSS; re-evaluate ongoing needs. |
| **Class III** | 30 – 40 | HR > 120 beats·min⁻¹, SBP decreased, PP decreased, CR delayed or absent, RR 30 – 40 breaths·min⁻¹, CNS confused | Rapidly infuse 2 L of BSS; re-evaluate; replace blood losses with 1:3 BSS or 1:1 with colloids (PRBCs, colloid, other blood products). Maintain urine output > 0.5 mL·kg⁻¹·hr⁻¹. |
| **Class IV** | > 40 | HR > 140 beats·min⁻¹, SBP decreased, PP decreased, CR absent, RR > 35 breaths·min⁻¹, CNS lethargic. | |

BSS = balanced salt solution; BV = blood volume; CNS = central nervous system; CR = capillary refill; DBP = diastolic blood pressure; HR = heart rate; PP = pulse pressure; PRBCs = packed red blood cells; RR = respiratory rate; SBP = systolic blood pressure.

signs and predicts the percent blood loss and appropriate initial therapy.

### Class I hemorrhage:

Class 1 hemorrhage is defined as the loss of as much as 15% of blood volume. It is associated with minimal physiologic changes.

### Class II hemorrhage:

Class II hemorrhage is defined as a 15 - 30% loss of blood volume. Class II hemorrhage is associated with modest elevations in heart rate and decreases in pulse pressure as diastolic pressures rise with smaller stroke volumes. Systolic pressures tend to be maintained, but digital capillary refill is slightly delayed. Urinary output is only mildly depressed. Postural hypotension and subtle central nervous system changes, such as fright and hostility, may be associated with class II hemorrhage.

### Class III hemorrhage:

Class III hemorrhage is defined as a 30 - 40% loss of blood volume. Patients with class III hemorrhage present with tachycardia, systolic and diastolic hypotension, delayed capillary refill (>2 sec), reduced urinary output, and an apprehensive, slightly clouded sensorium.

### Class IV hemorrhage:

Class IV hemorrhage is defined as a blood loss of ≥ 40% of the blood volume. The patient manifests signs of frank shock with cool, diaphoretic, ashen skin, tachycardia, hypotension or unobtainable blood pressure, anuria, and a reduced level of consciousness.

Patients with class III and IV hemorrhages will require immediate intravenous fluid administration to survive. Patients with class IV hemorrhage are likely to require blood transfusion to survive, but class III hemorrhage patients may tolerate post resuscitation

anemia if fluid resuscitation is accompanied with immediate control of the hemorrhage.

Hematocrits as low as 20 - 25% may be well tolerated if total blood volume is adequate. The use of clinical signs to estimate traumatic blood loss is very important because soft tissues and body cavities frequently conceal large quantities of blood with minimal external body changes.

### Other forms of shock

*Hypovolemic shock* is the most common type of shock. A low central venous pressure and low pulmonary capillary wedge pressure (PCWP) is characteristic of hypovolemia. Other forms of circulatory shock include distributive shock, obstructive shock, and cardiogenic shock. Table 22.6 characterizes the hemodynamic features of the different forms of shock.

*Distributive shock* is characterized by systemic vasodilation, relative hypovolemia, and an increase in cardiac output. The most common form of distributive shock is septic shock. Arteriovenous shunting at the tissue level results in an accumulation of lactic acid and tissue anoxia. Table 22.7 lists examples of the four classes of shock.

*Cardiogenic shock* results when the heart fails to perform its pumping function. This occurs as a result of a myocardial, valvular, or electrical problem. A myocardial infarction is the most common cause of cardiogenic shock. Characteristic findings include an increase in central venous pressure (CVP), PCWP, and SVR, with a cardiac index of < 1.8 $L·min^{-1}$ per $m^2$ and a systolic BP < 80 mm Hg (see Chapter 10: Tables 10.1 and 10.2 for derivations and normal values).

*Obstructive shock* occurs when there is an obstruction preventing cardiac filling or emptying. Two immediately treatable causes of obstructive shock include a tension pneumothorax and cardiac tamponade.

## Table 22.6 Hemodynamic parameters with various shock states

| Shock State | Blood Pressure | Central Venous Pressure | Pulmonary Capillary Wedge Pressure | Cardiac Output | Systemic Vascular Resistance |
|---|---|---|---|---|---|
| **Hypovolemic** | ↓ | ↓ | ↓ | ↓ | ↑ |
| **Cardiogenic** **LV dysfunction** **RV dysfunction** | ↓ ↓ | ↑ ↑ | ↑↑ ↓ | ↓ ↓ | ↑↑ ↑↑ |
| **Distributive** | ↓ | ↓ | ↓ | ↑ | ↓↓ |
| **Obstructive** | ↓ | ↑ | ↑ or ↓ | ↓ | ↑ |

Combinations of shock (e.g., hypovolemic and cardiogenic) may be present at the same time. LV = left ventricular; RV = right ventricular.

## Table 22.7 Classification and Etiology of Shock States

| **Hypovolemic shock** | |
|---|---|
| Most common cause of shock | Occult blood or fluid loss |

| **Cardiogenic Shock** | |
|---|---|
| Myocardial Relative drug overdose (anesthesia medications) Other drug effects (beta-blockers, Ca²⁺ channel blockers) Ischemia Infarction | Arrhythmias Cardiomyopathy (congestive, hypertrophic, restrictive, obliterative) Valvular disease (e.g., aortic and mitral regurgitation; especially important in the presence of stress) |

| **Distributive Shock** | |
|---|---|
| Anaphylaxis, anaphylactoid reaction Sepsis Drugs (vasodilators) High regional sympathetic block (e.g., high spinal or epidural anesthetic) | Addisonian crisis Transfusion reaction Severe liver disease Arteriovenous fistulas Thyrotoxicosis Hypothyroidism |

| **Obstructive Shock** | |
|---|---|
| Tension pneumothorax Pericardial tamponade Pulmonary embolism (blood clot, fat, air, tumor) Aortocaval compression (gravid uterus) Inferior vena cava (IVC) or heart compression by surgical instruments | Aortic dissection Aortic cross-clamping Atrial myxoma Idiopathic hypertrophic subaortic stenosis (IHSS) Valvular heart disease (e.g., aortic or mitral stenosis; especially important in the presence of stress) |

## Nausea and Vomiting

Postoperative nausea and vomiting (PONV) has a profound and lasting negative effect on a patient's perception of the quality of care received. PONV is associated with an increase in health care costs, prolonged hospital stay, increased patient dissatisfaction, and unanticipated admission to hospital. Surveys indicate that patients are willing to pay up to $100 to avoid PONV. Numerous high-quality studies published over the last 20 years have provided clinicians with a much better understanding of the factors contributing to PONV. Recent evidence-based guidelines have identified effective strategies in the prevention and treatment of this problem.

Historically, numerous factors were believed to contribute to PONV, including anxiety, obesity, use of cholinesterase inhibitors, and others. We now recognize that the risk of PONV is closely tied to patient, anesthesia, and factors related to surgery. The only consistent independent patient-related risk factors for PONV are female sex, non-smoking status, a history of PONV, or a history of motion sickness (Table 22.8).

## Table 22.8 Risk Factors for Postoperative Nausea and Vomiting in Adults

| Patient | Anesthesia | Surgical |
|---------|-----------|----------|
| Female sex<br>Non smoker<br>History of PONV or motion sickness | Use of volatile anesthetics<br>Use of nitrous oxide<br>Use of intraoperative and postoperative opioids | Duration of surgery<br>For every 30 min, the risk of PONV increases by 60% of the baseline risk<br>Type of surgery<br>Abdominal, breast, eye, middle ear, plastic, gynecologic, neurologic |

Without antiemetic prophylaxis and with no identified risk factors for PONV, 20 – 30% of patients undergoing a general anesthetic with inhalational agents will experience nausea and or vomiting in the postoperative period. This number increases to 70 – 80% when several risk factors for PONV are identified.

Apfel developed a simple scoring system for PONV in adults using identified risk factors.[2] The presence of each risk factor was given a value of 1, with the total score ranging from 0 – 4. The risk of developing PONV based on the Apfel score was 10, 20, 40, 60, and 80% in patients with 0, 1, 2, 3, and 4 risk factors, respectively.

| Risk Factors | Points |
|--------------|--------|
| Female sex | 1 |
| Non smoker | 1 |
| History of PONV | 1 |
| Postoperative opioids | 1 |
| Total score | 0 – 4 |

Patients most likely to benefit from prophylactic antiemetic therapy can be identified using a combination of the Apfel score, the type of anesthetic used, and the surgical procedure. Current guidelines do not support the routine use of antiemetic prophylaxis in patients at low risk of PONV. Prophylaxis may be appropriate in patients at risk of complications from vomiting (e.g., wired jaw, neurosurgical cases, gastric, or esophageal surgery) or when the patient expresses a strong preference to avoid PONV.

Monotherapy with a serotonin (5-HT3) receptor antagonist, such as ondansetron, is recommended for patients who require a general anesthetic and have one risk factor for PONV. Combination therapy is recommended for patients with two or more risk factors for PONV. The recommended available classes of drugs include 5-HT3 receptor antagonists, steroids, phenothiazine, butyrophenones, antihistamines, and anticholinergics (Table 22.9).

Children from age 3 yr to puberty have a heightened risk of POV that is unrelated to sex. Nausea in children can be difficult to assess due to limitations in their ability to describe their feelings. The independent risk factors for POV in children include an age from 3 years to puberty, strabismus surgery, duration of surgery ≥ 30 min, and a positive history of PONV in the patient, parent, or sibling. The baseline risk of PONV in children without any of these risk factors is 10%, and this increases to 70% when all four risk factors are present.[2]

When using prophylactic antiemetic therapy, the cost of the treatment, the number of patients needed to treat (NNT), and the number of patients needed to harm (NNH)

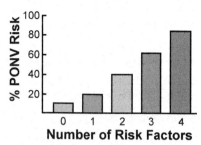

Fig. 22.1 Simplified risk score for PONV in adults. The risk is approximately 10, 20, 40, 60 and 80 percent respectively when the number of independent risk factors for PONV increases from 0 to 4. Adapted from Apfel CC et. al. Anesthesiology 1999;91: 693-700

should be considered. The NNT is defined as the number of patients who need to receive a particular antiemetic to prevent one emetic event that would have occurred without treatment. The NNT for a patient at low risk of PONV increases, while the NNT for a patient at high risk of PONV decreases. The NNH refers to the number of patients who need to receive the treatment to result in one patient experiencing unintended harm from the treatment.

## Table 22.9 Drug classes of perioperative antiemetics

| 5-HT3 receptor antagonists | ondansetron*, granisetron, dolasetron, tropisetron |
| --- | --- |
| steroid | dexamethasone |
| butyrophenone | haloperidol, droperido'¶ |
| phenothiazine | promethazine, prochlorperazine |
| antihistamine | dimenhydrinate |
| anticholinergic | transdermal scopolamine |

*Ondansetron is the most extensively studied 5-HT3 receptor antagonist. It has a similar safety profile and efficacy of other 5-HT3 antagonists, and it is the only 5-HT3 receptor antagonist approved for use in infants as young as one month of age. ¶Droperidol's use has declined following the 2001 U.S. Food and Drug Administration (FDA) black box warning (see text).

## Table 22.10 Strategies to reduce the risk of PONV[1,2,3,9]

| | |
|---|---|
| Use of regional or local anesthesia rather than general anesthesia | 9 to 11-fold reduction with RA |
| Use of propofol for induction and maintenance of anesthesia | 19% - 25% reduction in PONV |
| Avoid nitrous oxide | 12% reduction* in PONV |
| Avoid volatile anesthetic agents | Up to 25% reduction in PONV |
| Minimize opioid use | |
| Ensure adequate hydration | |

*Nitrous oxide's effect is observed primarily in PONV occurring < 2 hr after procedures. Avoiding nitrous oxide ($N_2O$) has little impact when the risk of PONV is low. $N_2O$ and volatile anesthetics are the primary cause of early PONV (0 – 6 hr) and do not influence delayed PONV (6 – 24 hr). The emetic effect of $N_2O$ may be less than volatile anesthetic agents and is independent and additive to the volatile anesthetic agent contribution. There is no difference between isoflurane, sevoflurane, and desflurane in the tendency to produce PONV.[9] PONV = postoperative nausea and vomiting; RA = regional anesthesia.

### Ondansetron

Ondansetron is a serotonin 5-HT3 receptor antagonist with efficacy and safety profiles similar to other drugs in the same class. It is better for preventing and treating vomiting than it is for nausea. The NNT to prevent one case of nausea is 6 – 7 patients (0 – 24 hr) and one case of vomiting is 5 – 6 patients (0 – 24 hr). Ondansetron has a short duration of action (approximately 4 hr); therefore, administration is recommended at the end of surgery. The prophylactic dose is 4 – 8 mg *iv*, although the recommended rescue treatment dose is only ¼ of this (1 – 2 mg). The drug is approved for use in infants as young as one month; the pediatric dose is 50 – 100 $\mu g \cdot kg^{-1}$ *iv*. The NNH to produce a headache, increase liver enzymes, or cause constipation is 36, 31, and 23 patients, respectively. It may be repeated after 6 hr; however, if early PONV develops (< 6 hr) despite prophylaxis, a different class of antiemetic should be used, as repeat dosing of ondansetron has been shown to be ineffective.[2] Ondansetron results in a similar prolongation of the QTc interval (i.e., QT interval / square root of R-R interval) when compared with droperidol.[9]

### Dexamethasone

Dexamethasone has a relatively slow onset (up to 2 – 4 hr); hence, administration is recommended at the start of surgery, and it is not recommended as a rescue drug. Several studies suggest that dexamethasone is safe as a single dose; however, repeat dosing is not recommended more frequently than q8hr. The NNT is 4 patients (0 – 24 hr) to prevent nausea and vomiting using a dose of 4 – 8 mg *iv*. Dexamethasone results in a significant reduction in PONV and pain when used for molar extractions, adenotonsillectomy, and jaw surgery. There are limited data to determine if a single dose of dexamethasone is in fact harmless. Side effects, such as an increased risk of hyperglycemia, bleeding, perineal pain, impaired wound healing, and possibly infection challenge current opinion that a single dose of dexamethasone is innocuous.[4,5,6,8,10] Steroids in the perioperative period have been

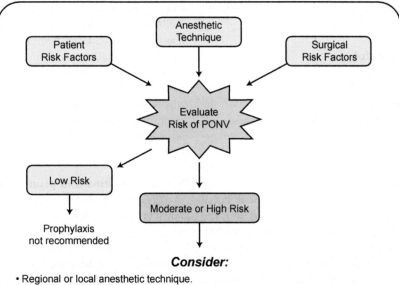

Fig. 22.2 Postoperative nausea and vomiting (PONV) risk assessment.

## Table 22.11 Antiemetic doses, trade names, and timing of administration to prevent PONV in adults[2,9]

| Drug | Trade name | Dose | Timing |
|------|-----------|------|--------|
| Ondansetron | Zofran® | 4 mg *iv* | End of surgery |
| Dexamethasone | Decadron® | 4 – 8 mg *iv* | Start of surgery |
| Haloperidol | Haldol® | 0.5 – 1 mg *im iv* | Any time during surgery |
| Dimenhydrinate | Gravol® | 1 mg·kg⁻¹ *iv* | |
| Prochlorperazine | Stemetil® | 5 – 10 mg *im iv* | End of surgery |
| Promethazine | Phenergan® | 6.25 – 25 mg *iv* | Start of surgery |
| Scopolamine | Transderm Scop® | Transdermal patch | At least 2 – 4 hr prior to surgery |

Recommendations based on pooled randomized controlled trials (RCTs) or systematic reviews. *iv* = intravenous; *im* = intramuscular; PONV = postoperative nausea and vomiting.

shown to increase the risk of anastomotic leaks in bowel surgery from 7 to 19%.[7]

## Haloperidol

Low-dose droperidol (0.25 – 1.25 mg *iv*) was studied extensively in relation to the prevention and treatment of PONV. In 2001, the FDA issued a black box warning for the use of droperidol due to a risk of QTc prolongation, torsade-de-pointes arrhythmias, and cardiac arrest. The evidence supporting this decision has been repeatedly challenged. The latest guidelines for the prevention of PONV state that droperidol would have been the overwhelming first choice for PONV prophylaxis if it were not for the black box warning.[2] Following the release of the black box warning, the use of droperidol declined. Haloperidol, another butyrophenone, has been identified as an alternative to droperidol. In doses of 0.5 – 1 mg iv, it is an effective non-sedating antiemetic that can be repeated as needed *q*8hr. Although it can cause a prolongation of the QTc interval, there have been no reports of associated cardiac arrhythmias or extra-pyramidal effects when used in this dose range. It has a long duration of action (half-life of up to 18 hr) and may be administered at any time during surgery for PONV prophylaxis.[11] Its efficacy in the prevention of PONV is equal to that of dexamethasone, and it is safe to administer with dexamethasone and/or ondansetron.[12,13] Administration of haloperidol with ondansetron provided more effective and longer lasting protection for PONV than ondansetron alone.[13] A study in geriatric patients sustaining hip fractures demonstrated its safety as well as a 50% decrease in the duration of postoperative delirium in this high-risk population.[14]

## Dimenhydrinate

Dimenhydrinate is an antihistamine with anticholinergic properties, and it has an antiemetic efficacy similar to ondansetron, dexamethasone, and droperidol. Up to 1 mg·kg[-1] *iv* doses have been recommended. The anticholinergic side effects can result in a dry mouth, difficulty with urinating, blurred vision, sedation, and tachycardia and may contribute to postoperative delirium. Caution is recommended in patients with an enlarged prostate (due to the risk of urinary retention), glaucoma (increased intraocular pressure), and heart disease as well as in patients at risk of delirium.

## Prochlorperazine and promethazine

These two phenothiazine drugs have been shown to have antiemetic properties in doses of 5 – 10 mg *iv* and 12.5 – 25 mg *iv*, respectively, when administered at the end of surgery. Dizziness, dry mouth, and sedation limit the use of these drugs in an ambulatory setting. Extrapyramidal side effects increase with repeated doses. As such, these drugs are not recommended for use as first or second-line antiemetics.

## Transdermal scopolamine

Transdermal scopolamine has been shown to be an effective antiemetic with a prolonged duration of action (72-hr patch). It has a slow onset of action, requiring up to 4 hr to be effective, and as such, it should be applied either the night before surgery or 4 hr before the end of surgery. Its anticholinergic side effects may result in blurred vision (18%), dry mouth (8%), dizziness (2%), or agitation (1%).

## Propofol

Small doses of propofol (20 mg *iv*) may have an antiemetic effect, and the drug has been used as a rescue treatment for PONV. Its effect is limited by its short duration of action.

## P6 Electro-acupoint stimulation

Several non-pharmacologic techniques have been used to prevent PONV. Perhaps the most promising is the stimulation of the P6 acupuncture point, which has been shown to decrease the incidence of PONV comparable with that of ondansetron (NNT = 5).

**Ineffective treatments** A systematic review has shown metoclopramide in doses of 10 mg *iv* to be ineffective when used for PONV prophylaxis. The use of supplemental oxygen has also been shown to be ineffective in reducing the incidence of PONV.

Table 22.12 outlines the extensive differential diagnosis for nausea and vomiting.

## Postoperative Agitation and Delirium

*Agitation* is a non-specific descriptor of excessive motor activity resulting from an internal discomfort, such as pain, anxiety, fear of death, etc.

*Anxiety* describes an unpleasant alteration in mood or emotion that does not impair the patient's normal ability to think or comprehend.

*Delirium* refers to an acute confusional state accompanied by cognitive or perceptual impairment. The state evolves over a short period of time (hours to days) and typically fluctuates with intermittent lucid intervals. It results in a reduced ability to focus or sustain attention that is not otherwise accounted for by a pre-existing dementia. It may result in a hyperactive agitated state or a hypoactive lethargic state. Hypoactive delirium is often not appreciated or diagnosed and may be associated with a worse long-term outcome compared with an agitated delirium.

*Postoperative cognitive dysfunction (POCD)* refers to subtle declines in cognitive function lasting for weeks, months, or longer. It typically impairs memory, learning, and concentration. Neuropsychological testing is needed for verification. An in-depth discussion of POCD is beyond the scope of this primer.

The diagnosis of delirium in a patient in the postoperative or Intensive care unit (ICU) can be made using the Confusional Assessment Method[15] (CAM-ICU) when a patient is identified as having:

1. An acute onset or fluctuating impairment in cognition,
2. Inattention, and
3. Disorganized thinking or an altered level of consciousness

Two-thirds of patients admitted to the ICU will have an episode of delirium. Postoperative delirium typically develops 2 – 7 days postoperatively. As this period corresponds to the time course of the systemic inflammatory response following surgery, it has been postulated that increases in oxidative and inflammatory mediators along with psychological stress produce inflammatory cytokines and neurotoxins responsible for the delirium state.[16] The development of delirium in the postoperative period is associated with unintended extubation, removal of catheters (intravenous, urinary), as well as requirements for physical and chemical restraints and prolonged ICU and hospital stays. Delirium is also associated with increased hospital costs, increased risk of death, and a greater long-term functional decline

Nowadays, the agitated, delirious, or aggressive patient is rarely seen in the postanesthetic care unit (PACU). Perhaps this is due to a combination of our improved understanding of pain management, the availability of shorter-acting anesthesia agents, and improvements in our monitoring equipment (oximetry, peripheral nerve stimulator, and end-tidal carbon dioxide monitoring). The Richmond Agitation-Sedation Scale has been used to objectify and quantitate the severity of agitation and sedation.

Preoperative geriatric consultation for patients at high risk of delirium is the most effective means of preventing delirium in the perioperative period.[17] Interventions used to prevent delirium include maintenance of a normal sleep-wake cycle, ensuring adequate hydration, involving family members, providing

## Table 22.12 Etiology of perioperative nausea and vomiting

| Neurologic | Acute neurologic event | Acute withdrawal (drugs, alcohol) |
|---|---|---|
| | Increased ICP | Acute intoxication |
| | Pain | |
| Cardiac | Hypotension | Ischemia |
| | Bradycardia | |
| GI / Urinary | Bowel distension | Gastroenteritis |
| | Ileus | Renal failure |
| | Hepatitis | Pregnancy, |
| Endocrine | Ketoacidosis | Hypothyroidism |
| | Hyponatremia (post TURP) | Adrenal failure |
| | Hypercalcemia (cancer) | |
| Medications | Anesthesia medications | Drug toxicity |
| | Opioids | ASA |
| | Volatile anesthetic agents | Acetaminophen |
| | Cholinesterase inhibitors | Alcohol |
| | | Digoxin |

Gi = gastrointestinal; ICP = intracranial pressure; TURP = trans-urethral resection of prostate; ASA = acetylsalicylic acid.

hearing and visual aids (glasses, hearing aids, clocks), frequently reorienting the patient, and early mobilization. Other measures include minimizing attachments (e.g., surgical drains, intravenous catheters, urinary catheters, endotracheal tube, etc.), and prompt treatment of infection, hypoxemia, and pain. The use of regional anesthesia does not reduce the incidence of delirium when compared with general anesthesia.[18] Also, there is no evidence that neuraxial anesthetica techniques are superior to general anesthesia with opioid pain management in reducing the risk of postoperative delirium.[19] Elderly patients at risk of delirium who were undergoing surgery for repair of a hip fracture under spinal anesthesia had a 50% reduction in the incidence of delirium with light sedation (bispectral Index [BIS] > 80) compared with deeper sedation (BIS = 50).[19,20] There are many causes of postoperative agitation and delirium in the perioperative period. Possible causes are listed in Table 22.14.

An initial ABC approach is used to manage the agitated or delirious patient. Physical or medication restraints may be required to protect both the patient and the medical team.

These should be removed as soon as the offending cause of agitation is identified and treated.

An upper airway obstruction, residual paralysis, hypercarbia, hypoxemia, hypoglycemia, pain, and fear are all potent stimulants that can produce an agitated state. A gross neurological examination should be quickly performed (e.g., pupillary assessment, movement of arms and legs, Glasgow Coma Scale [GCS] score) while communicating reassuringly with the patient.

Elderly patients are particularly prone to postoperative confusion and agitation. Common causes of agitation include pain as well as bladder or bowel distension. Patients recovering from anesthesia may be unable to recognize and communicate that the cause of their distress is pain or a full bladder.

Following clinical evaluation, appropriate investigations may include a measurement of the patient's glucose, electrolytes, calcium, arterial blood gas, and tests of neuromuscular strength. Some of the organic causes of altered cognition in the perioperative period are listed in Table 22.14.

## Table 22.13 Risk factors for postoperative delirium

| | |
|---|---|
| Age > 70 | Anemia |
| Depression | Vascular surgery |
| Alcohol abuse | Hip fracture surgery |
| Pre-existing cognitive deficit | Thoracic surgery |
| Poor functional status | Prolonged operative time |
| Markedly abnormal Na, K, glucose | Substantial blood loss |
| Low albumin | |

### Treatment

Benzodiazepines are commonly used to treat anxiety, agitation, and delirium; however, the duration of action in the elderly and critically ill is unpredictable. There is no evidence to support the use of benzodiazepines in the treatment of delirium when it is not associated with alcohol withdrawal. The use benzodiazepines may increase the risk and duration of delirium in the postoperative period.

The American Psychiatric Association (APA) guidelines support the use of haloperidol for the treatment of delirium[21]. Low-dose haloperidol may reduce the severity, duration, and hospital length of stay in elderly patients suffering from delirium. Extrapyramidal side effects are relatively uncommon in critically ill patients. Like droperidol, haloperidol may prolong the QTc interval and result in serious arrhythmias (torsade-de-pointes). The APA guidelines recommend that consideration should be given to discontinuing haloperidol if the QTc interval is > 450 msec or is prolonged > 25% of the baseline QTc interval. The starting dose of haloperidol is 0.5 – 1 mg $iv$, similar to that used for antiemetic prophylaxis. In patients with mild, moderate, and severe agitation, haloperidol doses of 2, 5, and 10 mg $iv$, respectively, are often required. Elderly patients typically require approximately one-third of this dose. As the onset of action of haloperidol is 11 min, repeat dosing is recommended after 20 min as required. Supplementary analgesics or anxiolytics may also be required. The half-life of haloperidol ranges from 14 – 24 hr, with intravenous administration being twice as potent as the oral formulation. Intravenous administration is preferred in critically ill patients as absorption is guaranteed and side effects may be reduced compared with oral administration. Once a calm state is achieved for 24 hr, the dose is reduced by 50% every 24 hr and tapered off over the next 3 – 5 days. More recent trials using second-generation antipsychotic medications, such as olanzapine, risperidone, ziprasidone, and quetiapine in the treatment of postoperative delirium have been encouraging.

Small doses of naloxone (0.04 - 0.08 mg $iv$ increments), flumazenil (0.2 - 0.6 mg $iv$), or physostigmine (0.5 - 2 mg $iv$) may be appropriate if excessive sedation is considered secondary to opioids, benzodiazepines, or anticholinergic agents, respectively.

## Table 22.14 Possible causes of postoperative agitation and delirium

| | | |
|---|---|---|
| Neurologic | Pain<br>Anxiety<br>Hypothermia<br>Meningitis<br>Encephalitis<br>Acute intoxication<br>Acute withdrawal (drugs or alcohol) | Glycine or water toxicity<br>(Surgical fluid absorption syndrome)<br>Hypertensive encephalopathy<br>Wernicke's encephalopathy<br>Acute intracranial event<br>Thrombosis, bleed<br>Increased ICP |
| Respiratory | Airway obstruction<br>Residual paralysis | Hypoxia<br>Hypercarbia |
| Cardiac | Hypotension<br>Bradycardia | Ischemia<br>Arrhythmia |
| GI / Urinary | Bowel distension<br>Ileus<br>Hepatitis<br>Hepatic failure | Viral illness<br>Bladder distension<br>Renal failure |
| Endocrine | Hypoglycemia<br>Ketoacidosis<br>Hypercalcemia (cancer)<br>Hypothyroidism | Hyponatremia<br>(Surgical fluid absorption syndrome)<br>Adrenal failure |
| Medications | Drugs with anticholinergic effects<br>(e.g., atropine, dimenhydrinate (Gravol®), diphenhydramine (Benadryl®),<br>scopolamine, olanzapine (Zyprexa®)<br>quetiapine (Seroquel®)<br>TCAs (e.g., amitriptyline)<br>Other medications<br>(e.g., opioids, street drugs, alcohol) | |

ICP = intracranial pressure; GI = gastrointestinal; TCAs = tricyclic antidepressants.

## References:

1. Gan TJ, Meyer TA, Apfel CC et al. Consensus Guidelines for Managing Postoperative Nausea and Vomiting. Anesth Analg 2003; 97: 62-71.
2. Gan TJ, Meyer TA, Apfel CC et al. Society for ambulatory anesthesia guidelines for the management of postoperative nausea and vomiting. Anesth Analg 2007;105:1615-1628.
3. Apfel CC, Kortila K, Abdalla M et al. A Factorial Trial of Six Interventions for the Prevention of Postoperative Nausea and Vomiting. N Engl J Med 2004;350;2441-2451.
4. Ho KM. Editorial. Dexamethasone for postoperative nausea and vomiting: time for a definitive phase IV trial. Anaesth Int Care 2010;38:619-620.
5. Corcoran TB, Truyens A, Moseley AR. Anti-emetic dexamethasone and postoperative infection risk: a retrospective cohort study. Anaesth Int Care 2010;38:654-660.
6. Percival VG, Riddell J, Corcoran TB. Single dose dexamethasone for postoperative nausea and vomiting – a matched case-control study of postoperative infection risk. Anaesth Int Care 2010;38:661-666.
7. Slicker JC, Comen NA, Mannaerts GH et al. Long term and perioperative corticosteroids in anastomotic leakage. Arch Surg Jan 2012.
8. Henzi I, Walder B, Tramèr MR. Dexamethasone for the prevention of postoperative nausea and vomiting: a quantitative systematic review. Anesth Analg 2000;90:186-194.
9. Miller RD. Millers Anesthesia 7th edition 2009. Churchill Livingstone.
10. Jakobsson J. Preoperative single-dose intravenous dexamethasone during ambulatory surgery: update around the benefit versus risk. Curr Opin Anesth 2010;23:682-686.
11. Habib AS, Gan TJ. Editorial. Haloperidol for postoperative nausea and vomiting: are we reinventing the wheel? Anesth Analg 2008;106:1343-1345.
12. Chu CC, Shieh J-P, Tzeng J-I. The prophylactic effect of haloperidol plus dexamethasone on postoperative nausea and vomiting in patients undergoing laparoscopically assisted vaginal hysterectomy. Anesth Analg 2008;106:1402-1406.
13. Grecu L, Bittner EA, Kher J et al. Haloperidol plus ondansetron versus ondansetron alone for prophylaxis of postoperative nausea and vomiting. Anesth Analg 2008;106:1410-1413.
14. Kalisvaart KJ, de Jongha JFM, Bogaards MJ et al. Haloperidol prophylaxis for elderly hip-surgery patients at risk for delirium: a randomized placebo-controlled study. J Amer Ger Soc 2005;53:1658-1666.
15. Wong CL, Holroyd-Leduc J, Simel DL, et al. Does this patient have delirium? Value of beside instruments. JAMA 2010;304:779-786.
16. Van Munster BC, Korevaar JC, Zwinderman AH, et al. Time course of cytokines during delirium in elderly patients with hip fractures. J Am Geriatr Soc 2008;56:1704-1709.
17. Chaput AJ, Bryson GL. Postoperative delirium: risk factors and management: Continuing professional development. Can J Anesth 2012;59:304-320.
18. Fong HK, Sands LP, Leung JM. The role of postoperative analgesia in delirium and cognitive decline in elderly patients: a systematic review. Anesth Analg 2006;102:1255-1266.
19. Sieber FE, Zakriya KJ, Gottschalk A, et al. Sedation depth during spinal anesthesia and the development of postoperative delirium in elderly patients undergoing hip fracture repair. Mayo Clin Proc85:18-26.
20. Williams-Russo P, Urquhart BL, Sharrock NE, et al. Post-operative delirium: predictors and prognosis in elderly orthopaedic patients. J Am Geriatr Soc 1992;40:759-767.
21. Practice guideline for the treatment of patients with delirium. American Psychiatric Association. Am J Psychiatry 1999;156:1-20. Access through Guideline watch: Practice guideline for the treatment of patients with delirium. Cook IA, Psychiatry online.org

# CHAPTER 23

# Managing the Circulation

Melanie Toman MD, Viren Naik MD and Christopher Hudson MD

## Learning Objectives

1. To understand the phases of the cardiac cycle.
2. To identify the determinants of cardiac output and blood pressure.
3. To understand the effect of anesthesia on cardiac physiology.
4. To become familiar with current ACLS algorithms and gain an interest in a formal ACLS training course.

## Key Points

| | |
|---|---|
| 1 | The cardiac cycle is composed of systole and diastole phases. Ventricular relaxation is an active process of energy consumption. |
| 2 | Heart rate and stroke volume determine cardiac output. |
| 3 | Stroke volume is determined by preload, afterload, and contractility. |
| 4 | Cardiac output and systemic vascular resistance determine blood pressure. |
| 5 | Hypotension in the operating room is common, and treatment should be directed at correcting the underlying cause. |
| 6 | The purpose of ACLS is to provide a standardized approach to manage abnormal heart rhythms, to restore normal circulation, to optimize tissue perfusion, and to minimize ischemic injury. |

## Introduction

The heart is composed of four chambers; the right atrium, right ventricle, left atrium, and left ventricle. Deoxygenated blood returns from the body via the superior vena cava and the inferior vena cava to the right atrium. It then passes through the tricuspid valve into the right ventricle. From there, the blood is pumped through the pulmonic valve into the pulmonary arteries. Once in the lungs, the blood is oxygenated and carbon dioxide is removed. The blood then returns to the left atrium of the heart via the pulmonary veins. From here it travels through the mitral valve into the left ventricle where it is then pumped through the aortic valve into the systemic circulation via the aorta.

The systemic circulation is composed of an arterial tree (arteries, arterioles, and capillaries) and a venous tree (venules and veins). The arterial tree is a high-pressure system that carries oxygenated blood away from the heart to the tissues, while the venous tree is a low-pressure system that returns the deoxygenated blood to the heart. A normal adult has approximately 5,000 mL of blood; 15% is in the arterial system and 60% is in the venous system. The remaining 25% of blood is found in the heart and pulmonary circulation (i.e., pulmonary veins, arteries, and capillaries).

## Cardiac Cycle

The cardiac cycle refers to the mechanical events of the ventricle that occur from the beginning of one heartbeat to the beginning of the next. The cardiac cycle is regulated by the heart's intrinsic conduction system. Action potentials arise from the sino-atrial (SA) node; they spread throughout the atria, cross into the ventricles via the atrio-ventricle (AV) node, and are finally transmitted across the ventricles via the bundle of His and Purkinje fibers. The cardiac cycle is divided between the systolic and diastolic phases (see Fig. 10.4).

*Systole*

Systole is the period of ventricular contraction. As the left ventricle contracts, the pressure generated within the left ventricular cavity causes the mitral valve to close, preventing blood from flowing back into the left atrium. Isovolumetric contraction refers to the period of time where the ventricular pressure continues to increase without any change in ventricular volume. Eventually, the pressure generated by the ventricle exceeds that in the aorta, causing the aortic valve to open and blood to eject. Blood continues to be propelled forward until the pressure equalizes between the left ventricle and aorta at the beginning of diastole.

Diastole is the period of ventricular relaxation. Equalization of pressure between the left ventricle and aorta causes the aortic valve to close. Initially, there is a period of ventricular relaxation with no change in volume (termed isovolumetric relaxation). Eventually, the pressure in the left atrium overcomes that of the left ventricle resulting in the opening of the mitral valve and filling of the left ventricle (see Fig. 23.1). Early diastolic filling is passive, secondary to the pressure gradient between the left atria and ventricle, while late diastolic filling is due to left atrial contraction.

## Cardiac Output

Cardiac output (CO) is defined as the volume of blood that enters the systemic circulation per minute. It is expressed as the product of heart rate (HR) multiplied by the stroke volume (SV).

Cardiac Output (L·min$^{-1}$) = Heart Rate (beats·min$^{-1}$) x Stroke Volume (mL)

A normal CO for an adult is 4.5 – 6.0 L·min$^{-1}$. Since cardiac output is associated with patient size, i.e., larger patients require greater cardiac output, we typically index CO by dividing it by total body surface area (BSA). Cardiac index (L·min$^{-1}$·m$^2$) = CO (L·min$^{-1}$) / BSA (m$^2$). A normal cardiac index is 2.5 - 3.5 L·min$^{-1}$·m$^2$.

## Stroke Volume

Stroke volume is the amount of blood that is pumped out of the ventricle with each heart beat. A normal stroke volume is 0.5 – 1.0 mL·kg$^{-1}$ and is calculated by subtracting end-systolic volume (ESV) from end-diastolic volume (EDV).

Stroke volume (mL) = EDV (mL) – ESV (mL)

The three principal determinants of stroke volume are the preload, afterload, and contractility.

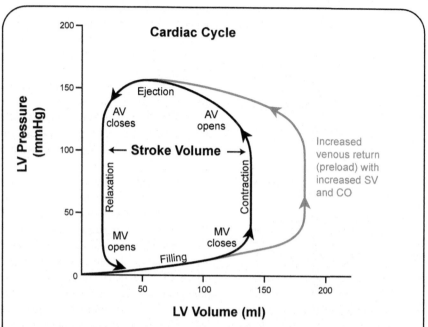

Fig. 23.1 Ventricular pressure-volume loop during a cardiac cycle. The mitral valve opens (lower left) initiating the cardiac cycle. The ventricle fills to the end-diastolic volume (lower right). Isovolumetric contraction results in closure of the mitral valve. Ventricular ejection begins (upper right curve) as the aortic valve opens. As the ventricle empties (end-systolic volume; upper left curve) the aortic valve closes and the ventricle fills during isovolumetric relaxation completing the loop. Changes in contractility, preload, afterload, heart rate and rhythm can be manipulated to improve stroke volume (SV) and cardiac output (CO).

Preload is defined as the end-diastolic ventricular wall stress. It is the stretch on ventricular fibers at the end of diastole immediately before the onset of contraction. Changes in ventricular preload dramatically affect stroke volume (Frank-Starling relationship, Fig. 23.2).

As preload increases, left ventricular work, cardiac output, blood pressure, and stroke volume also increase. Excessive increases in end-diastolic stretch can result in a decline in cardiac performance as the left ventricle becomes over distended. This can result in heart failure and pulmonary edema. An accurate assessment of preload and the need for intravenous fluids is challenging and is commonly based on clinical assessments, such as heart rate, blood pressure, blood loss, and urine output. Information obtained from a peripheral arterial catheter (pulse pressure variation), central venous catheter, pulmonary artery catheter, or from echocardiography may

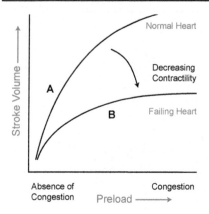

Fig. 23.2 Frank-Starling relationship for ventricular function of the normal and failing heart. A: Initial increases in the end diastolic volume (preload) result in large increases in stroke volume. B: In the failing heart, overdistension of the ventricle may result in a reduction in the stroke volume.

be used to assess whether additional fluid administration would be beneficial. Refer to Chapter 10 for a discussion on the assessment of preload and an advanced assessment of techniques used to predict whether additional fluids may be beneficial.

The University of Ottawa Departments of Anesthesia and Emergency Medicine have developed a Web-based instructional module that discusses the anatomy, indications, preparation, technique, complications, and pitfalls regarding insertion of a central venous catheter. The module can be accessed at http://www.med.uottawa.ca/courses/cvc/e_index.html.

*Afterload*

Afterload is the resistance the heart must overcome to propel blood forward. Afterload can be estimated by wall stress, which is a product of ventricular pressure (P) and the radius (r) of the ventricular cavity divided by ventricular wall thickness (h), i.e., LaPlace's Law.

Wall stress= Pr/2h

Wall stress increases when the ventricle needs to generate higher pressures (e.g.,

hypertension) or when the ventricle becomes distended (e.g., dilatation secondary to heart failure). Wall stress decreases when the ventricle hypertrophies. In the absence of aortic stenosis, afterload depends on the elasticity of the large arteries and on the systemic vascular resistance (SVR). The SVR can be estimated using a calculation incorporating the mean arterial pressure, central venous pressure, and cardiac output (see Chapter 10).

Contractility, or inotropy, is the myocardium's intrinsic ability to perform work at any given level of end-diastolic fiber length. Substances that increase contractility are termed positive inotropes, and those that decrease contractility are termed negative inotropes. All agents that increase myocardial contractility produce an increase in intracellular calcium. The most important mechanism regulating inotropy is the autonomic nervous system. The sympathetic nervous system increases contractility while the parasympathetic nervous system decreases contractility. Common conditions that decrease contractility include hypoxia, acidosis, myocardial ischemia or infarction, and the use of beta or calcium channel blockers. Increases in preload, heart rate, and contractility or decreases in afterload all promote forward flow and increase cardiac output.

Ejection fraction (EF) is commonly used as an index of contractility. It is the ratio of blood that leaves the ventricle during systole to the total blood present in the ventricle at the end of diastole.

EF (%) = SV (mL) /EDV (mL)

A normal EF is 55 – 70%. The ejection fraction may be misleading because it is a ratio. A patient may have a normal ejection fraction but have a very small stroke volume, as occurs in mitral regurgitation. Conversely, a patient may have a low EF, but a normal stroke volume, such as in dilated cardiomyopathy.

## Table 23.1 Normal Hemodynamic Parameters

| Measure | Normal Range |
|---------|-------------|
| Heart rate | 60 – 100 beats·min⁻¹ |
| Stroke volume | 55 – 100 mL |
| Cardiac output | 4.0 – 6.0 L·min⁻¹ |
| Cardiac index | 2.5 – 3.5 L·min⁻¹·m² |
| Ejection fraction | 55 – 70% |

### Heart Rate

The heart rate is the number of times the heart beats per minute. The primary determinant of heart rate is the balance of sympathetic and parasympathetic nervous stimulation. Normal adult heart rates vary from 60 - 100 beats·min⁻¹. Bradycardia is defined as a heart rate < 60 beats·min⁻¹, and tachycardia is defined as a heart rate > 100 beats·min⁻¹. Medications that affect heart rate are known as chronotropes.

### Blood Pressure

Blood pressure is the pressure generated by the blood against the walls of the blood vessels. As blood flow is more difficult to measure, we often, though inaccurately, use blood pressure as a surrogate measure for cardiac output.

Blood pressure is the product of cardiac output and systemic vascular resistance (SVR) (Fig. 23.3). Systemic vascular resistance is the resistance to forward flow caused by the arterial vasculature, and it is regulated by changes in vascular tone. Arterial constriction will increase the SVR and increase blood pressure. Arterial vasodilation will decrease SVR and decrease blood pressure.

When measuring blood pressure, we typically look at systolic blood pressure (maximum pressure generated), diastolic blood pressure (minimum pressure generated), and mean blood pressure (average pressure over the entire cardiac cycle).

## Table 23.3 Blood Pressure Classification

| Category | Systolic (mmHg) | Diastolic (mmHg) |
|----------|-----------------|------------------|
| Hypotension | < 90 | < 60 |
| Normotension | 90 – 119 | 60 – 79 |
| Pre-hypertension | 120 – 139 | 80 – 89 |
| Hypertension | 140 – 179 | 90 – 109 |
| Critical hypertension | ≥ 180 | ≥ 120 |

Hemodynamic abnormalities of the circulation may require interventions to maintain normal oxygen transport and organ perfusion. This may occur in the perioperative period as a result of pain, anxiety, hypoxia, hypercarbia, or abnormalities in intravascular volume or temperature (Chapter 22). Pharmacologic manipulation of both the parasympathetic and sympathetic nervous systems may be required to correct hypotensive, ischemic, or hypertensive emergencies. Table 23.4 lists the different classes of medications that may be used to restore circulatory homeostasis. The principle goal of circulatory support is to optimize tissue perfusion with oxygenated blood. To achieve this, it is necessary to assess and optimize preload, afterload, heart rate, oxygen transport, and organ perfusion. Refer to the additional resources for an advanced discussion on optimizing fluid and oxygen therapy in the perioperative period.

The heart rate and blood pressure are two easily measured vital parameters that provide information on a patient's physiologic well-being. The diagnosis and management of arterial hypotension requires a basic knowledge of the physiological principles that control blood pressure. Both the duration and severity of intraoperative hypotension have been linked to surgical mortality and are closely associated with perioperative myocardial ischemia and infarction. The end goal of a complex interaction of cardiovascular, neuroendocrine, and hematologic physiology is to provide adequate perfusion and oxygenation to the tissues. Persistent deficiencies in perfusion and oxygenation result in varying degrees of shock.

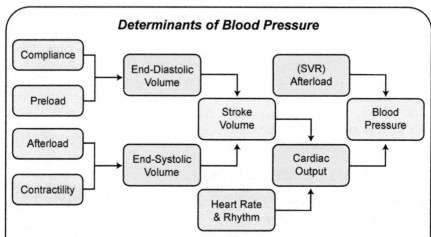

Fig. 23.3 The determinants of blood pressure. Preload, afterload and contractility are the primary determinants of stroke volume. The cardiac output is the product of the stroke volume and heart rate. The blood pressure is directly influenced by both the cardiac output and afterload.

## Table 23.4 Cardiorespiratory Effects of Receptor Stimulation

| Receptor | Agonist | Antagonist |
|---|---|---|
| Adrenergic | | |
| Alpha-1 | Vasoconstriction of the skin, gut, kidney, liver, and heart (e.g., phenylephrine). | Peripheral vasodilation, reflex tachycardia, hypotension (e.g., prazosin). |
| Alpha-2 | Reduces sympathetic outflow from the CNS inhibiting norepinephrine release (e.g., clonidine, dexmedetomidine). | CNS stimulation, increased sympathetic outflow, increased HR, contractility, and cardiac output. |
| Beta-1 | Increased HR, myocardial conduction, and contractility (e.g., isoproterenol). | Decreased HR, conduction, and contractility (e.g., metoprolol). |
| Beta-2 | Bronchodilation, peripheral vascular smooth muscle relaxation (e.g. salbutamol). | Bronchospasm, peripheral vasoconstriction. |
| Dopamine | Peripheral vasodilation of the renal and splanchnic vasculature. | |
| Cholinergic | Decreases HR, conduction, and cardiac output. Increases bronchial secretions (e.g., neostigmine). | Anticholinergics increase HR, conduction, and contractility. They also decrease bronchial secretions (e.g., atropine). |
| Calcium channel | Increases contractility, vasoconstriction (e.g., calcium). | Decreases contractility; increases vasodilation (e.g., diltiazem). |
| Other | Phosphodiesterase inhibitors produce a concentration-dependent increase in contractility with arterial and venous dilation (e.g., milrinone). Cardiac glycosides result in an increase in intracellular calcium and increase the force of contraction and cardiac output (e.g., digoxin). | |

CNS = central nervous system; HR = heart rate.

## Effect of Anesthesia

Hypotension in the operating room is common and may result from changes in any of the determinants of blood pressure. Thus, a change in heart rate, rhythm, preload, afterload, contractility, or systemic vascular resistance may be the cause.

## General Anesthesia

Most intravenous and inhalational anesthetics are negative inotropes and will decrease myocardial contractility and cause peripheral vasodilation. Furthermore, they may depress baroreceptor reflexes and inhibit compensatory tachycardia. Sympathetic outflow from the medulla is also reduced under anesthesia.

The decrease in blood pressure seen during induction and maintenance of anesthesia is multifactorial. If the hypotension is significant, treatment should be directed at the underlying cause.

*Preload*

Reductions in preload may be corrected with a fluid bolus or by raising the patient's legs to increase venous return to the right side of the heart.

*Afterload*

If hypotension persists despite optimization of preload status, vasopressors may be used to increase afterload and peripheral vascular resistance. Vasopressors stimulate alpha-adrenergic receptors (alpha agonists) and cause arterial constriction. Commonly used agents include phenylephrine (Neo-Synephrine®) and norepinephrine (Levophed®).

*Contractility*

Inotropes stimulate beta-adrenergic receptors (beta agonists) and are used to improve cardiac contractility.

## Table 23.5 Manipulating Determinants of Cardiac Output

| Determinants of Cardiac Output | Hemodynamic Disturbance (With common vasoactive agents and Interventions used to treat the disturbance) | |
| --- | --- | --- |
| Preload | **Increased Preload**<br><br>Venous vasodilators<br>- nitroglycerine,<br>- nitroprusside<br>Diuretics<br>- furosemide<br>Phlebotomy | **Decreased Preload**<br><br>Crystalloid or colloid infusion<br>(see Chapter 21) |
| Heart Rate | **Increased Heart Rate**<br><br>Beta blockers<br>- metoprolol<br>- esmolol<br>Calcium channel blockers<br>- diltiazem, verapamil | **Decreased Heart Rate**<br><br>Anticholinergics<br>- atropine<br>Beta agonists<br>- ephedrine<br>Pacemaker |
| Contractility | **Increased Contractility**<br><br>General anesthetics<br>- desflurane<br>- sevoflurane<br>- propofol<br>Beta blockers<br>Calcium channel blockers | **Decreased Contractility**<br><br>- ephedrine<br>- dopamine<br>- dobutamine<br>- epinephrine<br>Aortic balloon pump<br>Surgery |
| Afterload | **Increased Afterload**<br><br>Arterial vasodilators<br>- nitroprusside<br>- hydralazine<br>- labetalol<br>ACE inhibitors<br>- dobutamine | **Decreased Afterload**<br><br>Alpha agonists<br>- phenylephrine<br>- norepinephrine<br>Crystalloid or colloid infusion |

ACE = angiotensin-converting-enzyme.

## Regional Anesthesia

Spinal and epidural anesthesia (i.e., neuraxial anesthesia) block nerves entering and exiting the spinal cord. The blockade of sympathetic output from the spinal cord causes peripheral vasodilation and thus a reduction in systemic vascular resistance and blood pressure. The degree of hypotension associated with neuraxial anesthesia is dependent on many variables. Some of the most common factors include the height of the spinal block, the

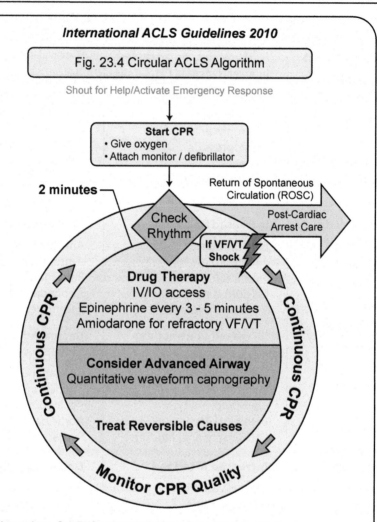

**International ACLS Guidelines 2010**

Fig. 23.4 Circular ACLS Algorithm

Shout for Help/Activate Emergency Response

**Start CPR**
• Give oxygen
• Attach monitor / defibrillator

2 minutes

Return of Spontaneous Circulation (ROSC)

Check Rhythm

If VF/VT Shock

Post-Cardiac Arrest Care

**Drug Therapy**
IV/IO access
Epinephrine every 3 - 5 minutes
Amiodarone for refractory VF/VT

**Consider Advanced Airway**
Quantitative waveform capnography

**Treat Reversible Causes**

Continuous CPR

Continuous CPR

Monitor CPR Quality

ABC changed to a C-A-B (Compression, Airway, Breathing) approach

2010 AHA Guidelines emphasize the need for high quality CPR, including
• a compression rate of at least 100/min
• a compression depth of at least 2" in adults
• allowing for complete chest recoil after each compression
• minimizing interruptions in chest compressions

No change in the recommendation for a compression-to-ventilation ratio of 30:2 for single rescuers. Inspiration time should be approximately 1 second. Once an advanced airway is in place, chest compressions are continuous and no longer interrupted by ventilation. Ventilation is provided every 6 to 8 seconds (8 - 10 breaths per minute).

Adapted with permission AHA 2010 Guidelines

## International ACLS Guidelines 2010

### Fig. 23.5 Circular ACLS Algorithm

**CPR Quality**
- Push hard (≥ 2 inches) and fast (≥ 100/min) and allow complete chest recoil
- Minimize interruptions in compressions
- Avoid excessive ventilation
- Rotate compressor every 2 minutes
- If no advanced airway, 30:2 compression-ventilation ratio
- Quantitative waveform capnography
  - If PETCO$_2$ < 10 mm Hg, attempt to improve CPR quality
- Intra-arterial pressure
  - If relaxation phase (diastolic) pressure < 20 mm Hg, attempt to improve CPR quality

**Return of Spontaneous Circulation (ROSC)**
- Pulse and blood pressure
- Abrupt sustained increase in PETCO$_2$ (typically ≥ 40 mm Hg)
- Spontaneous arterial pressure waves with intra-arterial monitoring

**Shock Energy**
- **Biphasic:** Manufacturer recommendation (120 - 200 J); if unknown use maximum available. Second and subsequent doses should be equivalent, and higher doses should be considered.
- **Monophasic:** 360J

**Drug Therapy**
- **Epinephrine IV/IO Dose:** 1 mg every 3 - 5 minutes
- **Vasopressin IV/IO Dose:** 40 units can replace first or second dose of epinephrine
- **Amiodarone IV/IO Dose:** First dose: 300 mg bolus.
  Second dose: 150 mg

**Advanced Airway**
- Supraglottic advanced airway or endotracheal intubation
- Waveform capnography to confirm and monitor ET tube placement
- 8 - 10 breaths per minute with continuous chest compressions

**Reversible Causes**
- Hypovolemia
- Hypoxia
- Hydrogen ion (acidosis)
- Hypo-/hyperkalemia
- Hypothermia
- Tension pneumothorax
- Tamponade, cardiac
- Toxins
- Thrombosis, pulmonary
- Thrombosis, cardiac

Adapted with permission AHA 2010 Guidelines

## International ACLS Guidelines 2010

Fig. 23.6 Ventricular Fibrillation / Pulseless Ventricular Tachycardia

Shock **First** x 1
(If defibrillator is not immediately available, start CPR then shock ASAP;
200 J Biphasic, 360 J Monophasic)

↓

**High Quality CPR\* x 2 mins**
(prior to rhythm or pulse check;
Ventilate, IV or IO access)

↓

Shock

↓

**CPR x 2 mins**
(Intubate, give drugs during CPR,
Treat reversible causes)

↓

**Epinephrine 1 mg IV** (may be given after 1st or 2nd shock)
(Repeat every 3 - 5 mins; **Vasopressin 40 U IV**
may be an alternate to 1st or 2nd dose of epinephrine)

↓

Shock

↓

**CPR x 2 mins**

↓

**Amiodarone 300 mg** IV bolus (1st choice)
(may give 2nd dose of 150 mg IV)
or
**Lidocaine 1.5 mg/kg** IV
(repeat in 3 - 5 mins; max. 3 mg/kg)
or
**Magnesium Sulfate 2 g** IV
(with torsades)

↓

Shock

**\*High Quality CPR:** Push hard (≥ 2 inches) and fast (≥ 100/min), complete chest recoil, minimize interruptions, avoid excessive ventilation (8 - 10 / min), change compressors every 2 mins, monitor end-tidal CO2.

**Hypothermia** (32 - 34 C) recommended for resuscitated V. Fib. patients who remain comatose and intubated with a BP > 90.

**Treat Reversible Causes:** Hypovolemia, hypoxia, acidosis, K, hypothermia, toxins, ischemia

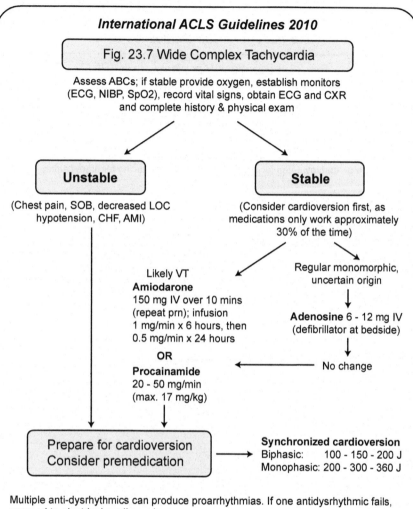

**International ACLS Guidelines 2010**

Fig. 23.7 Wide Complex Tachycardia

Assess ABCs; if stable provide oxygen, establish monitors (ECG, NIBP, SpO2), record vital signs, obtain ECG and CXR and complete history & physical exam

**Unstable**

(Chest pain, SOB, decreased LOC hypotension, CHF, AMI)

**Stable**

(Consider cardioversion first, as medications only work approximately 30% of the time)

Likely VT
**Amiodarone**
150 mg IV over 10 mins (repeat prn); infusion 1 mg/min x 6 hours, then 0.5 mg/min x 24 hours

**OR**

**Procainamide**
20 - 50 mg/min (max. 17 mg/kg)

Regular monomorphic, uncertain origin

**Adenosine** 6 - 12 mg IV (defibrillator at bedside)

No change

**Prepare for cardioversion Consider premedication**

**Synchronized cardioversion**
Biphasic:     100 - 150 - 200 J
Monophasic: 200 - 300 - 360 J

Multiple anti-dysrhythmics can produce proarrhythmias. If one antidysrhythmic fails, proceed to electrical cardioversion.

If Ventricular tachycardia is polymorphic (torsades); consider 2 g magnesium IV, overdrive pacing, amiodarone, isoproterenol, lidocaine or phenytoin.

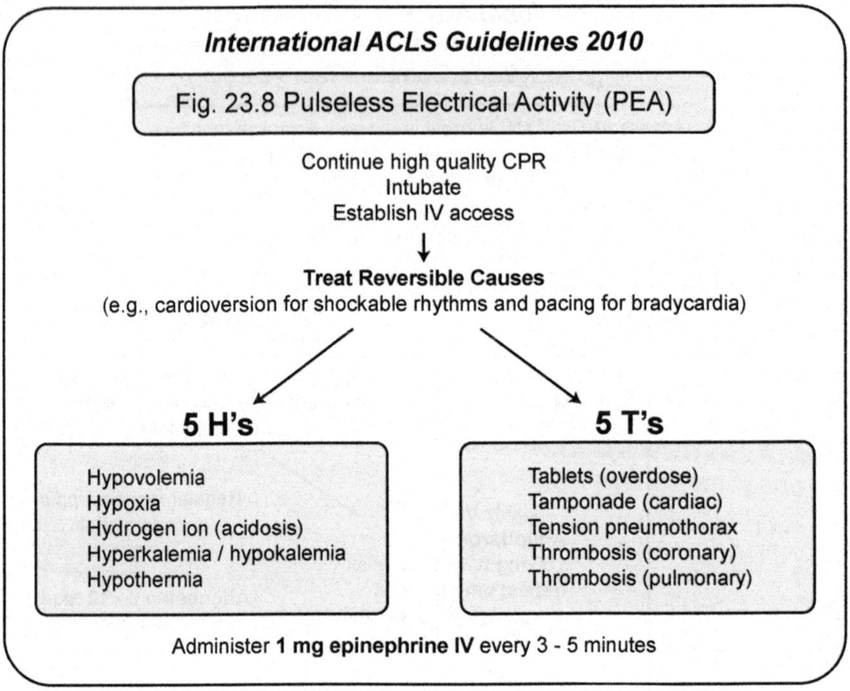

**International ACLS Guidelines 2010**

Fig. 23.8 Pulseless Electrical Activity (PEA)

Continue high quality CPR
Intubate
Establish IV access

↓

**Treat Reversible Causes**
(e.g., cardioversion for shockable rhythms and pacing for bradycardia)

**5 H's**

Hypovolemia
Hypoxia
Hydrogen ion (acidosis)
Hyperkalemia / hypokalemia
Hypothermia

**5 T's**

Tablets (overdose)
Tamponade (cardiac)
Tension pneumothorax
Thrombosis (coronary)
Thrombosis (pulmonary)

Administer **1 mg epinephrine IV** every 3 - 5 minutes

**International ACLS Guidelines 2010**

Fig. 23.9 Bradycardia (Slow HR < 60 bpm)

Assess ABCs, provide Oxygen, establish IV and monitors

Bradycardia (HR < 60 bpm)

Serious Signs or Symptoms?

(Hypotension, Chest pain, dyspnea, CHF, ischemia, LOC)

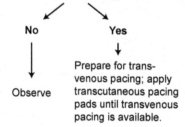

**No**

Type II 2nd degree block
or 3rd degree block

**No**          **Yes**

Observe

Prepare for trans-
venous pacing; apply
transcutaneous pacing
pads until transvenous
pacing is available.

**Yes**

Atropine 0.5 mg q 3 - 5 mins
Maximum 3 mg (0.04 mg/kg)

(Atropine is not effective for 3rd heart
block with wide complex escape
idioventricular rhythm).

Consider:
Transcutaneous Pacing
Prepare for IV Pacing
Dopamine 2 - 10 mcg/kg/min
Epinephrine 2 - 10 mcg/min.

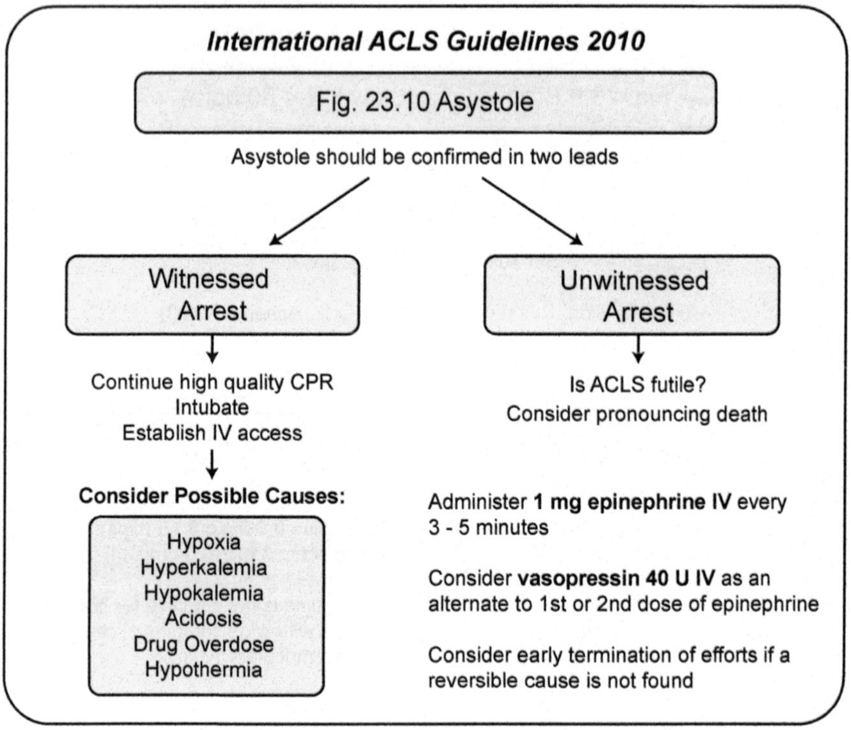

**International ACLS Guidelines 2010**

Fig. 23.10 Asystole

Asystole should be confirmed in two leads

| Witnessed Arrest | Unwitnessed Arrest |
|---|---|

Continue high quality CPR
Intubate
Establish IV access

**Consider Possible Causes:**

Hypoxia
Hyperkalemia
Hypokalemia
Acidosis
Drug Overdose
Hypothermia

Is ACLS futile?
Consider pronouncing death

Administer **1 mg epinephrine IV** every 3 - 5 minutes

Consider **vasopressin 40 U IV** as an alternate to 1st or 2nd dose of epinephrine

Consider early termination of efforts if a reversible cause is not found

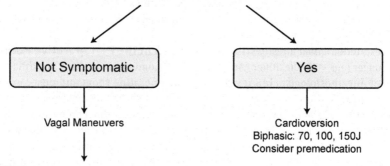

**International ACLS Guidelines 2010**

Fig. 23.11 Paroxysmal Supraventricular Tachycardia

Assess ABCs, provide Oxygen, establish IV and monitors

Serious Signs or Symptoms?

(Hypotension, Chest pain, dyspnea, CHF, ischemia, LOC)

Not Symptomatic

Yes

Vagal Maneuvers

Cardioversion
Biphasic: 70, 100, 150J
Consider premedication

**Class I:**
**Adenosine** 6 mg IV over 3 seconds, may repeat 12 mg in 1 - 2 minutes
or **Diltiazem** 20 mg IV over 2 minutes, may repeat in 15 minutes
or **Verapamil** 2.5 - 5 mg IV over 2 minutes, may repeat 5 - 10 mg in 10 mins
or **Metoprolol** 5 mg IV, may repeat x 2; maximum total = 15 minutes

Consider (Class IIa evidence)
Procainamide 30 mg/min to 17 mg/kg
Amiodarone 150 mg IV over 10 minutes

intravascular volume status of the patient, and the concomitant use of vasoactive medications (e.g., beta blockers, ACE inhibitors, diuretics).

Cardiac arrest associated with neuraxial anesthesia has been reported since the early 1990s. Severe bradycardia (HR 20 – 40 beats·min⁻¹) or asystolic arrest is more likely to occur with spinal anesthesia (approximately 6 per 10,000 cases) compared with epidural anesthesia (0.8 per 10,000 cases). In comparison, arrests associated with a general anesthetic occur with a frequency of approximately 5.5 per 10,000 cases. Patients suffering a cardiac arrest under spinal anesthesia are typically younger (age < 50), healthier (American Society of Anesthesiologists [ASA] physical status 1), and have a lower resting heart rate compared with the general anesthesia group. Other associated risk factors include the use of beta blockers and a prolonged PR interval. The mechanism of cardiac arrest associated with spinal anesthesia is not completely understood, but it does not appear to be related to hypoventilation, hypoxia, or oversedation. An increase in vagal tone and reflexes, initiated with a reduction in vascular volume, has been implicated. Severe progressive bradycardia associated with hypotension precedes the arrest and can occur during the operative procedure or in the recovery phase. Prompt intervention, administration of vasoactive medications (rapidly escalating doses of atropine, ephedrine, epinephrine, or vasopressin) and oxygen, and discontinuation of sedative medications are required to treat bradycardia and prevent the progression to a full arrest.[1,2]

## Advanced Cardiac Life Support (ACLS)

Advanced Cardiac Life Support provides a standardized approach to resuscitation for cardiac arrest and other cardiac rhythm disturbances. The goal of ACLS is to restore normal circulation to optimize tissue perfusion and minimize ischemic injury. The American Heart Association (AHA) updates the ACLS guidelines every five years, with the last update in 2010. Algorithms based on the 2010 guidelines are included for reference (Tables 23.3 – 23.10).

### ACLS in the Perioperative Period

Conditions resulting in cardiac arrest in the operating room and post-surgical care phase differ in etiology from a cardiac arrest that occurs in the community or in a non-surgical hospitalized patient.[4] Myocardial ischemia rarely evolves into cardiac failure or ventricular fibrillation in the operating room. The most common dysrhythmia in the operating room is bradycardia and asystole (45%), followed by ventricular tachycardia and ventricular fibrillation (14%) and pulseless electrical activity (7%).

### Clinical Pearl:

*Severe prolonged hypoxemia will universally result in progressive bradycardia that devolves into asystole when not corrected. When managing a difficult airway, progressive bradycardia should be considered to be secondary to hypoxemia until proven otherwise. Always activate the pulse oximeter's audible tone when providing care in remote locations.*

Table 23.6 Properties of Cardiovascular Drugs

| Drug | Receptor Activity | | | | Single bolus dose | Infusion rate and preparation | Comments |
|---|---|---|---|---|---|---|---|
| | α-1 | α-2 | β-1 | β-2 | | | |
| epinephrine¶ (Adrenalin®) | 2+ | 3+ | 1+ | 2+ | Anaphylaxis: 3 – 5 µg·kg⁻¹ Arrest: 1 mg | 0.01 - 0.2 µg·kg⁻¹·min⁻¹ 4 mg in 500 mL (8 µg·mL-1) | Inotropic beta effects at 0.02 – 0.09 µg·kg⁻¹·min⁻¹; pressor alpha effects at > 0.09 µg·kg⁻¹·min⁻¹. Used for hypotension with myocardial depression. |
| aminrinone¶ (Inocor®) | Phosphodiesterase inhibitor with positive inotropic action independent of adrenergic receptors. | | | | 0.75 mg·kg⁻¹ over 2 – 3 min | 2 – 10 µg·kg⁻¹·min⁻¹ | CO increased, HR unchanged, BP may decrease. PAP, PCWP, SVR all decrease. Used as an inotrope in patients with end-stage heart disease. Produces arterial and venous vasodilation and may decrease BP. |
| dopamine¶ (Inotropin®) | 1-4+ | 0 | 1+ | 2-4+ | | 1 – 10 µg·kg⁻¹·min⁻¹ 400 mg in 500 mL 800 µg·mL⁻¹ | Dopaminergic-1 receptors are the most sensitive at 1 – 4 µg·kg⁻¹·min⁻¹ and cause vasodilation. Beta effects start at 2 µg·kg⁻¹·min-1. At 5 – 10 µg·kg⁻¹·min⁻¹, beta effects predominate with an increase in HR and CO. Above 10 µg·kg⁻¹·min⁻¹, alpha effects predominate and effect mimics norepinephrine. |
| dobutamine¶ (Dobutrex®) | 0-1+ | 0 | 1+ | 3+ | | 1 - 20 µg·kg⁻¹·min⁻¹ 500 mg in 500 mL (1 mg·mL-1) | CO increases, SVR and PCWP decrease. At lower doses, CO increases without severe tachycardia or hypotension. At 10 – 15 µg·kg⁻¹·min⁻¹, HR and vasodilation become more prominent. BP may not change. |

¶ = invasive pressure monitoring mandatory; BP = blood pressure; CO = cardiac output; HR = heart rate; PAP = pulmonary artery pressure; PCWP = pulmonary capillary wedge pressure; SVR = systemic vascular resistance.

Table 23.7 Properties of Cardiovascular Drugs

| Drug | Receptor Activity | | | | Single bolus dose | Infusion rate and preparation | Comments |
|------|------|------|------|------|------|------|------|
| | α-1 | α-2 | β-1 | β-2 | | | |
| norepinephrine¶ (Levophed®) | 4+ | 4+ | 2+ | 0 | | $0.05 - 0.5\ \mu g \cdot kg^{-1} \cdot min^{-1}$ 4 mg in 500 mL ($8\ \mu g \cdot mL{-1}$) | Direct alpha and beta-receptor agonist. Decreases in renal blood flow occur even with low doses. At low doses, the alpha effects increase blood pressure causing vasoconstriction and reflex bradycardia. At higher doses, beta-receptor stimulation increases contractility. |
| phenylephrine¶ (Neo-Synephrine®) | 4+ | 0 | 1+ | 0 | $0.75\ mg \cdot kg^{-1}$ over 2 – 3 min | $2 - 10\ \mu g \cdot kg^{-1} \cdot min^{-1}$ | Phenylephrine represents an almost pure alpha-1 agonist. Beta stimulation occurs only at very high doses. Phenylephrine may be used to provide profound vasoconstriction temporarily while the underlying cause of hypotension is corrected. Reflex bradycardia may occur. May be useful in patients with hypotension associated with a decreased SVR and tachycardia. |
| ephedrine | 3+ | 0 | 2+ | 1+ | 5 – 10 mg iv 25 – 50 mg im | Onset within 1 min with a duration of 5 – 10 min. Generally not used as an infusion due to tachyphylaxis. (50 mg·mL⁻¹ 1 mL ampule) | Ephedrine is an indirect-acting alpha and beta agonist. It causes vasoconstriction and an increase in heart rate, blood pressure, and cardiac output. It is useful in patients with hypotension without tachycardia. |

¶ = invasive pressure monitoring mandatory; SVR = systemic vascular resistance.

Table 23.8 Properties of Cardiovascular Drugs

| Drug | Mechanism of Action | Single bolus dose | Infusion rate and preparation | Comments |
|---|---|---|---|---|
| milrinone (Primacor®) | Phosphodiesterase-3 inhibitor | 37.5 - 50 μg·kg⁻¹ loading dose iv | Loading dose is followed by a 0.375 – 0.5 μg·kg⁻¹·min⁻¹ infusion | Inotropic and vasodilator properties; useful in patients with congestive heart failure; causes a dose-dependent reduction in SVR, PAP, PCWP, and BP. |
| nitroprusside¶ (Nipride®) | Direct arterial and venous vasodilation | 1 – 2 μg·kg⁻¹ iv | 0.2 – 8.0 μg·kg⁻¹·min⁻¹ 50 mg in 500 mL (100 μg·mL⁻¹) | Useful in patients requiring minute-to-minute control of their blood pressure. A reflex tachycardia and increase in plasma renin levels may result from administration. Tachyphylaxis and cyanide toxicity may occur with infusions of > 6 μg·kg⁻¹·min⁻¹ for ≥ 2 hr. |
| nitroglycerin (Nitrostat®) | Direct venous vasodilation | 0.3 – 0.4 mg SL 10 – 200 μg iv | 0.1 - 5 μg·kg⁻¹min⁻¹¶ 50 mg in 500 mL (100 μg·mL⁻¹) | Direct venous vasodilation results in a reduction in preload and blood pressure. NTG improves LV performance and coronary blood flow. It is useful in treating congestive heart failure, coronary artery ischemia, and pulmonary hypertension. |
| labetalol (Trandate®) | 4 to 1 non-selective beta antagonist to alpha-1 antagonist properties | 0.05 – 2 mg·kg⁻¹ iv (5 – 20 mg iv over 2 min) | 2 amps (40 mL; 5 mg·mL⁻¹) with 160 mL saline(1 mg·mL⁻¹ concentration). Infusion 2 mg·min⁻¹. | Used in the treatment of hypertension and tachycardia. Reduces both blood pressure and heart rate. Labetalol has a relatively slow onset of 5 – 10 min and can be used without direct arterial monitoring. |

¶ = invasive pressure monitoring mandatory; BP = blood pressure; LV = left ventricular; NTG = nitroglycerin; PAP = pulmonary artery pressure; PCWP = pulmonary capillary wedge pressure; SL = sublingual; SVR = systemic vascular resistance.

Table 23.9 Properties of Cardiovascular Drugs

| Drug | Receptor Activity | Single bolus dose | Comments |
|---|---|---|---|
| calcium chloride | No beta-adrenergic activity. Rapid direct-acting inotrope with a duration of 5 – 10 min. | 1 – 10 mg·kg⁻¹ iv | Used to treat hypocalcemia, ECG changes of hypocalcemia in the presence of hypotension, and calcium channel blocker overdose. May also be useful in the treatment of hypermagnesemia, and to protect the myocardium from the effects of hyperkalemia. |
| metoprolol (Betabloc®) | Selective beta-1 antagonist | 1 – 5 mg iv every 2 – 5 min prn; may require up to 15 mg. | Useful in controlling hypertension, tachycardia, and reducing myocardial ischemia. Potential side effects include bradycardia, heart block, pulmonary edema, bronchospasm, and impaired insulin release resulting in hypoglycemia. |
| esmolol (Brevibloc®) | Selective beta-1 antagonist | Single bolus dose 0.5 – 1 mg·kg⁻¹ iv Infusion 1 mg·mL⁻¹ solution; 50 – 300 μg·kg⁻¹·min⁻¹ | Rapid onset in < 2 min with a duration of < 30 min. Indicated in the treatment of hypertension and tachycardia in patients at risk of hemodynamically induced myocardial ischemia. Also indicated in the control of the ventricular rate in acute atrial fibrillation and atrial flutter. |
| verapamil (Isoptin®) | Calcium channel antagonist | Single bolus 2.5 – 5 mg iv; Maximum 10 mg iv. | Useful in terminating a supraventricular dysrhythmia. Also used in controlling the ventricular rate in patients with atrial fibrillation and atrial flutter. Contraindicated in pre-excitation syndromes (e.g., Wolff-Parkinson–White [WPW] syndrome) as it may increase conduction in the accessory pathway. |

ECG = electrocardiography

Table 23.10 Properties of Cardiovascular Drugs

| Drug | Mechanism of Action | Single bolus dose | Comments |
|------|---------------------|-------------------|----------|
| atropine | Anticholinergic | 0.3 – 0.6 mg iv increments; maximum 3 mg | Most commonly used to treat bradycardia (heart rate < 45 beats·min-1). Also useful as an antisialagogue to dry oral secretions and aid oropharyngeal topical anesthesia for an "awake" fiberoptic intubation. |
| adenosine (Adenocard®) | Antidysrhythmic Adenosine-1 receptor agonist resulting in transient AV node block | 6 mg iv rapidly over 3 sec followed by a saline flush; may repeat x 1 after 1 – 2 min with 12 mg iv push. | Useful in treating paroxysmal supraventricular tachycardia (SVT). May be associated with significant hypotension, facial flushing, and shortness of breath. Does not convert atrial fibrillation, atrial flutter, or ventricular tachycardia to a sinus rhythm, but may be useful in distinguishing an SVT from other tachydysrhythmias. |
| enalapril (Vasotec®) | Angiotensin converting enzyme (ACE) inhibitor | 1.25 mg iv Maintenance 1.25 mg iv every 6 hr. | Useful in treating hypertension and heart failure. Onset within 15 min, with maximum effect from 1 – 4 hr. Use with caution in patients with renal insufficiency. Decrease in BP is exaggerated in patients on diuretics. Hypotension responds to volume expansion. |
| diltiazem | Calcium channel blocker | 10 – 20 mg iv over 2 min; may repeat in 15 min prn. | Useful in controlling the heart rate response in atrial fibrillation and flutter and in treating a paroxysmal supraventricular tachycardia. Potent vasodilator, negative inotrope, negative chronotrope depressing AV node conduction. Also useful in treating hypertension and angina. Contraindicated in CHF, WPW syndrome and hypotensive states. |

ACE = angiotensin-converting-enzyme; AV = atrioventricular; BP = blood pressure; CHF = congestive heart failure; WPW = Wolff-Parkinson-White.

## Table 23.11 Etiology of ACLS Events in the Perioperative Setting[4]

| Anesthesia | Respiratory |
|---|---|
| Intravenous anesthetic overdose | Hypoxemia |
| Inhalational anesthetic overdose | Auto PEEP |
| Neuraxial block with high sympathectomy | Acute bronchospasm |
| Medication error | Upper airway obstruction |
| Local anesthetic toxicity | |
| **Cardiovascular** | |
| Hypovolemic or hemorrhagic shock | Right or left ventricular failure |
| Vasovagal or oculocardiac reflex | Transfusion reaction |
| Pulmonary embolism (clot, cement, gas) | Hyperkalemia |
| Tension pneumothorax | Pacemaker failure |
| Anaphylaxis | Prolonged QT syndrome |
| Malignant arrhythmia | Acute coronary syndrome |
| Abdominal compartment syndrome | |

ACLS = Advanced Cardiac Life Support; PEEP = positive end-expiratory pressure.

Unlike an arrest in the community, an intraoperative arrest is relatively rare, generally witnessed, and often anticipated; furthermore, resources are immediately available and information about the patient is known. The anesthesia surgical team and not the medical team direct the management of an intraoperative arrest. If the clinical situation suggests possible progression to an arrest state, the arrest cart should be brought into the operating room (OR) and the transcutaneous pads should be positioned on the patient's chest ready for use should they be required for defibrillation or synchronized cardioversion. In a cardiac arrest or impending arrest, all anesthetic drugs should be immediately discontinued. A general call is announced in the ORs to summon any available help, and one person is designated to bring the arrest cart into the OR if this has not already been done. In a cardiac arrest, the surgeon and a designated health care provider take turns performing chest compressions by rotating between providers every two minutes. Importance is placed on high-quality compressions.

### Clinical Pearl:

*The 1977 Bee Gees disco hit "Stayin' alive" has 103 beats per minute. It's a song that everyone seems to know and can be used by the care-giver performing chest compressions to maintain a recommended rate of 100 compressions per minute.*

A number of circumstances determine how next to proceed. The surgical site may need to be packed and covered with a sterile drape to permit chest compressions. If the patient's chest is open, the surgeon initiates direct cardiac massage. If an endotracheal tube is present, its position must be confirmed. If the patient's trachea is not intubated, bag-mask ventilation should be initiated followed by expeditious endotracheal intubation and delivery of 100% oxygen. If the patient is in a prone or lateral position for surgery, the patient must immediately be placed in a supine position to permit chest compressions. If the patient has obstructive lung disease (COPD, asthma), consideration should be given to disconnecting (10 – 20 sec) the endotracheal tube from the circuit to diagnose and relieve any obstruction to exhalation (auto-PEEP). Ventilation with 8 – 10 breaths·min$^{-1}$ should be instituted, avoiding excessive ventilation. Advanced Cardiac Life Support algorithms should be instituted with modifications appropriate to the clinical case (e.g., rapid fluid and blood product resuscitation in hemorrhagic shock; calcium chloride/bicarbonate/dextrose-insulin for hyperkalemia-associated arrest; pleural decompression for tension pneumothorax). Point-of-care testing (e.g., hemoglobin, blood gases, electrolytes) may assist in diagnosing the cause of the arrest. All equipment and drugs should be secured for post-cardiac arrest analysis.

## References:

1. Pollard JB. Cardiac arrest during spinal anesthesia: common mechanisms and strategies for prevention. Anesth Analg 2001;92:252-256.
2. Kopp SL, Horlocker TT, Warner ME et al. Cardiac arrest during neuraxial anesthesia: frequency and predisposing factors associated with survival. Anesth Analg 2005;100:855-865.
3. Hazinski MF et al. Highlights of the 2010 American Heart Association Guidelines for CPR and ECC. www.anesthesiaprimer.com/AP/Ch23Circulation/ACLShighlights2010.pdf
4. Gabrielli A, O'Connor MF, Maccioli GA. Anesthesia advanced circulatory life support. Developed by the ASA Committee on Critical Care Medicine, currently awaiting approval as a practice parameter or policy statement by the ASA House of Delegates. www.anesthesiaprimer.com/AP/Ch23Circulation/Anesthesiology-CentricACLS.pdf

# CHAPTER 24

# Hypoxemia and Oxygen Therapy

Andy Roberts MD, Amy Fraser MD

## Learning Objectives:

1. To review the five causes of hypoxemia.
2. To gain an appreciation of the different methods of delivering oxygen to a patient and an understanding of their indications.
3. To gain awareness of the oxygen concentration delivered by the different devices.
4. To gain insight into the potential problems associated with the administration of oxygen.

## Key Points

| | |
|---|---|
| 1 | A patient with hypoxemia should be administered oxygen while being diagnosed and treated for the underlying cause. |
| 2 | Supplemental oxygen should be administered to maintain an oxygen saturation > 92%. |
| 3 | Most cases of hypoxemia have mixed causes. |
| 4 | An endotracheal tube or tracheostomy will protect against aspiration of gastric contents. |

### Hypoxemia

Oxygen is an essential and vital substrate required for life. It comprises about two-thirds of our mass (mostly in the form of water). As we breathe in oxygen, it diffuses across the alveolar cell membrane to the pulmonary capillaries where it is bound to hemoglobin, transported from the lungs to the heart, and transported from there to the different organ systems. The cytochrome c oxidase enzyme system in the mitochondria is responsible for > 90% of oxygen consumption in the body. This enzyme system is used for cellular respiration, a process that provides energy in the form of adenosine triphosphate (ATP) for aerobic metabolic functions through the oxidative phosphorylation of food products. If oxygen supply is limited or if oxygen demand is too great, the body switches to anaerobic metabolism to synthesize ATP temporarily. Anaerobic metabolism results in the accumulation of lactic acid. If a hypoxic state persists, a state of shock with cellular death and organ damage will ensue.

Organs differ in their sensitivity to the lack of oxygen (anoxia). Skeletal muscle can tolerate anoxia for up to two hours without

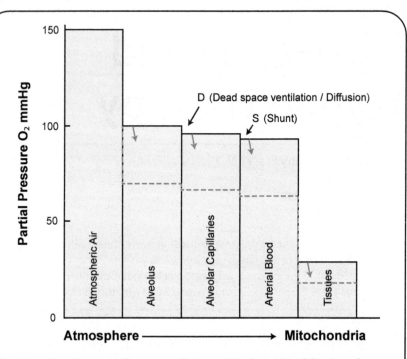

Fig. 24.1 The Oxygen Cascade. Schematic diagram of O₂ transfer from the atmosphere to the tissues. D represents the decrease in oxygen caused by either an increase in dead space ventilation or a decrease in oxygen diffusion. S represents a decrease in oxygen caused by a shunt. The decrease in oxygen secondary to D and S can be small (as depicted) or much larger in disease states. Hypoventilation (red dotted line) depresses the PO₂ in the alvelolus and therefore also the oxygen level in the tissues.
*Adapted from West JB. Respiratory physiology 3rd edition 1985.*

suffering irreversible damage. The brain is very susceptible to the lack of oxygen, with cellular injury occurring within one minute and irreparable damage after five minutes. The heart, liver, and kidneys have decreasing sensitivities to the effects of anoxia.

The concentration of oxygen in air is 21%. The partial pressure of oxygen is the product of the oxygen concentration and the atmospheric pressure. At sea level, the barometric pressure is approximately 760 mm Hg, and the partial pressure of oxygen is 160 mm Hg (760 x 0.21). Aerobic metabolism is dependent on an adequate partial pressure of oxygen. The decreased atmospheric pressure at the top of Mount Everest results in a decrease in the partial pressure of oxygen to 47 mm Hg (despite a concentration of 21% of oxygen), which can result in hypoxemia.

The oxygen cascade refers to the progressive decrease in the partial pressure of oxygen from the ambient air to the tissue level

(Fig. 24.1). At sea level, the partial pressure of oxygen decreases from 160 mm Hg to 4 - 23 mm Hg in the mitochondria. Fig. 24.1 depicts the progressive decrease in the partial pressure of oxygen from the inspired concentration to the alveolar, arterial, and cellular levels.

Table 24.1 lists the various factors influencing the oxygen partial pressure at each level of the cascade.

## Table 24.1 Factors influencing oxygenation at various levels in the oxygen cascade

| | Partial Pressure | Affected by: | | |
|---|---|---|---|
| I | Inspired oxygen ($P_iO_2$) | Barometric pressure ($P_B$) | Oxygen concentration ($F_iO_2$) |
| II | Alveolar gas ($P_AO_2$) | Oxygen consumption ($VO_2$) | Alveolar ventilation ($V_A$) |
| III | Arterial blood ($PaO_2$) | Dead space ventilation ($\uparrow$ V/Q*) | Shunt ($\downarrow$ V/Q) |
| IV | Cellular ($PO_2$) | Cardiac output (CO) | Hemoglobin (Hb) |

\* V/Q refers to the ratio of alveolar ventilation to perfusion

I. **Inspired oxygen partial pressure (PiO2)** A decrease in either the inspired oxygen concentration or the barometric pressure (e.g., high altitude environment) will lower the inspired oxygen partial pressure.

II. **Alveolar oxygen partial pressure (PAO2)** An increase in either the oxygen consumption (e.g., sepsis, shivering) or a decrease in alveolar ventilation will decrease the alveolar oxygen partial pressure.

III. **Arterial blood oxygen partial pressure (PaO2)** Arterial hypoxemia may occur as a result of ventilation perfusion abnormalities. This occurs when there is either an increase in dead space ventilation or an increase in shunt (Table 24.3).

IV. **Cellular oxygen partial pressure (PO2)** Tissue hypoxia will result

whenever any of the above factors result in a decrease in the $P_iO_2$, $P_AO_2$, or $PaO_2$. In addition, tissue hypoxia results either from inadequate cardiac output (with poor tissue perfusion) or from an insufficient amount of hemoglobin to carry the oxygen to the tissues.

"**Hypoxemia**" refers to a low partial *pressure* of oxygen in the arterial blood ($PaO_2$). A sample of blood can be analyzed to measure the partial pressure of oxygen (e.g., arterial blood gas). "**Hypoxia**" refers to a low *content* of oxygen in the blood or cellular tissues. The content of oxygen can be calculated using the saturation, hemoglobin concentration, and the partial pressure of oxygen (Chapter 10; Table 10.2). But how low is too low? Most experts would consider that a $PaO_2$ of 60 mmHg in a patient who is breathing room air would meet the criteria for hypoxemia. Hemoglobin-related problems, such as anemia, hemoglobinopathies, and carbon monoxide poisoning can lower blood oxygen *content.* Although these conditions can lead to tissue **hypoxia,** they are not considered causes of **hypoxemia,** as the $PaO_2$ in these cases is typically normal.

*Clinical Pearl:*

*Hypoxia is associated with an increase in cardiac and pulmonary work. Patients with heart and lung disease are especially vulnerable to hypoxemia, as their ability to increase cardiopulmonary output is limited.*

**Cyanosis** is a descriptive term used to describe a dark bluish or purplish coloration of the skin and mucous membranes accompanying hypoxemia. Cyanosis becomes evident when the reduced hemoglobin (deoxyhemoglobin) exceeds 5 g per 100 mL of blood. It may be detected with oxygen saturation as high as 85% provided the hemoglobin level is normal, there is no excessive pigmentation, and the lighting conditions are good. Cyanosis is generally readily detected at an oxygen saturation of 75% (corresponding to a $PaO_2$ of approximately 40 mm Hg (Chapter 10; Fig. 10.1). Anemia, poor lighting conditions, and dark pigmentation may mask cyanosis.

*Clinical Pearl:*

*The inner lip is a reliable site to examine for the presence of cyanosis.*

## Oxygen therapy

Postoperative surgical patients, patients with pneumonia, and patients with postoperative atelectasis are common candidates for supplemental oxygen therapy. These patients do not necessarily require mechanical ventilatory support (see Chapter 7; Criteria for Ventilation, Tables 7.1 and 7.2). A general goal of oxygen therapy is to achieve an oxygen saturation of at least 90%. At our institution, the minimal acceptable saturation is 92% for post-surgical patients who are being transferred to a hospital ward bed.

## Oxygen Delivery Systems

A number of oxygen delivery systems can be used to provide supplemental oxygen to patients. Some systems are suitable for low-flow $O_2$, while others are intended for high-flow $O_2$. A clinical decision regarding which method of delivery is best for a patient is based on many factors, including the patient's oxygen requirements, mode of ventilation (spontaneous, assisted, or controlled), and need for airway protection. Table 24.2 lists six modes of delivering supplemental oxygen as well as common indications for each.

## Table 24.2 Oxygen Delivery Systems

| Route | Mode of Ventilation | | | Indication |
|-------|:---:|:---:|:---:|-----------|
| | S | A | C | |
| Nasal prongs | + | | | Minimal oxygen requirements |
| Face mask[a] | + | | | High-flow oxygen requirements |
| CPAP / BiPAP | + | + | | Obstructive sleep apnea, hypoventilation |
| Bag valve mask | + | + | + | Used to assist or provide PPV |
| Supraglottic airway | + | + | + | Short surgical procedures |
| Endotracheal tube | + | + | + | Risk of aspiration, controlled ventilation |
| Tracheostomy | + | + | + | Emergency airway or long-term airway |

S = spontaneous; A = assisted; C = controlled ventilation; [a] = simple (Hudson), Venturi, and non-rebreathing face masks; CPAP = continuous positive airway pressure mask; BiPAP = bi-level positive airway pressure mask; PPV = positive pressure ventilation. Bag valve mask (e.g., AMBU® resuscitation bag unit). Supraglottic airway (e.g., LMA™; see Chapter 8).

### Nasal Prongs

Nasal prongs are ideally suited for the patient who requires minimal supplementary oxygen. Flow rates are generally restricted to 1 – 4 $L \cdot min^{-1}$, as higher flow rates frequently result in uncomfortable drying of the nasal mucosa. To estimate the concentration of oxygen delivered, multiply the flow rate (in $L \cdot min^{-1}$) by a factor of 4 and add this result to the concentration of oxygen in room air. For example, a patient on 3 $L \cdot min^{-1}$ of $O_2$ via nasal prongs is receiving approximately 33% $O_2$ (i.e., [3 x 4] + 21 = 33%). Nasal prongs are generally well tolerated and do not interfere with speaking, eating, or drinking.

### Face Masks

There are three basic types of masks that can be used to deliver oxygen: a "simple" or Hudson mask, a non-rebreathing mask, and a Venturi mask. A flow rate of 6 – 8 $L \cdot min^{-1}$ of oxygen is recommended for a simple Hudson face mask. This can provide an enriched oxygen supply of 40 – 60%. Flow rates < 6

$L \cdot min^{-1}$ are not recommended, as lower flows can lead to rebreathing of $CO_2$.

The Venturi face mask uses a flow rate of 4 – 12 $L \cdot min^{-1}$ to deliver a more accurate concentration of oxygen ranging from 24 to 40%. It is designed to deliver specific percentages of oxygen by varying the size of the air entrainment port and the oxygen flow rate. This mask is indicated when it is important to control the concentration of oxygen (e.g., a patient with chronic obstructive pulmonary disease [COPD] who requires oxygen to maintain a minimum acceptable saturation of 88% but is dependent on hypoxic drive to breathe).

A **non-rebreathing face mask** has an attached 1.5 L reservoir bag and is used to provide a high concentration of oxygen to a spontaneously breathing patient. The mask is filled with oxygen before being placed on the patient. One-third of the reservoir will typically be depleted with each breath when an oxygen flow rate of 15 $L \cdot min^{-1}$ of oxygen is used. The exhaled air is directed by a one-way valve, preventing the patient from inhaling room air or re-inhaling exhaled air. The reservoir fills again from the oxygen source during the exhalation phase. A concentration of approximately 60% can be delivered provided there is a good seal around the patient's nose and mouth. Concentrations of up to 80% may be achieved using higher oxygen flow rates with a tight-fitting mask and normal minute ventilation.

***Clinical pearl:***

*Simple face masks should not be used with flow rates < 6L·min⁻¹; lower flows can lead to rebreathing $CO_2$.*

The **puritan face mask** delivers the highest level of humidified oxygen compared with all of these systems and is indicated whenever an inspired concentration > 50% is required. Oxygen concentrations of 35 – 50% can be achieved with a flow rate of 15 L·min⁻¹. A double setup delivering 30 L·min⁻¹ of oxygen is capable of delivering oxygen in concentrations of up to 80%.

All of the above described delivery systems are susceptible to entrainment of room air, resulting in a decrease in the inspired oxygen concentration. In general, the higher the patient's minute ventilation (respiratory rate and tidal volume), the greater the reduction in the inspired oxygen concentration. Nasal prongs and a simple face mask are two examples of low-flow oxygen delivery systems. These devices have a limited reservoir to store oxygen, and they are unable to deliver a consistent inspired oxygen concentration in the setting of a high respiratory rate and tidal volume. The Venturi, non-rebreathing, and puritan face masks are examples of high-flow oxygen delivery systems.

A manual resuscitation unit, such as the AMBU® bag and mask, is used to provide positive pressure ventilation and oxygenation (Fig. 24.3). It can be used to support respiratory efforts or for positive pressure ventilation in a patient who is not breathing. If tracheal intubation is required, mask ventilation should be maintained until all the equipment is available and prepared. The mask should fit over the bridge of the patient's nose and produce an airtight seal around the nose, cheeks, and chin. Consider changing the size of the mask or inserting an oral or nasal airway if difficulty is encountered ventilating the patient's lungs. Fig. 24.3 shows the hand and finger positioning used to provide positive pressure ventilation with an AMBU® bag and mask. The thumb is positioned over the nasal bridge of the mask. The index finger exerts downward pressure on the base of the mask over the chin. The middle finger lifts the mandible forward into the base of the mask. The little finger is hooked around the angle of the mandible and displaces the mandible forward to create an open airway.

## CPAP/BiPAP

Use of continuous positive airway pressure (CPAP) and bi-level positive airway pressure (BiPAP) is increasing as a means of non-invasive ventilatory support in critical care areas. CPAP is most often used to relieve upper airway obstructive symptoms typically associated with obstructive sleep apnea. CPAP masks deliver a constant inspiratory and expiratory pressure, which reduces the work of breathing, splints the airway open, and prevents small airway collapse during sleep or after anesthesia. Lung units are recruited, increasing the functional residual capacity (FRC). The increased airway pressure (not the airflow) is responsible for splinting the upper airway open to permit unobstructed breathing and reduce or prevent apnea. CPAP pressures of 6 - 14 cm $H_2O$ are required for most patients with sleep apnea. Higher levels may be required in patients with severe obstructive symptoms. Non-compliance is a common problem as some patients find the mask and machine

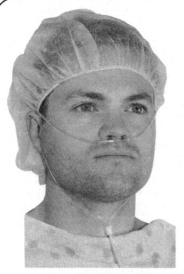

Nasal Prongs

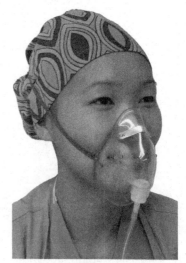

Simple (Hudson) Face Mask

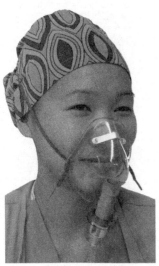

Venturi Face Mask

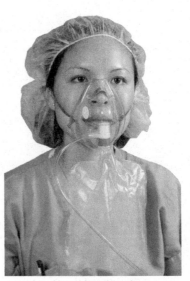

Non-rebreathing face
mask with reservoir bag

Fig. 24.2 Oxygen delivery systems for spontaneously breathing
patients.

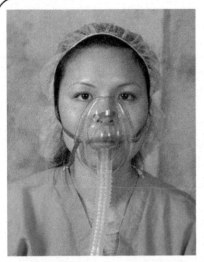
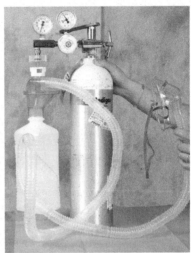

Fig. 24.3 The Puritan face mask provides high level humidity and predictable concentrations of oxygen. Shown here with a single bottle set up for delivering inspired $O_2$ concentrations up to 60%.

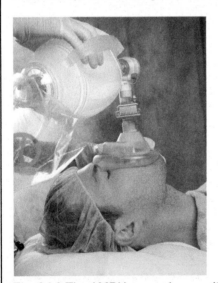
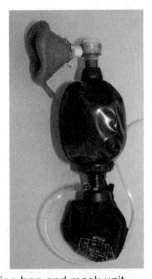

Fig. 24.3 The AMBU manual resuscitation bag and mask unit. Used for providing primary airway management in patients requiring positive pressure ventilation and oxygenation. Note the hand and finger positioning on the mask. The fingers are used to displace the mandible forward and create a seal between the mask and the patient's face.

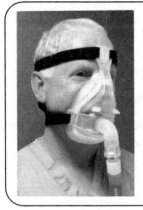
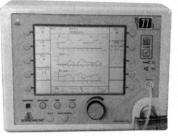

Fig. 24.4 Bi-level positive airway pressure (BiPAP) mask and machine.

cumbersome and uncomfortable or experience claustrophobia with the mask. Patients are unable to eat or speak when wearing the mask. BiPAP provides an inspiratory positive airway pressure and a lower expiratory pressure for easier exhalation. BiPAP provides a baseline CPAP and senses the patient's inspiratory efforts, which trigger a predetermined support pressure to augment inspiration. BiPAP is indicated in patients who hypoventilate and require short-term ventilatory support.

A trial of noninvasive positive pressure ventilation (NIPPV) is increasingly being used to treat patients with either a severe exacerbation of COPD or cardiogenic pulmonary edema. A trial of NIPPV may be appropriate as an alternative to tracheal intubation in treating patients with acute respiratory distress or hypoxemia or in managing critical care patients after a trial of tracheal extubation.[1]

## Supraglottic Airways

The laryngeal mask airway (LMA™) is the classic supraglottic airway that revolutionized the delivery of anesthesia in the 1990s (Chapter 8).This supraglottic device allows the provider to administer 100% oxygen, with spontaneous, assisted, or controlled ventilation. Supraglottic airways are ideally suited for shorter surgical procedures. They

are relatively contraindicated in patients with gastroesophageal reflux or obesity or in procedures that are prolonged or performed in the non-supine position. It is important to bear in mind that a risk of aspiration remains despite their proper placement.

### Endotracheal Tube

An endotracheal tube (ETT) can be used to deliver 100% oxygen and protect the airway from aspiration both during the short and long-term period (Chapters 6 & 7). There are many varieties of ETTs. The most commonly used ETT is a single lumen tube with a single cuff at its distal end. Once the cuff is inflated, it creates an infraglottic seal that allows for delivery of enriched oxygen concentrations with increased airway pressure if required. Spontaneous, assisted, or controlled modes of ventilation are possible with the use of an ETT.

### Tracheostomy

This is the only airway that requires surgical insertion. Cuffed tracheostomy tubes permit delivery of up to 100% oxygen. Tracheostomies are not routinely used in the operating room (OR).

### Causes of Hypoxemia

Hypoxemia results from one or more of five conditions (Table 24.3).

## Table 24.3 Causes of Hypoxemia

| I | Decreased inspired oxygen | Decreased inspired oxygen concentration |
|---|---|---|
| II | Decreased alveolar ventilation | Hypoventilation |
| III | Increased dead space ventilation | Increased zone I |
| IV | Increased shunt | Intrapulmonary, cardiac, or peripheral (liver, AV fistula) |
| V | Decreased diffusion | Interstitial pulmonary pathology, severe anemia |

AV = arteriovenous.

### I. Decreased Inspired Oxygen Concentration ($F_iO_2$)

A low $F_iO_2$ is not a common cause of hypoxemia in clinical practice. Atmospheric air contains 21% oxygen. For a healthy person, this is more than enough oxygen to saturate the circulating hemoglobin. Generally, we do not have to consider the effects of atmospheric pressure, as the vast majority of anesthetics are delivered at or near sea level. Historically, it was possible to inadvertently deliver oxygen from an anesthesia machine in a concentration of < 21%. Modern anesthetic machines have integrated safety features and alarms preventing the delivery of low concentrations of oxygen. It is still possible to dispense a hypoxic mixture of gas in the rare event that both central and portable oxygen supplies fail simultaneously. When a low-flow general anesthesia technique is used, a hypoxic mixture could also occur if the oxygen alarms are ignored and the patient's oxygen demand exceeds the oxygen volume delivered.

### II. Decreased Alveolar Ventilation

Hypoventilation can be thought of as low alveolar ventilation resulting from a decrease in the respiratory rate and / or the tidal volume. Prolonged hypoventilation will result in a hypoxemic and hypercarbic state.

Hypoventilation may result from an overdose or misuse of sedating medications (e.g., benzodiazepines, opioids), weakness (e.g., myopathy, residual muscle paralysis), or airway obstruction (e.g., foreign body aspiration or obstructive sleep apnea). The cause of hypoventilation must be identified and treated to correct the condition. Prior to correcting the underlying cause, a short period of intervention may be required with ventilatory support and an increase in the concentration of delivered oxygen.

### Clinical Pearl:

*An opioid overdose that results in hypoventilation can occur after procedural sedation. Definitive treatment includes administration of naloxone, an opiate antagonist (Chapter 14). Even if naloxone has already been given, the ventilation of a hypoxemic patient may still need support for several minutes with supplemental oxygen and or assisted ventilation. If the patient is hypoventilating, grab an Ambu® bag and mask and help the patient breathe!*

### III. Increased Dead Space Ventilation

The term *"ventilation-perfusion mismatching"* is commonly used to describe

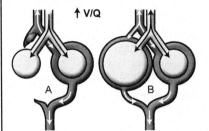
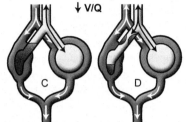

Fig. 24.5 Ventilation perfusion abnormalities.

A & B = Dead space ventilation
A = normal ventilation, no perfusion (e.g., pulmonary embolism).
B = normal ventilation, low perfusion (e.g., arterial hypotension, high airway pressure)
C & D = Pulmonary Shunt
C= no ventilation, normal perfusion (e.g., endobronchial intubation)
D = hypoventilation, normal perfusion (e.g., asthma, pneumonia)

either an increase in dead space ventilation or an increase in pulmonary shunting. It is perhaps the most common cause of hypoxemia in the perioperative setting. Optimized gas exchange occurs when the oxygen supplied to an alveolus "matches" adjacent capillary blood flow. When alveolar ventilation exceeds the capillary perfusion, a portion of the ventilation is directed to non-perfused alveoli. This ventilated but non-perfused lung is useless for gas exchange and is referred to as dead space ventilation. JB West originally described three zones of the lung, where zone I of the lung represents the non-perfused alveoli. Zone I only exists in the setting of arterial hypotension (e.g., severe hemorrhage) or increased alveolar pressure (e.g., positive pressure ventilation, positive end-expiratory pressure [PEEP], auto-PEEP, asthma). Anything that increases zone I in the lung will increase dead space ventilation and impair oxygenation. Other examples of increased dead space ventilation include emphysema, where there is a physical destruction of the alveolar capillaries, and pulmonary emboli, where the alveoli are not perfused because of the emboli.

### IV. Increased Shunt

Intrapulmonary shunting of blood is at the other end of the ventilation perfusion mismatch spectrum. Intrapulmonary shunting occurs when the alveoli are perfused but not ventilated. An extreme example of a pulmonary shunt occurs when an ETT is passed beyond the trachea into a mainstem bronchus creating an endobronchial intubation. In this case, a large shunt will occur in the lung that is not being ventilated. Other examples of pulmonary shunts include congestive heart failure, pneumonia, aspiration, mucous plugging, or infiltrative lung disease. Both dead space ventilation and pulmonary shunting can exist in a patient at the same time.

A shunt can be physiological or pathological. Even healthy patients do not typically have an oxygen saturation of 100% on room air. Approximately 2% of our left ventricular output is composed of blood from the Thebesian veins of the left ventricle and the bronchial circulation. This blood is deoxygenated and is therefore referred to as our physiological shunt. Some patients have pathological intracardiac shunts. This occurs when blood flows from the right side of the heart to the left without undergoing oxygenation (e.g. atrial septal defect [ASD] or ventricular septal defect [VSD]).

### V. Decreased Diffusion

Diffusion abnormalities occur when there is an increase in the tissue distance between alveoli and pulmonary capillaries or a shortened pulmonary transit time for gas exchange. Problems with oxygen diffusing across the alveolar capillary membrane are rare, but they may occur with severe exercise, anemia, or high altitude. Pulmonary fibrosis, emphysema, and interstitial pulmonary processes, such as sarcoidosis, may also result in a decrease in diffusion of oxygen and result in hypoxemia.

### Tissue Hypoxia

Tissue hypoxia can result from a decrease in circulating hemoglobin, a decrease in the arterial oxygen partial pressure ($PaO_2$), a decrease in tissue perfusion, or from a cellular toxin, such as cyanide (Table 24.4).

## Table 24.4 Causes of Tissue Hypoxia

| | |
|---|---|
| Decreased functional hemoglobin | Anemia, hemoglobinopathies |
| Decreased $PaO_2$ | Hypoxemia (Table 24.3) |
| Decreased tissue perfusion | Shock states (Chapter 22; Table 22.7) |
| Cellular hypoxia | Histotoxic hypoxia (e.g., cyanide poisoning) |

### Oxygen Toxicity

Although oxygen was discovered in the late18[th] century, it has been used for clinical purposes only in the last 150 years. Prior to this, humans had never before been exposed to concentrations of oxygen > 21%. While oxygen is an invaluable tool for treating many conditions, indiscriminate and excessive or inappropriate concentrations of oxygen can be detrimental to patients. Supranormal concentrations of oxygen can produce cellular injury mediated by reactive oxygen species. Free oxygen radicals, such as superoxide anions, hydroxyl radicals, and hydrogen peroxide, can overwhelm cellular antioxidant defenses and result in an inflammatory response mimicking an adult respiratory distress syndrome (ARDS). High concentrations of oxygen increase atelectasis, impair mucociliary clearance, and promote mucous plugging. Healthy volunteers experience retrosternal discomfort, heaviness, pleuritic pain, and dyspnea within 24 hr of breathing 100% oxygen.[2]

Adults may experience detrimental effects from even brief periods of exposure to 100% oxygen. Exposure to 100% oxygen for as little as 5 min rapidly promotes the formation of atelectasis.[3,4] Atelectasis develops rapidly in obese patients following induction of anesthesia with100% oxygen and no PEEP. The use of PEEP has been shown to limit or reverse the formation of atelectasis when high concentrations of oxygen are used.[3] High concentrations of oxygen are still commonly used for the induction of and emergence from general

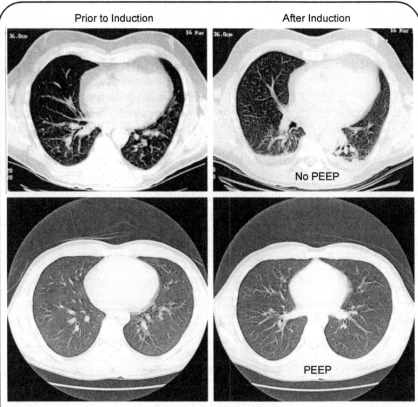

Fig. 24.6 CT Scan before and after induction of anesthesia with 100% $O_2$ with and without PEEP. Adapted from Rusca M. Anesth Analg 2003;97:1835-9.

anesthesia, as the time to desaturation in the apneic patient is increased with higher concentrations of oxygen.[5] The intraoperative use of 30% oxygen rather than 80% oxygen appears to have no effect on the incidence of atelectasis following bowel surgery.[6]

*Clinical Pearl:*

*When administering 100% oxygen during anesthesia, the use of PEEP will limit or reverse atelectasis.*

The deleterious effects of oxygen for the newborn infant (i.e., retinopathy of prematurity and bronchopulmonary dysplasia) have radically challenged traditional thinking for neonatal resuscitation. This has led to more conservative recommendations for the use of oxygen in the 2010 Neonatal Resuscitation Guidelines (see Chapter 20 Neonatal Resuscitation).

The administration of oxygen to patients with COPD may be followed by hypercapnia. The mechanisms involved include an increase in ventilation perfusion mismatching (secondary to impaired hypoxic pulmonary vasoconstriction), a decreased binding of $CO_2$ to hemoglobin, and a depression of the minute ventilation. Nevertheless, oxygen therapy should not be withheld from patients with COPD who have significant hypoxemia.[4]

The *e*Primer clinical case discussion on perioperative hypoxemia can be accessed at: http://www.ottawaanesthesiaprimer.com/AP/Ch24oxygen/ClinicalCasePresentation.pdf

**Test your knowledge:**
1. What are the five causes of hypoxemia?
2. What are the advantages and disadvantages of nasal prongs compared with a face mask for the delivery of oxygen?
3. What is the difference between a shunt and dead space?
4. How might sedating medications contribute to hypoxemia?

**Resources**
1. Merck Manual
   www.merckmanuals.com/professional/critical_care_medicine/approach_to_the_critically_ill_patient/oxygen_desaturation.html.
2. Miller RD, Eriksson LI, Fleisher LA, Wiener-Kronish JP, Eds. Miller's Anesthesia, Seventh Edition. Chapter 15: Respiratory Physiology. Churchill Livingstone Elsevier, Philadelphia: 2010.

**References**
1. Keenan SP, Sinuff T, Burns KEA, et al. Clinical practice guidelines for the use of noninvasive positive-pressure ventilation and noninvasive continuous positive airway pressure in the acute care setting. CMAJ 2011;183:E195-E214.
2. Malhotra A, Schwartz DR, Schwartzstein RM. Oxygen toxicity. www.uptodate.com (literature review current to February 2012, last updated March 2009.
3. Rusca M, Proietti S, Schnyde P et al. Prevention of atelectasis formation during induction of general anesthesia. Anesth Analg 2003;97:1835-9.
4. Magnusson L, Spahn DR. New concepts of atelectasis during general anesthesia. B J Anaesth 2003;91:61-72.
5. Edmark L, Kostova-Aherdan K, Enlund M et al. Optimal oxygen concentration during induction of general anesthesia. Anesthesiology 2003;98:28-33.
6. Akça O, Podolsky A, Eisenhuber E. Comparable postoperative pulmonary atelectasis in patients given 30% or 80% oxygen during and 2 hours after colon resection. Anesthesiology 1999;91:991-998.

# CHAPTER 25

# Unusual Anesthesia Complications

Kim Walton MD, PhD, Alan Chaput MD

## Learning Objectives:

1. To identify the triggers, clinical presentation, and management of malignant hyperthermia.
2. To become familiar with other causes of a perioperative rise in temperature.
3. To understand the key strategies used to reduce the risk of perioperative aspiration pneumonitis.
4. To gain an understanding of negative pressure pulmonary edema and an awareness of strategies used to reduce the incidence and treat the symptoms of this complication.
5. To review the management of allergic and anaphylactic reactions.

## Key Points

| | |
|---|---|
| 1 | Malignant hyperthermia is an inherited disorder that is triggered by succinylcholine and volatile anesthetics. |
| 2 | Early recognition and treatment of malignant hyperthermia with dantrolene play a key role in preventing the high mortality associated with this disorder. |
| 3 | Prophylaxis with strict fasting guidelines is the best strategy to avoid aspiration in the perioperative period. |
| 4 | The severity of aspiration is closely associated with the volume and pH of the aspirate, the type of aspirate (solid *vs* liquid), and the underlying health of the patient. |
| 5 | Negative pressure pulmonary edema is most often caused by laryngospasm or biting on the airway (endotracheal tube or laryngeal mask airway device) during emergence. |
| 6 | Perioperative anaphylaxis and anaphylactoid reactions are clinically indistinguishable, potentially life-threatening, and fortunately rare. Muscle relaxants and latex are the two most common triggers of a perioperative allergic reaction. |
| 7 | The most important steps in the management of anaphylaxis are to remove the triggering agent and to administer epinephrine. |

## I. Malignant Hyperthermia (MH)

### What is MH?

Malignant hyperthermia is a rare (approximately 1 in 10,000 general anesthetics) life-threatening clinical syndrome that occurs in genetically susceptible patients upon exposure to a triggering agent. The triggering agent typically occurs during general anesthesia with exposure to a volatile anesthetic agent or the depolarizing muscle relaxant, succinylcholine. Once exposed to these triggers, the key features of MH include a rise in the end-tidal $CO_2$ ($ETCO_2$), muscle rigidity, rhabdomyolysis, hyperthermia, acidosis, hypoxemia, and hyperkalemia. The rise in temperature can be dramatic and as much as 1°C every 5 minutes (Table 25.1; Fig. 25.1). Malignant hyperthermia may occur at any time during general anesthesia (from induction to emergence), or it may be delayed, presenting within the first few hours following a general anesthetic.

## Table 25.1 Clinical Features of Malignant Hyperthermia

| Hypermetabolism | Muscle Rigidity | Rhabdomyolysis |
|---|---|---|
| Increased oxygen consumption<br>Dark blood in surgical field<br>Cyanosis | Masseter muscle spasm (unable to open mouth) | Hyperkalemia |
| Increased CO2 production Increased ETCO2<br>Tachypnea | Chest wall rigidity (Difficulty ventilating) | Painful, tender, swollen muscles |
| Tachycardia | Abdominal and limb rigidity | Elevated creatine kinase (CK) |
| Unstable blood pressure (BP) | | Myoglobinemia and myoglobinuria |
| Metabolic acidosis<br>Increased lactic acid production | | |
| Elevated temperature | | |

### How serious is it?

The mortality of MH has decreased from > 80% in the 1960s to < 5%. Only about 10% of MH episodes are fulminant with rapid onset and severe physiological derangements and complications.

### Who is susceptible?

Malignant hyperthermia is an inherited disorder of skeletal muscle. History and physical examination are usually not helpful in the preoperative diagnosis of MH susceptibility. A history of uneventful anesthetics is no guarantee that the patient does not have

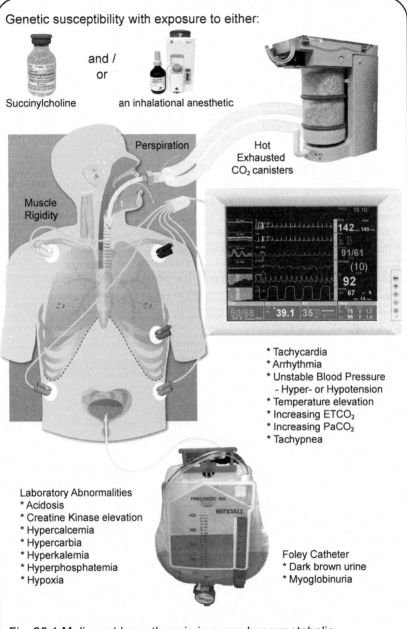

Genetic susceptibility with exposure to either:

and /
or

Succinylcholine          an inhalational anesthetic

Perspiration          Hot
Exhausted
$CO_2$ canisters

Muscle
Rigidity

* Tachycardia
* Arrhythmia
* Unstable Blood Pressure
  - Hyper- or Hypotension
* Temperature elevation
* Increasing $ETCO_2$
* Increasing $PaCO_2$
* Tachypnea

Laboratory Abnormalities
* Acidosis
* Creatine Kinase elevation
* Hypercalcemia
* Hypercarbia
* Hyperkalemia
* Hyperphosphatemia
* Hypoxia

Foley Catheter
* Dark brown urine
* Myoglobinuria

Fig. 25.1 Malignant hyperthermia is a rare hypermetabolic syndrome observed in genetically susceptible patients under general anesthesia when exposed to triggering agents such as succinylcholine and / or volatile anesthetic gases.

the disorder. A history of intraoperative cardiac arrest, muscle rigidity or stiffness and high fever, or the unexpected death of a family member under anesthesia warrants further investigations and a review of medical records. Patients with certain rare forms of myopathies have been observed to have an increased association with MH. In addition, it was long thought that patients with muscular dystrophy had an increased association with MH. It is now known that these patients develop life-threatening disturbances and muscle destruction when exposed to the triggering agents for MH, but this is not considered "true" MH. These changes usually result from hyperkalemia and muscle destruction following the administration of succinylcholine, and therefore, succinylcholine should never be administered to patients with muscular dystrophy.

The pattern of inheritance is autosomal dominant. In most cases, MH-susceptible patients have a defective calcium channel in the sarcoplasmic reticulum. This channel has been identified as the ryanodine receptor (RYR). To date, more than 100 defects have been identified in the RYR gene, and 30 of these have been recognized in 70% of the families with MH. It should be noted, however, that not all genetic defects causing MH have been identified, and work in this area is ongoing. Due to the complicated genetics involved, a simple screening blood test to identify all patients at risk is not available and likely won't be available for the next several years. Although genetic testing has begun in some centers, thus far this test lacks sensitivity and only checks for the mutations that are most frequently found. The gold standard for MH testing remains the *in vitro* contracture test (IVCT). This procedure involves taking a muscle biopsy from a patient's quadriceps muscle and exposing it to caffeine and halothane gas. Muscle from a patient with MH is noted to develop an abnormally strong response when exposed to either of these agents. Unfortunately, this test is performed only at certain special testing centers and cannot be used for screening patients.

## What anesthetic agents trigger MH?

The triggers for MH include the depolarizing muscle relaxant, succinylcholine, and **any** of the volatile anesthetic agents, such as sevoflurane, desflurane, isoflurane, and halothane.

## What anesthetic agents are safe?

Intravenous agents, including propofol, benzodiazepines (e.g., midazolam), ketamine, and opioids can all be used safely to induce and/or maintain anesthesia. The only safe inhalational agent is nitrous oxide as it is unrelated to the fluorinated hydrocarbons listed above. Nondepolarizing muscle relaxants, such as rocuronium, can be used, and their action can be reversed with a combination of an anticholinesterase and anticholinergic agents (e.g., neostigmine and glycopyrrolate). Local anesthetic agents, including the amide class (e.g., bupivacaine, ropivacaine, lidocaine) and ester class (e.g., tetracaine, chlorprocaine), with or without epinephrine, are safe to use in MH patients.

## What is the pathogenesis of MH?

Exposure of a patient with genetic susceptibility to an anesthetic triggering agent leads to MH. On a cellular level, the genetic defects that lead to MH are just beginning to be elucidated, and the ryanodine receptor (RyR1) has been shown to be an important mediator of this process. The ryanodine receptor is a critical transporter of calcium out of the sarcoplasmic reticulum (SR) during muscle depolarization. Normally, the RyR1 receptor is open for a limited time preventing sustained contraction and release of excess calcium. In MH, however, the RyR1 opening is easier and more sustained in the presence of volatile

## Table 25.2 Treatment of a Suspected Malignant Hyperthermia Crisis*

| Problem | Treatment |
|---|---|
| Emergency situation with lots to do. | CALL FOR HELP.<br>Get MH cart into the room.<br>Inform surgeon and attempt to complete the procedure ASAP. |
| Sustained muscle contraction and rhabdomyolysis. | Dantrolene 2.5 mg·kg$^{-1}$ up to 30 mg·kg$^{-1}$.<br>Place Foley catheter and monitor for myoglobinuria.<br>• Maintain urinary output (U/O) > 1mL·kg$^{-1}$·hr$^{-1}$.<br>• If U/O < 0.5 mL·kg$^{-1}$·hr$^{-1}$, start alkalinizing the urine by administering intravenous sodium bicarbonate treatment to prevent myoglobin-induced renal failure.<br>Cold intravenous fluid (see below) to maintain urine output. |
| Hypermetabolic State | |
| Increased O2 consumption and CO2 production. | 100% O2.<br>Increase minute ventilation (hyperventilate to ≥10L·min$^{-1}$).<br>Change CO2 absorber frequently to avoid exhaustion. |
| Temperature rise | Place temperature probe to monitor treatment (rectal or esophageal).<br>Cool patient to 38°C (over vigorous cooling can result in hypothermia).<br>Effective techniques include:<br>• Iced saline 15 mL·kg$^{-1}$ iv q 15 min x 3.<br>• Lavage stomach, bladder, rectum, and open cavities with iced saline .<br>• Surface cool with ice and hypothermia blanket. |
| Acidosis | Sodium bicarbonate 1-2 mEq·kg$^{-1}$ iv while awaiting blood gas, then guide therapy based on arterial blood gas (ABG).<br>Place arterial line for frequent ABG assessment. |
| Hyperkalemia | Hyperventilation<br>Insulin and glucose (10 units of regular insulin and 1 amp (50 mL) of dextrose in water 50% [D50W]).<br>Calcium chloride 10 mg·kg$^{-1}$ iv if life-threatening hyperkalemia. |
| Arrhythmias | Most resolve with correction of acidosis and hyperkalemia.<br>Treat as per Advanced Cardiac Life Support (ACLS) guidelines and avoid calcium channel blockers. |

* Based on the Malignant Hyperthermia Association Guidelines (revised 2010)

anesthetics, which allows for a sustained rise of $Ca2+$ in the myoplasm. This increase in muscle cytoplasmic calcium overwhelms the capacity of the reuptake protein to carry calcium back into the SR, resulting in unrelenting muscle contraction and uncontrolled aerobic and then anaerobic metabolism. This then leads to the clinical manifestations of respiratory and metabolic acidosis, muscle rigidity, and hyperthermia. If this process is allowed to continue without treatment, it will lead to systemic muscle hypoxia and cell death. The lysis of myocytes releases muscle cell contents, including potassium and myoglobin, into the bloodstream (known as rhabdomyolysis), manifesting as hyperkalemia and myoglobinuria and an increase in serum creatine kinase. Dantrolene has been shown to bind to RyR1, which is postulated to limit the time the receptor stays in the open state and thereby to decrease the amount of calcium that spills into the muscle cytoplasm.

## How do you treat an MH crisis?

Early diagnosis and administration of dantrolene are of critical importance in treating and reversing the hypermetabolic abnormalities of MH. Measures, such as cooling, treating hyperkalemia, and arrhythmias, focus on dealing with the consequences of the MH reaction (see Table 25.2). Dantrolene is classified as a skeletal muscle relaxant and is used occasionally in patients with disorders of skeletal muscle spasticity. It may result in skeletal muscle weakness, but typically, it does not result in muscle paralysis. It is supplied as a yellow powder in vials containing 20 mg dantrolene and 3 gm mannitol. Each vial of dantrolene is mixed with 60 mL of sterile water, which can be a time-consuming task because dantrolene is so insoluble. In fact, during an MH crisis, 1 or 2 people are needed to reconstitute the dantrolene! Every hospital that provides general anesthetic services is required to keep a current stock (minimum 36 vials) of dantrolene available for immediate use.

## Post MH crisis treatment.

Following the initial treatment of an MH suspected crisis, the patient should be observed in a critical care setting for at least 24 hr, since recrudescence of MH may occur, especially in fulminant cases.

1. Administer dantrolene 1 mg·kg⁻¹ *iv* every 6 hr for 24 - 48 hr after the episode.
2. Follow ABG, creatine phosphokinase (CPK), potassium, ionized calcium, urine and serum myoglobin, clotting studies, and core body temperature until such time as they return to normal values. Central temperature (e.g. rectal, esophageal) should be continuously monitored until stable.
3. Educate the patient and family regarding MH and further precautions. Refer the patient to the MH North American registry and biopsy center. Patients susceptible to MH should wear a medical alert bracelet.

## Postoperative fever:

An increase in body temperature above 38.5°C in the perioperative period is the result of:

1. An increase in body heat production,
2. A decrease in body heat elimination, or
3. The result of active warming measures.

Postoperative fevers are rarely due to malignant hyperthermia; however, MH must be considered in a patient with metabolic acidosis, rhabdomyolysis, tachycardia, rigidity, and hyperthermia occurring within 24 hr of exposure to succinylcholine and or an inhalational anesthetic. Table 25.3 lists a number of other clinical conditions that may also be associated with tachycardia, hyperthermia and/or rigidity, acidosis, and rhabdomyolysis in the immediate postoperative period.

## Table 25.3 Differential Diagnosis of Malignant Hyperthermia

| Cardiorespiratory | | |
|---|---|---|
| Atelectasis | Sepsis[a d] | |
| **Neurologic** | | |
| Meningitis[b] | Intracranial bleed[b] | Traumatic brain injury[b] |
| **Toxicology** | | |
| Amphetamine toxicity[a c] Serotonin syndrome[d] | Salicylate toxicity[a c] Anticholinergic syndrome[bd] | Cocaine toxicity[a c] |
| **Miscellaneous** | | |
| Iatrogenic overheating | Heat stroke[a c] | Neuroleptic malignant syndrome[d] |

[a] = metabolic acidosis, likely manifestation; [b] = metabolic acidosis, possible manifestation; [c] = rhabdomyolysis, likely manifestation; [d] = rhabdomyolysis, possible manifestation. Thyrotoxicosis and pheochromocytoma may be associated with perioperative tachycardia, hypercarbia, and hyperthermia, but they are not generally associated with metabolic acidosis or rhabdomyolysis.

## II. Aspiration Syndrome

### How common is aspiration syndrome and what are the risk factors?

Aspiration occurs as a complication in approximately 1 in 3,000 anesthetics, but the incidence can be up to four times higher in emergency cases. Aspiration can occur both on induction AND emergence from general anesthesia.

In Chapter 9, the concept of a rapid sequence induction was introduced, and factors were identified that placed a patient at risk for gastric aspiration (Table 9.1).

### What can we do to prevent aspiration?

1. Ensure an appropriate preoperative fasting period has been observed[1] (see Chapter 3).
2. Consider local or regional anesthesia to avoid the loss of airway reflexes associated with general anesthesia.
3. Consider a rapid sequence induction technique (Chapter 9) in patients with an increased risk of aspiration.
4. Place a nasogastric tube (NG) tube in high-risk patients (e.g., bowel obstruction) to drain and decompress the stomach prior to induction of anesthesia.
5. Perform tracheal extubation with the patient in the lateral position, once airway reflexes have returned with the patient awake and obeying commands.
6. Treat high-risk patients with medications to reduce stomach pH (e.g., 0.3M sodium citrate 30 mL if < 30 min prior to induction of anesthesia; or an $H_2$ receptor blocker or proton pump inhibitor if > 45 min prior to induction of general anesthesia). Consider motility agents (e.g., metoclopramide 10 mg *iv*) to increase gastric motility and promote gastric emptying.

### What are some factors that predict the severity of the aspiration?

1. Volume > 0.4 mL·kg$^{-1}$
2. pH < 2.4
3. Type of aspirate (solid worse than liquid)
4. Health of the patient

### What are the consequences of gastric aspiration?

Aspiration of a liquid causes a vigorous cough accompanied by a transient period of hypoxemia in the normal awake adult. When gastric acid is aspirated, surfactant is destroyed and the alveoli collapse, resulting in hemorrhage and exudation into the alveoli and interstitium. Severe bronchospasm usually accompanies a significant aspiration. Lung compliance decreases as alveoli collapse, and areas of shunt occur, resulting in severe hypoxemia.

Aspiration of particulate (food or fecal) matter may result in blockage of distal bronchi, resulting in large areas of collapse, edema formation, and shunting. Due to the initial infiltration by macrophages, the immune response to the aspiration is often worse than the aspiration itself. At its worst, aspiration can trigger an acute respiratory distress syndrome (ARDS)-like scenario that requires mechanical ventilation and admission to the intensive care unit (ICU).

### Diagnosis of aspiration

Early diagnosis and treatment may reduce the severity of the aspiration syndrome. The detection of aspiration may be difficult during mask anesthesia with either a face or laryngeal mask. Sudden laryngospasm, coughing, or stridor may be the first indication of aspiration. Bronchospasm may also occur, and the compliance of the chest may decrease, resulting in increased airway pressures during mechanical ventilation. Alternatively, desaturation with hypoxemia and the need for higher concentrations of oxygen may be the only indication of aspiration. Gastric aspiration may occur without the presence of gastric contents in the mouth.

### Treatment of aspiration

The first few minutes following an aspiration are critical, and attempts must be made to remove as much material as possible from the patient's mouth, pharynx, and trachea. As the most common site for aspiration is the apical posterior segment of the right lung, the patient should be positioned head down in the right lateral position to limit spread to the left lung and to aid drainage by way of gravity. Immediate bronchoscopy is performed to remove any particulate matter that has been aspirated.

With a significant aspiration, it is expected that severe hypoxemia accompanied by decreased lung compliance and difficulty providing positive pressure ventilation will occur within the first 30 - 60 min. Positive pressure ventilation with continuous positive airway pressure (CPAP) or positive end-expiratory pressure (PEEP) are used to prevent alveolar collapse, limit the reduction in residual volume, and prevent further atelectasis and shunting.

Steroids are not generally indicated and may promote granuloma formation in cases of aspirated food particles. Antibiotics are also not indicated unless there is evidence of gross aspiration of bowel contents. Bronchodilators are used in treating bronchospasm. Prolonged positive pressure ventilation and critical management of intravascular volume status, oxygenation, and ventilation are the principles of treating a significant aspiration. Invasive monitoring and frequent blood gas analysis may be required. Mortality and morbidity usually result from the initial severe hypoxemia that occurs at the time of aspiration. This emphasizes the need for initial aggressive treatment.

## III. Negative Pressure Pulmonary Edema (NPPE)

### What is NPPE and how does it occur?

Negative pressure pulmonary edema occurs as a result of marked inspiratory efforts by the patient against an upper airway obstruction. It occurs in approximately 1 in 1,000 patients receiving a general anesthetic. The most common cause of the airway obstruction is the patient involuntarily biting on the endotracheal tube (ETT) or laryngeal mask airway device (LMAD) during emergence from anesthesia. The negative inspiratory pressures generated (referred to as a "reverse Valsalva" maneuver) can exceed 100 cm $H_2O$ in young healthy adults. The negative pressure generated results in an acute increase in blood flow to the right heart. The pulmonary intravascular fluid moves into the interstitium, resulting in acute hypoxemia and triggering a catecholamine surge manifested by systemic and pulmonary hypertension.

In severe cases, the alveolar capillary membrane is disrupted, resulting in pink frothy sputum, frank hemoptysis, and chest infiltrates on pulmonary imaging (chest x-ray [CXR], computed tomography [CT] scan). Unlike cardiogenic pulmonary edema, NPPE is not typically associated with volume overload and high ventricular filling pressures. Pulmonary imaging typically reveals alveolar infiltrates in the middle lung zones in contrast to basilar infiltrates associated with cardiogenic pulmonary edema. Negative pressure pulmonary edema also lacks Kerley B lines, peribronchial cuffing, an enlarged heart, or fluid in the pleura commonly seen with cardiogenic pulmonary edema.

Laryngospasm, an involuntary closure of the vocal cords, can also result in an acute severe upper airway obstruction and subsequent NPPE. Laryngospasm may occur when a patient's trachea is extubated in a relatively light plane of anesthesia. It can also occur when the patient has a supraglottic airway device (e.g., LMAD) in place and there is a sudden increase in surgical stimulation.

## Who is at risk of NPPE?

Typically, young healthy muscular patients with a full set of teeth have an increased risk of biting on the ETT or LMAD during emergence. The risk of the patient forcefully biting on the airway increases when the patient rapidly emerges from a deep inhalational anesthetic in the presence of stimulation, hypothermia, and pain.

## How can it be prevented?

In patients requiring general anesthesia, care must be exercised to avoid laryngospasm, which can be challenging particularly in children. Any airway device should be placed or removed only when there is an adequate depth of anesthesia. For children, a quiet environment with a "no touch" technique may be used to avoid stimulation during emergence and minimize the risk of laryngospasm at tracheal extubation. Alternatively, tracheal extubation can be carried out with the patient deeply anesthetized and breathing spontaneously to minimize the risk of laryngospasm. Laryngeal secretions may also be a cause of laryngospasm, and the oropharynx should be gently suctioned prior to extubation. An oral airway or, alternatively, a bite block fashioned using a tightly rolled piece of gauze, can be placed next to the ETT or LMAD to prevent the patient from biting and occluding the airway on emergence. Adequate analgesia, measures to prevent hypothermia and shivering, gradually weaning the patient off the inhalational agent, and refraining from stimulating the patient during the emergence may also decrease the risk of the patient biting on the airway

on emergence. Some LMADs (e.g., AMBU®, LMA™) incorporate an integrated bite block with the LMAD to prevent the patient from biting and occluding the airway on emergence. Patients should be closely observed during the emergence phase of anesthesia. If the patient is observed to bite on the airway and attempts to breathe against an occluded airway, the anesthesiologist must act quickly to prevent NPPE. An oral bite block should be quickly placed or the depth of anesthesia quickly increased with intravenous anesthetic agents such as propofol. Occasionally, a small dose of succinylcholine (e.g., 0.25 mg·kg⁻¹) may be required to permit placement of an oral airway or to relieve laryngospasm in the patient with a non-intubated trachea.

## Treatment of NPPE

The treatment of NPPE is primarily supportive. Most patients will recover within 24 hr; however, severe persistent hypoxemia may require re-intubation, admission to an ICU, and ventilatory support with PEEP and supplemental oxygen. The most effective therapy is positive pressure ventilation and the use of PEEP, which may be delivered with a mask (CPAP, BiPAP) or ETT. Diuretics have been used to minimize the pulmonary pressures; however, unlike cardiogenic pulmonary edema, NPPE is generally not associated with volume overload.

## Anaphylactic Reactions

Anaphylactic reactions during anesthesia are acute and dramatic adverse events that often result in significant morbidity and mortality. In the operating room, they are most commonly caused by exposure to muscle relaxants and latex, producing anaphylactic shock in approximately 1 in every 6,000 anesthetics.[2]

## What is the difference between an anaphylactoid and anaphylactic reaction?

Anaphylaxis is an immune-mediated allergic reaction that results from the cross-linking of IgE antibodies on the surface of mast cells and basophils. In order to have this reaction, individuals must have had previous exposure to the offending agent or a substance that is immunologically similar. In essence, the body mounts a non-protective response to an antigen, which accounts for the Greek origin of the word ("ana" meaning opposite and prophylaxis meaning "protection"). An anaphylactoid reaction occurs through a direct non-immunoglobulin-mediated release of mediators from mast cells or via complement activation. IgE antibodies are NOT involved in an anaphylactoid response. The clinical manifestations of anaphylactoid and anaphylactic reactions are indistinguishable.

## How does anaphylaxis present in the perioperative period?

Anaphylaxis is a clinical syndrome that affects multiple organ systems. Pre-formed IgE antibodies cross-linked on the surface of mast cells (and basophils) recognize the triggering agent and disrupt the cell surface releasing vasoactive mediators (i.e., histamine, prostaglandins, and leukotrienes). These agents act quickly to produce rash, bronchospasm, and cardiovascular collapse (See Table 25.4). The most common clinical presentation during anesthesia involves the cardiovascular system (74%), skin (70%), and respiratory system, with 44% of reactions associated with bronchospasm.

## Table 25.4 Clinical Signs of Anaphylaxis under Anesthesia

| Organ system | Signs and Symptoms |
|---|---|
| Skin | Pruritis, flushing, urticaria, and angioedema |
| Eyes | Conjunctivitis |
| Cardiovascular | Tachycardia, hypotension, arrhythmias, shock, cardiovascular collapse, death |
| Upper Airway | Rhinitis, sneezing, laryngeal edema |
| Lower Airway | Bronchospasm, wheezing, dyspnea, decreased saturation, increased $ETCO_2$, increased airway pressures, respiratory arrest |
| Intestinal | Abdominal pain, nausea, vomiting, and diarrhea |
| Renal | Decreased urine output (acute tubular necrosis) |
| Hematologic | DIC |

DIC = disseminated intravascular coagulation. Skin changes may be difficult to appreciate during anesthesia if the skin is covered.

## How do we treat anaphylaxis once it is recognized?

The management of anaphylaxis consists of discontinuing the offending drug, blocking the effect of the mediators that have been released, and preventing further mast cell degranulation. Removal of the triggering agent and aggressive pulmonary and cardiovascular support with oxygen, fluids, and epinephrine is essential in averting cardiorespiratory

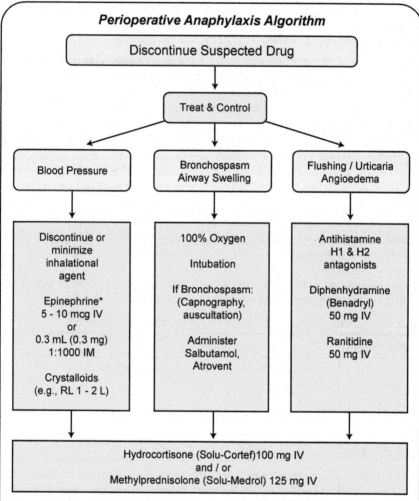

Fig. 25.2 Adult Algorithm for Perioperative Anaphylaxis

\* Epinephrine: 5 - 10 mcg IV initial boluses, up to 100 - 500 mcg for vascular collapse; start infusion at 1 mcg/min. Patients on beta blockers are resistant to the effects of epinephrine; administer 1 mg glucagon IV or IM. Start epinephrine infusion and repeat crystalloid bolus for persistent hypotension.

collapse. Removal of the offending allergen (e.g., drug or latex) and the administration of epinephrine is the mainstay of treatment. Epinephrine is the drug of choice because of its combined α-adrenoceptor and β-adrenoceptor effects, resulting in correction of the associated hypotension and in relaxation of bronchial smooth muscles to reverse bronchospasm, respectively.

Intravenous crystalloids are administered to counter the peripheral vasodilation and hypotension that results from anaphylaxis. The airway is supported with 100% oxygen as well as inhaled $\beta_2$-agonists. An $H_1$ receptor antagonist (e.g., diphenhydramine 0.5 mg·kg$^{-1}$ iv) is used in the early phase of anaphylaxis when there is urticaria and angioedema. An $H_2$ receptor antagonist (e.g., ranitidine 50 mg iv) is added to the $H_1$ antagonist to counteract the allergic vasodilation and hypotension. Inhalational therapy (e.g., salbutamol [Ventolin®] and ipratropium bromide [Atrovent®] nebulizers) is indicated in the setting of bronchospasm. Corticosteroids (e.g., hydrocortisone 1 – 5 mg·kg$^{-1}$ iv and methylprednisolone 0.5 – 1 mg·kg$^{-1}$ iv) are used to decrease airway edema and prevent further mast cell degranulation. Hydrocortisone is the initial preferred steroid as it has a rapid onset. Methylprednisolone has a prolonged duration of action and is used to prevent a recurrence of symptoms.

**Test your knowledge:**

1. A 45-yr-old obese woman is scheduled for an elective laparoscopic cholecystectomy. She believes her aunt developed malignant hyperthermia after an anesthetic. What are the anesthetic agents that should be avoided, and how would you provide anesthesia for this patient?

2. On induction of anesthesia, you notice some green-tinged fluid in the patient's mouth and airway as you are preparing for tracheal intubation. What should you do next?

3. On emergence, the endotracheal tube is removed before the patient is responding. You observe that she is attempting to breathe, but her chest is not moving with her attempts, and a high pitch sound is coming from her airway. What do you suspect, and how would this best be managed?

4. In the recovery room, the patient is noted to have a heart rate of 120 beats·min$^{-1}$ and a temperature of 38.7°C. What is your differential diagnosis?

5. The surgeon initiates treatment with a broad-spectrum antibiotic in the recovery room. A few minutes after administration of the antibiotic, the patient becomes agitated and complains of feeling nauseated and itchy. What is your differential diagnosis and how would you confirm it? How would you manage this patient?

**References:**
1. Warner MA, Caplan RA, Gibbs CP et al. Practice guidelines for perioperative fasting and the use of pharmacologic agents to reduce the risk of pulmonary aspiration: Application to healthy patients undergoing elective procedures. Anesthesiology 1999;90:896-905.
2. Broccard AF, Liaudet L, Aubert J-D et al. Negative pressure post-tracheal extubation alveolar hemorrhage. Anesth Analg 2001;92:273-5.

**Additional Resources:**
1. Cote CJ et al. A Practice of Anesthesia for Infants and Children, 4$^{th}$ Edition 2009. Elsevier.
2. HepnerDL, Castells MC. Anaphylaxis during the perioperative period. Anesth Analg 2003; 97:1381-95.
3. http://www.mhaus.org: Malignant Hyperthermia Association of the United States.

# CHAPTER 26

# Pediatric Anesthesia

Jarmila Kim MD

## Learning Objectives

1. To gain an appreciation of the basis of pediatric anesthesia practice.
2. To gain an understanding of the important features of the anatomy and physiology of pediatric patients.
3. To develop insight into commonly encountered preoperative issues in children undergoing anesthesia.
4. To acquire knowledge of common anesthesia-related problems in the recovery room.
5. To become informed of recent research in anesthetic neurotoxicity in the developing brain.

## Key Points

1. As the induction period in a child may be associated with significant anxiety, preoperative preparation, both psychological and anxiolytic, is an important part of anesthesia.

2. Anatomical and physiological differences in children and neonates necessitate specific training and technical skills for the safe provision of anesthesia.

3. A child with a recent upper respiratory tract infection (URI) is at an increased risk for perioperative respiratory complications.

4. Adenotonsillar hypertrophy is the leading cause of obstructive sleep apnea syndrome (OSAS) in children.

5. There is overwhelming experimental evidence that anesthesia causes neurodegeneration in a variety of animal species, including primates. The clinical relevance of these findings in children undergoing anesthesia remains unclear.

## Introduction:

The pediatric years represent a time of significant growth and change in both form and function. As the human organism progresses through fetal life, infancy, childhood, and adolescence toward adulthood, tremendous physical, cognitive, and emotional maturation occurs. Differences amongst the age groups have specific implications for the assessment, therapy, and monitoring of patients. Pediatric anesthesiologists must have a thorough understanding of the different developmental stages to provide optimal care. Although the anesthetic approach to a procedure in a child is similar in principle to that in an adult, there are significant differences in the physiology and behavior of children that distinguish them from being merely small adults. As an infant's response to most oral, inhalational, and intravenous medications differs from that of an adult, the concentrations of inhalation agents should be modified, medications should be diluted, and the respective doses should be carefully titrated.

## Preparation for Anesthesia and Surgery:

A thorough medical and surgical history, family history, chart review, and physical examination should be performed on every patient requiring anesthesia care. Laboratory investigations should be performed when indicated, and the emotional state of the child and the family must be considered.

## Preoperative Sedation

Hospitalization may have profound emotional consequences for children. Children undergoing anesthesia and surgery can experience significant anxiety and distress during the preoperative period. Depending on the age of the child, this anxiety may be exhibited verbally and/or behaviorally. Crying, silence, pallor, agitation, deep breathing, trembling, urinary retention, violent actions, tense muscles, and other behaviors may be signs and symptoms of the anxious child. Preoperatively, this stress peaks at the time of induction of anesthesia. Current available interventions to aid with preoperative anxiety in children fall into three major categories: (1) hospital-based preparation programs, (2) administration of sedatives and anxiolytics, and (3) parental presence at induction of anesthesia. There are numerous routes of administration of premedications. Oral and rectal routes are most commonly used; however, they are not always predictable because of marked fluctuations in bioavailability and a substantial first-pass effect. The oral route is the most acceptable route, and midazolam is the most commonly used agent (90% of cases). A midazolam dose of 0.5 $mg \cdot kg^{-1}$ by mouth to a maximum of 15 - 20 mg produces consistent preoperative anxiolysis in children with a wide margin of safety. Midazolam is usually mixed with a flavored solution to mask its unpleasant taste. A common solution is to use a flavored acetaminophen elixir in an age-appropriate dose that is mixed with the oral midazolam and administered together. Sedation and anxiolysis occur in the majority of children within 20 min, with a peak effect at 30 min. Risks of preoperative sedation include respiratory depression, loss of protective reflex control, and a paradoxical response.

## Table 26.1 Childhood conditions requiring careful preoperative assessment and postoperative monitoring.

| |
|---|
| Central or obstructive sleep apnea syndrome |
| Adenotonsillar hypertrophy |
| Functional macroglossia due to hypertrophy of the tongue (Down's syndrome, Beckwith-Weidemann syndrome) or relative hypomandibularism (Pierre-Robin syndrome) |
| Neurological impairment, including dysphagia and impaired cough |
| Muscular dystrophy |
| Infants < 10 kg |
| Cyanotic heart disease (they may become increasingly cyanotic or develop hypercarbia) |

### Preoperative Fasting

Appropriate preoperative fasting should always be ordered. Infants must receive special consideration, as a prolonged fasting period may lead to dehydration or hypoglycemia. A 2-hr fast from clear fluids is acceptable for healthy children. In practice, it is simpler to extend these guidelines to 3 hr in order to facilitate the operating room (OR) schedule.

## Table 26.2 Preoperative Fasting Recommendations

| Food | Patient | Recommendation |
|---|---|---|
| **Clear Fluids** | healthy patient | minimum of 3 hr |
| | ill patient | minimum of 4 hr |
| | emergency surgery | individualized care |
| **Milk** | breast milk | minimum of 4 hr |
| | non-human milk (formula) | minimum of 6 hr |
| **Solids** | elective surgery | no solids on day of surgery |
| | emergency surgery | individualized care |

### OR Monitoring

The degree of monitoring must be adjusted according to a child's underlying clinical condition and the planned surgical procedure. The basic principles for monitoring are the same as for adult anesthesia; however, the monitors must be size appropriate. With increased sophistication in monitoring, the anesthesiologist has become more distant than ever from the patient. It can be dangerous to rely totally on electronic monitoring devices to detect clinical abnormalities. The focus must always be on the child and the surgical field, and the anesthesiologist must maintain full concentration throughout the procedure. Ongoing communication between the anesthesiologist and surgeon is always important to allow the anesthesiologist to anticipate and troubleshoot potential problems.

### Induction and Maintenance of Anesthesia

A smooth anesthetic induction can be achieved in a variety of ways. The most appropriate induction technique should be selected for each child based on their clinical history and the proposed surgical procedure. To minimize anxiety, clinicians should proceed without undue delay once the patient is positioned on the OR table. It is helpful to talk to the child throughout the induction period in order to explain or distract the child.

## Table 26.3 Normal Age-Dependent Values of Common Hemodynamic Parameters.

| Age | Mean Heart Rate (beats·min⁻¹) |
|---|---|
| 0-24 hr | 120 |
| 1-7 days | 135 |
| 8-30 days | 160 |
| 3-12 mo | 140 |
| 1-3 yr | 126 |
| 3-5 yr | 100 |
| 8-12 yr | 80 |
| 2-16 yr | 75 |

| Age | Normal Blood Pressure (mmHg) | |
|---|---|---|
| | Average Systolic | Average Diastolic |
| 0-12 hr (preterm) | 50 | 35 |
| 0-12 hr (full term) | 65 | 45 |
| 4 days | 75 | 50 |
| 6 wk | 95 | 55 |
| 1 yr | 95 | 60 |
| 2 yr | 100 | 65 |
| 9 yr | 105 | 70 |
| 12 yr | 115 | 75 |

## Table 26.4 Normal Age-Dependent Values of Common Respiratory Parameters

| Age | Frequency (breaths·min-1) | Tidal Volume mL (mL·kg-1) | PaO2 (mmHg) | PaCO2 (mmHg) |
|---|---|---|---|---|
| newborn | 50 | 21 (6-8) | 60-90 | 30-35 |
| 6 mo | 30 | 45 | 80-100 | 30-40 |
| 12 mo | 24 | 78 | 80-100 | 30-40 |
| 3 yr | 24 | 112 | 80-100 | 30-40 |
| 5 yr | 23 | 270 | 80-100 | 30-40 |
| 12 yr | 18 | 480 | 80-100 | 30-40 |
| >16 yr | 12 | 575 (6-7) | 80-100 | 37-42 |

## Pediatric Induction Methods

### Inhalational Induction

This technique is commonly used to facilitate an induction with sevoflurane and is based on stepwise increments of 1 – 2% of inspired concentration every two to three breaths until an adequate depth of anesthesia has been achieved. Induction may be preceded by inhalation of a $N_2O:O_2$ (60:40%) mixture in a cooperative child to achieve a state of hypnosis prior to introducing sevoflurane. Inhalation induction is generally rapid, pain free, and well tolerated. A "high-dose" inhalation induction technique starts with a circuit primed with 8% sevoflurane in 100% oxygen. After loss of consciousness, the sevoflurane is decreased to 1 minimum alveolar concentration (MAC). This technique speeds the onset of anesthesia and reduces patient struggling. Desflurane and isoflurane have a very pungent smell and are unsuitable inhalation induction agents because of a high incidence of coughing, breath holding, and laryngospasm.

### Intravenous Induction

With the use of a sedative premedication and local anesthetic agents, such as EMLA® and Ametop™, intravenous induction has become increasingly simple. Propofol is the most common intravenous induction agent for infants and children. It has a rapid onset and ultra-short duration of action. The worst side effect is pain on injection. Other, less commonly used intravenous agents include ketamine, etomidate, and thiopental (Chapter 13).

### Intramuscular Induction Agents

In the uncooperative child or adolescent, ketamine 3 - 7 $mg·kg^{-1}$ intramuscular (*im*) is used when intravenous access cannot be accomplished safely or the child rejects attempts at an inhalational mask induction. General anesthesia with spontaneous ventilation is achieved within 3 - 5 min, at which point intravenous access can be obtained. Once anesthesia has been induced, maintenance is accomplished either with an inhalational agent, an intravenous agent, or a combination of both.

## Basic Pediatric Anatomy and Physiology

### Airway and Respiratory:

Changes in the respiratory system continue to occur from infancy to 12 yr of age. The architecture of the major conducting airways is established by the 16th week of gestation, and the alveoli continue to mature after birth and increase in number until 8 yr of age. The newborn's muscles of ventilation are subject to fatigue, as the type I muscle fibers (slow-twitch, highly oxidative, fatigue resistant) compose only 30% of the diaphragm in a newborn. The number of slow-twitch muscle fibers doubles in the first year of life. The chest wall of infants is composed mainly of cartilage and deforms easily. Also, the closing volume is higher in infants and young children and may exceed the functional residual capacity (FRC), thus encroaching on the tidal volume even during normal respiration. Alveolar ventilation is 3 - 4 times larger in a neonate, and the oxygen consumption is also higher. All these factors predispose a neonate to rapid desaturation during periods of apnea. Premature infants are particularly susceptible to postoperative apnea due to their immature respiratory center.

### *Clinical Pearl:*

*Preterm infants, who were born prior to 37 weeks post-conceptual age (PCA) and are less than 60 weeks of age (PCA), should have cardio-respiratory apnea monitoring after anesthesia pending a minimum 12- hour apnea-free period.*

*Clinical Pearl:*

Full-term infants, who were born after 37 weeks PCA and are less than 44 weeks PCA, should also be monitored for postoperative apnea after anesthesia.

*Clinical Pearl:*

For many years, it has been commonly accepted knowledge that the larynx in infants and children is "funnel shaped with the narrowest point at the cricoid cartilage". Recent findings suggest that the pediatric larynx is more cylindrical in shape and the glottis is the narrowest part.

## Table 26.5 Anatomic Characteristics of the Upper Airway in Infants and Children

| 1 | Comparatively large head with small mouth and short neck |
|---|---|
| 2 | Narrow nares and choanae |
| 3 | Large and relatively short tongue |
| 4 | Long, stiff, and narrow U-shaped epiglottis |
| 5 | Larynx positioned more cephalad and anterior |
| 6 | Short trachea requiring careful endotracheal tube (ETT) positioning to avoid tracheal extubation or endobronchial intubation |
| 7 | Soft tracheal cartilage that can be easily compressed by external pressure on the neck |

## Table 26.6 Endotracheal Tube Sizes*

| Age | ETT Size (mm) (Internal diameter) |
|---|---|
| Preterm 1,000 g<br>1,000 - 2,500 g | 2.5<br>3.0 |
| Neonate – 6 mo | 3.0 - 3.5 |
| 6 mo – 1 yr | 3.5 - 4.0 |
| 1 - 2 yr | 4.0 - 4.5 |
| Older than 2 yr | age/4 + 4 |

* When using a cuffed ETT, decrease the size by 0.5 mm

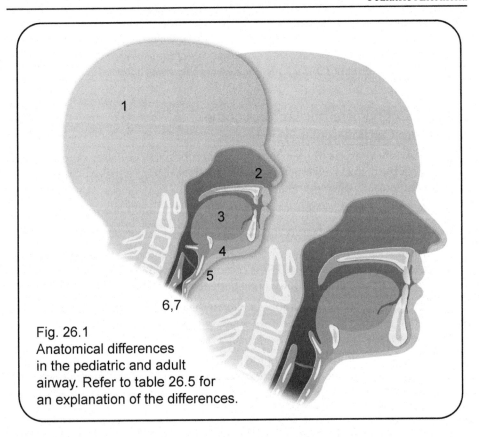

Fig. 26.1
Anatomical differences
in the pediatric and adult
airway. Refer to table 26.5 for
an explanation of the differences.

## Should a cuffed or uncuffed endotracheal tube (ETT) be used in children?

Historically, there was a higher incidence of airway complications, such as subglottic edema and tracheal stenosis, with the use of cuffed red rubber ETTs. Improvements in ETT design have significantly increased the safety of cuffed ETTs in children. There is no increased incidence of airway complications with a cuffed ETT compared with an uncuffed ETT provided the appropriate size is used and cuff over-inflation is avoided. Advantages of cuffed ETTs include fewer tube exchanges, reliable ventilation, the use of low fresh gas flows, and reduced OR pollution.

## Cardiac:

The transition to a normal neonatal circulation occurs after the umbilical cord is clamped and spontaneous breathing begins (Chapter 20). Changes in oxygen concentration and decreasing levels of prostaglandins lead to closure of the patent foramen ovale (PFO) and patent ductus arteriosus (PDA) shunts. However, under certain conditions resulting in hypoxemia or acidosis, these shunts can reopen and result in a "persistent fetal circulation" (PFC).

*Clinical Pearl:*

*Always make sure that your intravenous tubing is free of any bubbles as these may be shunted across the foramen ovale or PDA and enter the cerebral circulation or other key organs*

## Table 26.7 Characteristic Features of the Newborn Cardiovascular System

| | |
|---|---|
| 1 | The right ventricle (RV) exceeds the left ventricle (LV) in wall thickness. After birth, the LV enlarges disproportionately, reaching the adult ratio of ventricular size at 6 months of age. |
| 2 | At age 2 - 3 yr, the electrocardiogram (ECG) has an adult-like appearance. |
| 3 | Sinus arrhythmia is common in children. |
| 4 | The myocardium of the newborn contains less contractile tissue and more connective tissue and thus is less compliant. This limits the size of the stroke volume, thus cardiac output is rate dependent. |
| 5 | Reduced compliance and contractility of the ventricles predispose the infant heart to failure when challenged with a volume load. Ventricular interdependence leads to biventricular failure. |
| 6 | The autonomic innervation of the heart is incomplete with a relative lack of sympathetic elements. Neonates exposed to hypoxemia suffer pulmonary and systemic vasoconstriction, bradycardia, and a decrease in cardiac output. |
| 7 | A slow progressive reduction in pulmonary vascular resistance occurs during the first 3 months of life. |
| 8 | Most (>75%) of hemoglobin (Hb) at term birth is of fetal type (HbF), which has a greater affinity for $O_2$ and releases it to tissues less readily. |
| 9 | Physiologic anemia of infancy reaches a low point at 3 months of age with Hb levels of 80-100g·$L^{-1}$. |

**Cardiac Murmurs:**

The vast majority of children found to have a murmur preoperatively have an "innocent" murmur. An innocent murmur is characterized as a soft, early systolic murmur with no thrill or abnormal cardiac impulses, and it is not associated with cardiac signs or symptoms. Cardiology consultation is indicated if the child with a murmur is younger than 1 year, if the murmur fits pathological criteria, or if there is evidence of left ventricular hypertrophy (LVH) or right ventricular hypertrophy (RVH).

*Clinical Pearl:*

*Criteria for a pathological murmur include all diastolic, pansystolic, late systolic, and very loud murmurs.*

## Table 26.8 Normal Blood Volume in Children

| Age | Blood Volume (mL·kg⁻¹) |
|---|---|
| Preterm | 80-90 |
| Newborn | 80-85 |
| 6 wk – 2 yr | 75 |
| 2 yr - puberty | 70 |

## Renal:

The kidneys are very active *in utero*, and fetal urine output contributes to the volume of amniotic fluid. The glomerular filtration rate (GFR) and tubular function are lower at birth but quickly mature by the end of the first year of life. The newborn infant cannot readily handle a large water load and may be unable to excrete excess electrolytes. Due to limited tubular function, sodium losses may be large, especially in the preterm infant.

## Hepatic:

At term, the neonate has stores of glycogen that are located mainly in the liver and myocardium. Preterm infants and small-for-gestational age infants may have inadequate glycogen stores and fail to establish adequate gluconeogenesis. Hypoglycemia is common in the stressed and sick neonate. Blood glucose levels should be measured in these neonates and hypoglycemia should be corrected promptly.

### *Clinical Pearl:*

*Serious hypoglycemia leading to irreversible neural damage can occur in a sick infant with minimal symptoms. Symptoms, when present, may manifest as lethargy, somnolence, or jitteriness.*

Albumin levels are lower in infants than in adults, and this may alter the binding and activity of some anesthetic drugs. Physiologic jaundice (unconjugated hyperbilirubinemia) is due to an increased bilirubin load, limited hepatic uptake of bilirubin, and deficient hepatic conjugation. The preterm infant may sustain neurologic damage at lower serum bilirubin levels due to an immature blood-brain barrier and therefore should be carefully monitored for increased serum bilirubin levels.

## Temperature regulation:

Due to a large surface area relative to body weight and a lack of heat-insulating subcutaneous fat, infants tend to lose heat rapidly when placed in a cool environment. When heat loss occurs, infants rely primarily on non-shivering thermogenesis to generate heat. This occurs in the brown adipose tissue and is a catecholamine response. Hydrolysis of triglyceride to fatty acids and glycerol occurs with associated increased oxygen consumption and heat production. Brown fat deposits decline during the first weeks of life.

### *Clinical Pearl:*

*The majority of children undergoing surgery will become hypothermic during anesthesia unless active preventative steps are taken. Increasing ambient temperature, draping the child and covering the head can make a significant contribution to reducing heat loss.*

## Common Preoperative Problems

### Upper Respiratory Tract Infection (URI) and Surgery

One of the most controversial issues in pediatric anesthesia has revolved around the decision to proceed with anesthesia and surgery for the child who presents with a URI. Typically, children experience 6 - 8 URIs per year. Approximately 95% of these infections are of viral etiology. Although most viral URIs are self-limiting, they may produce airway hyperreactivity that persists for up to 8 wk. This has important implications for children requiring anesthesia in the acute and convalescent periods, particularly when the child requires tracheal intubation. Children with an URI are at an increased risk of perioperative respiratory complications, including breath holding, arterial oxygen desaturation, coughing, laryngospasm, and bronchospasm. Independent risk factors for adverse respiratory events in children with an active URI include the use of an ETT, prematurity, age < 5 yr, history of reactive airway disease, paternal smoking, surgery involving the airway, presence of copious secretions, and presence of nasal congestion with purulent discharge.

*Clinical Pearl:*

*In general, otherwise healthy children with an uncomplicated URI (afebrile, clear secretions) can safely undergo anesthesia and surgery. Children with more severe symptoms, including mucopurulent secretions, productive cough, fever > 38°C, lethargy, or signs of pulmonary involvement, should have their elective surgery postponed for a minimum of 2 - 4 wk.*

### Obstructive Sleep Apnea

Obstructive sleep apnea syndrome (OSAS) is a sleep-disordered pattern of breathing characterized by periodic, partial, or complete obstruction of the upper airway during sleep. In children, the airway obstruction occurs primarily during rapid eye movement (REM) sleep. It leads to sleep fragmentation, nocturnal intermittent hypoxia, and episodic hypercapnia and has an effect on multiple organ systems, including cardiovascular, neurocognitive, and endocrine systems. Diagnosis of OSAS may be difficult based on clinical grounds alone. Children may present with failure to thrive, behavioral problems, and poor school performance. Polysomnography is considered the gold standard but is not routinely available. Overnight oximetry can provide some indication of the severity of OSAS. There is a 2% incidence of OSAS in children, and adenotonsillar hypertrophy is considered the leading cause. For the majority of children, tonsillectomy and adenoidectomy (T&A) is curative. Resolution of the obstructive symptoms may require at least 6 wk after the adenotonsillectomy.

*Clinical Pearl:*

*Children with severe OSAS who experience profound nocturnal desaturation during sleep are at increased risk for postoperative respiratory morbidity after T&A, with up to a 20% reported incidence. Children with severe OSAS show a blunted response to hypercarbia and greater opioid-induced respiratory depression.*

Children at particular risk are the very young (< 3 yr of age) and those with a significant comorbidity. Following T&A, morphine requirements are decreased in children who show recurrent episodic desaturation during sleep. Children who undergo T&A and have severe OSAS are at risk for airway obstruction and are best cared for in a hospital setting with cardiorespiratory monitoring and supportive management, which may include continuous positive airway pressure (CPAP), reintubation, and ventilation.

## Sickle Cell Disease

Sickle cell disease represents an inherited group of disorders ranging in severity from the common benign sickle cell trait (Hb AS) to the rarer debilitating and often fatal sickle cell anemia (Hb SS). Variants include hemoglobin SC disease (Hb SC) and sickle-beta thalassemia trait (Hb SThal). Variants of sickle cell disease have varying quantities of Hb S. The deoxygenated forms of Hb S result in deformation of the erythrocytes into sickle shapes. These abnormal erythrocytes bond with each other forming long aggregates. This abnormal aggregation of cells results in stasis of blood flow leading to infarctive crisis. Clinical manifestations include acute chest syndrome, splenic sequestration, aplastic crises, infections with encapsulated organisms (parvovirus B19), renal failure, cholelithiasis, painful vaso-occlusive crises, stroke, and retinopathy.

*Clinical Pearl:*

*Infants under the age of 4 months do not suffer from sickle cell crises due to an abundance of fetal HbF.*

The Canadian Anesthesiology Society (CAS) guidelines recommend sickle cell screening in genetically predisposed patients. Up to 20% of patients with SS anemia are not of African ancestry. Screening is recommended for patients with a positive or unknown family history, anemia, or high-risk procedure.

## Exposure to Chicken Pox

Chickenpox or varicella-zoster virus is a disease predominantly of early childhood with approximately 90% of individuals infected in the first decade of life. The average incubation period is 14 days, with a range of 7 - 21 days.

The contagious period is considered to be at least 48 hr prior to the development of the rash and at least 5 days after the skin rash appears.

*Clinical Pearl:*

*To avoid infecting other children or immune-compromised patients, children exposed to chicken pox are best kept out of the hospital for a period of 21 days from their exposure.*

Patients recovering from chickenpox should have all of their lesions crusted over prior to elective surgery.

# Problems Commonly Encountered in the Recovery Room

## Emergence Delirium (ED)

Emergence delirium, also referred to as emergence agitation, is defined as a dissociated state of consciousness in which the child is inconsolable, irritable, uncompromising, or uncooperative, typically thrashing, crying, moaning, or incoherent. The incidence of postoperative ED in children who recieve a volitile anesthetic is 12%. Although generally self-limiting (5 - 15 min), it can be severe and may result in physical harm to the child and, in particular, the site of surgery. Possible etiological factors include rapid emergence, intrinsic characteristics of an anesthetic (more commonly recognized with the newer, less soluble, inhaled anesthetics when compared with halothane), postoperative pain, type of surgery, younger age (with ages 2 - 5 yr being the most susceptible), preoperative anxiety, child temperament, and adjunct medications. Treatment of ED may include the use of opioids, midazolam, propofol, and dexmedetomidine. Flumazenil may be used in those cases where paradoxical reaction to midazolam is suspected to contribute to the negative behavior.

**Clinical Pearl:**

*Several serious physiologic abnormalities, such as hypoxia, hypercarbia, hypotension, hypoglycemia, bladder distension, and increased intracranial pressure, may manifest as an altered mental status. These entities must be recognized and treated promptly.*

## Laryngospasm

Laryngospasm is defined as an involuntary glottic closure due to a reflex constriction of the laryngeal muscles. It occurs more commonly in children than in adults, with an estimated incidence of 17 events in 1,000 anesthetics. It can be partial or complete. In complete laryngospasm, there is chest movement but no ventilation is possible. In partial laryngospasm, chest movement is accompanied with a stridorous, high-pitched crowing noise and a mismatch between the patient's strenuous respiratory efforts and the lack of effective air movement. Laryngospasm occurs during anesthesia due to a lack of inhibition of glottic reflexes. Typical causes include a light depth of anesthesia, a sudden noxious stimulus (e.g., premature tracheal extubation), irritation of the vocal cords with secretions and/or blood, placement of an artificial airway, laryngoscopy, or oral suctioning during a light stage of anesthesia. Initial treatment of laryngospasm should include jaw thrust and chin lift. Gentle positive pressure should be administered with 100% oxygen, however, positive pressure will not break laryngospasm in the presence of complete airway obstruction. Attempts to ventilate with high airway pressures in the presence of a complete airway obstruction may result in gastric insufflation and distension and will increase the risk of gastric regurgitation and pulmonary aspiration. Gastric distension

will also make ventilation more difficult. The gold standard for treatment of complete laryngospasm is succinylcholine 0.1 mg·kg$^{-1}$ *iv* and atropine 20 μg·kg$^{-1}$. A small dose of propofol 0.5 - 1.0 mg·kg$^{-1}$ *iv* can also be used to facilitate a rapid increase in anesthetic depth and has been used successfully to treat laryngospasm. When intravenous access is not available, succinylcholine 3 – 4 mg·kg$^{-1}$*im* can be administered with atropine 20 μg·kg$^{-1}$.

**Clinical Pearl:**

*Untreated laryngospasm can progress to desaturation, hypoxia, bradycardia, and, in some cases, negative pressure pulmonary edema.*

## Post-intubation Croup

The incidence of post tracheal intubation croup in children can be as high as 1%. Factors associated with an increased risk of croup include a tight endotracheal tube, overinflation of the tracheal cuff, repeat attempts at tracheal intubation, traumatic tracheal intubation, a lengthy procedure, and younger age. Initial treatment is humidified oxygen by mask, nebulized racemic epinephrine, and intravenous dexamethasone, although the use of steroids in this setting is controversial.

**Clinical Pearl:**

*Patients must be observed for rebound airway edema and croup after the effects of racemic epinephrine wear off. Patients requiring a second dose of racemic epinephrine should be observed in hospital overnight.*

## Postoperative Nausea and Vomiting

Postoperative vomiting (POV) is approximately twice as frequent amongst children as adults, with an incidence of up to 40% in pediatric patients. Severe POV can result in a range of complications, including wound dehiscence, dehydration and electrolyte imbalance, and pulmonary aspiration. It is one of the leading causes of parental dissatisfaction after surgery and is the leading cause of unanticipated hospital admission following ambulatory surgery.

## Table 26.9 Factors associated with an increased risk of POV

| Patient Factors | • POV risk increases markedly > 3 yr of age and continues to rise throughout early childhood into adolescence<br>• Previous history of motion sickness<br>• Previous history of POV<br>• Post-pubescent girls |
|---|---|
| Surgical Procedures | • Strabismus surgery<br>• Adenotonsillectomy (T&A)<br>• Procedures > 30 min duration |
| Anesthetic Factors | • Volatile anesthetics<br>• Opioids<br>• Anticholinesterase agents |

Recommendations for prophylaxis of POV (see Chapter 22):

1. Children at increased risk should receive ondansetron 0.15 mg·kg⁻¹ *iv.*
2. Children at high risk of POV should receive ondansetron 0.05 mg·kg⁻¹ *iv* and dexamethasone 0.15 mg·kg⁻¹ *iv.*
3. Consider intravenous anesthesia and alternatives to opioid analgesia.

### Postoperative Pain Management

Children of all ages experience pain. The provision of optimal postoperative analgesia for every infant and child should be an integral part of the perioperative management. Inadequately treated pain has an impact on outcome and may trigger long-term behavioral changes. Unsatisfactory acute postoperative pain management is one of the most common medical reasons for delayed discharge after ambulatory surgery. A multimodal approach using regional anesthesia, opioids, and non-steroidal anti-inflammatory agents (NSAIDs) or acetaminophen is now being widely accepted.

Non-opioids (acetaminophen and NSAIDs) are used for treatment of mild to moderate pain or as adjuvants. They provide an opioid sparing effect in multimodal therapy in patients with more severe pain. Acetaminophen is the most used analgesic for children.

### Clinical Pearl:

*Prolonged administration of ordinary doses of acetaminophen can cause toxicity and hepatic failure in children who are febrile, dehydrated, and have a reduced caloric intake.*

## Table 26.10 Guidelines for acetaminophen dosing for analgesia in healthy children

| Age | Oral Initial Dose (mg·kg⁻¹) | Rectal Initial Dose (mg·kg⁻¹) | Maintenance Oral/Rectal Dose (mg·kg⁻¹) | Dosing Interval (hr) | Maximum Daily Dose (mg·kg⁻¹) | Duration of Maximal Dose (hr) |
|---|---|---|---|---|---|---|
| Preterm | 20 | 20 | 15 | 12 | 60 | 48 |
| 0 – 3 months | 20 | 20 | 15 | 8 | 60 | 48 |
| > 3 months | 20 | 40 | 15 | 4 - 6 | 90 | 72 |

The NSAIDs are a heterogeneous group of compounds that share common antipyretic, analgesic, and anti-inflammatory effects. Neonatal clearance increases with age, and dosing should take into account the weight and age of the infant. Cyclo-oxygenase-2 inhibitors alleviate pain without the adverse effects mediated by nonselective NSAIDs, such as the risk of perioperative bleeding and gastric ulcer.

## Table 26.11 Dosage recommendations for commonly administered NSAIDs in children

| Drug | Dosing |
|---|---|
| IBUPROFEN (Advil®, Motrin®) | 5-10 mg·kg⁻¹ po q 6hr<br>Max 40 mg·kg⁻¹ per day or 2,400 mg |
| KETOROLAC (Toradol®) | 0.5 mg·kg⁻¹ iv q 6hr<br>Max 15 mg per dose < 16 yr and 30 mg per dose > 16 yr |
| CELECOXIB (Celebrex®) | 2-4 mg·kg⁻¹ po q 12 hr<br>Max 400 mg per day |

Opioids are still the drug of choice, but their use is limited by adverse events, such as nausea and vomiting, respiratory depression, pruritus, and urinary retention. Morphine remains a cornerstone of pharmacologic analgesia in children. It has been suggested that up to 35% of pediatric patients are inefficient in hepatic conversion of codeine to morphine and thus get incomplete pain relief from codeine. Similarly, up to 30% of the population are rapid converters of codeine to morphine, which can result in dangerously high levels of morphine. At the Children's Hospital of Eastern Ontario, we have eliminated codeine from the formulary.

## Table 26.12 Dosages for commonly used intravenous opioids in children

| Drug | Dosing |
|---|---|
| **FENTANYL** | 1-2 µg·kg⁻¹ bolus<br>0.5-2 µg·kg⁻¹·hr⁻¹ as an infusion |
| **HYDROMORPHONE** | 10-20 µg·kg⁻¹ bolus $q$ 2-4hr<br>4-8 µg·kg⁻¹·hr⁻¹ as an infusion |
| **MORPHINE** | 25-100 µg·kg⁻¹ bolus $q$ 2-4hr<br>10-40 µg·kg⁻¹·hr⁻¹ as an infusion<br>**5-10 µg·kg⁻¹·hr⁻¹ in premature babies and neonates < 6 months** |
| **SUFENTANIL** | 0.5-1 µg·kg⁻¹ bolus<br>0.2 – 0.5 µg·kg⁻¹·hr⁻¹ as an infusion |

*Clinical Pearl:*

*Newborns, and especially premature babies, are thought to be more sensitive to opioids due to hepatic and renal immaturity, and they are at risk of developing respiratory depression. They should be placed in a monitored setting that permits rapid intervention for airway management.*

## Caudal Blockade

This block represents the most commonly used regional technique in children and can be used successfully for all subumbilical procedures. Typical indications include herniorrhaphies; operations on the urinary tract, anus, and rectum; and orthopedic procedures on the pelvic girdle and lower extremities. The caudal block consists of injecting local anesthetic within the caudal part of the epidural space, below the conus medullaris and cauda eqina, and through the sacral hiatus and the sacrococcygeal membrane. Administration of **1 mL·kg⁻¹ of 0.25% bupivicaine or 0.2% ropivicaine** produces adequate postoperative analgesia with minimal risk for postoperative motor block. The procedure must be carried out with strict aseptic technique.

Complications are rare and usually minor. They are related to misplacement of the needle (1) into superficial soft tissue, resulting in a failed block, or (2) into the caudal epidural vessel or bony sacrum, resulting in intravascular or intraosseous injection and leading to systemic toxicity of local anesthetic or inadvertent spinal anesthesia. There is a 2% risk of urinary retention.

## Anesthetic Neurotoxicity in the Developing Brain

The safety of anesthetics administered to infants and young children is a growing public health concern. A number of rodent and primate studies have linked neurotoxicity in very young animals to that of human neonates with the exposure to clinically relevant doses of commonly administered anesthetic agents. The anesthetic community is currently conducting research to determine whether the same risks apply to humans. Developmental anesthetic neurotoxicity has largely been attributed to the combination of GABA agonist and N-Methyl-D-aspartate (NMDA) receptor antagonist actions of the anesthetic drugs.

To date, the best available evidence has failed to show that anesthesia has a negative impact on neural development in human

385

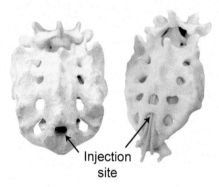

Injection
site

Fig. 26.2 Anatomy of the caudal
space.

infants. The studies have shown an association between the number of anesthetic expos-
ures and impaired neurocognitive development. To be clear, this association does not
prove causation. Nothing to date justifies a
change in clinical anesthetic practice in infants.
However, as the link between the animal and
human data is starting to emerge, physicians
should strive to minimize the length of time
a child is exposed to sedative and anesthetic
medications and weigh the risk of deferring the
surgery (until after 4 years of age) against the
need for more urgent surgery. More research
is urgently needed to determine whether anesthesia impairs neurodevelopment and brain
function in humans. If specific neurodevelop-
mental deficits are associated with anesthetic

and sedative medications, it will be important
to identify whether these deficits can be prevented or treated.

**Clinical Case:**

A 3-yr-old boy with Trisomy 21
(Down's syndrome) is scheduled for elective
adenotonsillectomy. He underwent a ventricular septal defect (VSD) repair in infancy. His
mom states that he snores at night. He has a
runny nose with occasional cough, but no fever.

How would you assess this patient
preoperatively?

Outline an anesthetic management plan
for his upcoming surgery.

**Test your knowledge:**

1. List 5 different reasons why infants
   desaturate rapidly under anesthesia.

2. Discuss the pros and cons of various
   anesthesia induction techniques for
   children.

3. How does a recent URI affect the child
   having anesthesia?

4. What are the anesthetic considerations
   for a child with obstructive sleep apnea
   syndrome?

5. What is laryngospasm and how is it
   managed?

6. What is emergence delirium and what
   would be your approach for treatment?

**References:**

1. Coté CJ, Todres ID, Nishan G et al. (editors). A Practice of Anesthesia for Infants and Children,
   3rd Edition. W.B. Saunders, 2001.
2. Bissonnette B, Dalens B. (editors). Pediatric Anesthesia: Principles and Practice. McGraw-Hill,
   New York 2001.

# Index

CPSIA information can be obtained
at www.ICGtesting.com
Printed in the USA
BVOW05s1627031216
469292BV00009B/183/P